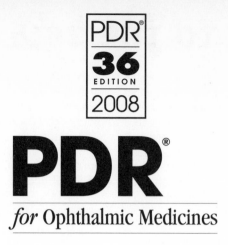

PDR 36 EDITION 2008

PDR®

for Ophthalmic Medicines

Editorial Consultants and Contributors

Douglas J. Rhee, MD, Assistant Professor of Ophthalmology, Massachusetts Eye and Ear Infirmary, Harvard Medical School, Boston, MA

Christopher J. Rapuano, MD, Co-Director and Professor of Ophthalmology, Cornea Service, Wills Eye Hospital, Jefferson Medical College of Thomas Jefferson University, Philadelphia, PA

George N. Papaliodis, MD, Instructor, Massachusetts Eye and Ear Infirmary, Harvard Medical School, Boston, MA

F.W. Fraunfelder, MD, Director, National Registry of Drug-Induced Ocular Side Effects; and Assistant Professor of Ophthalmology, Casey Eye Institute, Oregon Health & Science University, Portland, OR

Executive Vice President, PDR: Kevin D. Sanborn
Vice President, Product & Solutions: Christopher Young
Vice President, Clinical Relations: Mukesh Mehta, RPh
Vice President, Operations: Brian Holland
Vice President, Pharmaceutical Sales & Client Services:
  Anthony Sorce
Senior Director, Copy Sales: Bill Gaffney
Senior Product Manager: Ilyaas Meeran
Manager, Strategic Marketing: Michael DeLuca, PharmD, MBA
National Solutions Managers: Elaine Musco, Marion Reid, RPh
Senior Solutions Managers: Debra Goldman, Warner Stuart,
  Suzanne Yarrow, RN
Senior Director, Sales Operations & Client Services: Dawn Carfora
Sales Associate: Janet Wallendal
Sales Coordinator: Dawn McPartland

Senior Director, Editorial & Publishing: Bette LaGow
Senior Director, Client Services: Stephanie Struble
Directors, Client Services: Eileen Bruno, Patrick Price
Manager, Clinical Services: Nermin Shenouda, PharmD
Drug Information Specialists: Anila Patel, PharmD; Greg Tallis, RPh
Manager, Editorial Services: Lori Murray
Associate Editor: Sabina Borza

Director, Database & Vendor Management: Jeffrey D. Schaefer
Production Manager, PDR: Steven Maher
Manager, Production Purchasing: Thomas Westburgh
Senior Print Production Manager: Dawn Dubovich
Production Manager: Gayle Graizzaro
PDR Database Supervisor: Regina L. Dickerson
Index Supervisor: Noel Deloughery
Index Editor: Allison O'Hare
Format Editor: Eric Udina
Senior Production Coordinators: Gianna Caradonna,
  Yasmin Hernández
Production Coordinator: Nick W. Clark
Production Specialist: Jennifer Reed
Traffic Assistant: Kim Condon
Vendor Management Specialist: Gary Lew

Manager, Art Department: Livio Udina
Electronic Publishing Designers: Deana DiVizio, Carrie Faeth
  Jaime Pinedo
Production Associate: Joan K. Akerlind
Digital Imaging Manager: Christopher Husted

Digital Imaging Coordinator: Michael Labruyere

ISBN: 1-56363-663-8

FOREWORD TO THE 36th EDITION

Thomson Healthcare is pleased to provide eyecare professionals with this updated guide to ophthalmic pharmaceuticals. The *PDR® for Ophthalmic Medicines* includes FDA-approved guidelines for leading eyecare products, as well as information on newly released medications. In addition, the book's opening sections feature useful tables summarizing the major pharmaceutical alternatives currently available in ophthalmology, as well as a brief guide to suture materials and information on vision standards and low vision. There are also lens comparison and conversion tables and a directory of soft-contact lens manufacturers. Four detailed indices help you locate products by manufacturer, product name, product category, and active ingredient; and a full-color product identification section features photos of many leading ophthalmic medications.

The special reference sections near the beginning of *PDR for Ophthalmic Medicines* have been prepared with the assistance of Douglas J. Rhee, MD, and George N. Papaliodis, MD, of the Massachusetts Eye and Ear Infirmary, Harvard Medical School, in Boston; and Christopher J. Rapuano, MD, of Wills Eye Hospital, Jefferson Medical College of Thomas Jefferson University in Philadelphia. Our thanks also go to F.W. Fraunfelder, MD, of Oregon Health & Science University in Portland, who edited the section on ocular toxicology. The opinions expressed in these sections are those of the authors and are not necessarily endorsed by the publisher.

About This Book

PDR for Ophthalmic Medicines is published by Thomson Healthcare in cooperation with participating manufacturers. The *PDR* contains Food and Drug Administration (FDA)-approved labeling for drugs as well as prescription information provided by manufacturers for grandfathered drugs and other drugs marketed without FDA approval under current FDA policies. Some dietary supplements and other products may also be included. Each full-length entry provides you with an exact copy of the product's FDA-approved or other manufacturer-supplied labeling. Under the Federal Food, Drug and Cosmetic (FD&C) Act, a drug approved for marketing may be labeled, promoted, and advertised by the manufacturer for only those uses for which the drug's safety and effectiveness have been established. The Code of Federal Regulations Title 21 Section 201.100(d)(1) pertaining to labeling for prescription products requires that for *PDR* content "indications, effects, dosages, routes, methods, and frequency and duration of administration, and any relevant warnings, hazards, contraindications, side effects, and precautions" must be "*same in language and emphasis*" as the approved labeling for the products. The FDA regards the words *same in language and emphasis* as requiring VERBATIM use of the approved labeling providing such information. Furthermore, information that is emphasized in the approved labeling by the use of type set in a box, or in capitals, boldface, or italics, must be given the same emphasis in *PDR*.

The FDA has also recognized that the FD&C Act does not, however, limit the manner in which a physician may use an approved drug. Once a product has been approved for marketing, a physician may choose to prescribe it for uses or in treatment regimens or patient populations that are not included in approved labeling. The FDA also observes that accepted medical practice includes drug use that is not reflected in approved drug labeling. In the case of over-the-counter dietary supplements, it should be remembered that this information has not been evaluated by the Food and Drug Administration, and that such products are not intended to diagnose, treat, cure, or prevent any disease.

The function of the publisher is the compilation, organization, and distribution of this information. Each product description has been prepared by the manufacturer, and edited and approved by the manufacturer's medical department, medical director, and/or medical consultant. In organizing and presenting the material in *Physicians' Desk Reference*, the publisher does not warrant or guarantee any of the products described, or perform any independent analysis in connection with any of the product information contained herein. *Physicians' Desk Reference* does not assume, and expressly disclaims, any obligation to obtain and include any information other than that provided to it by the manufacturer. It should be understood that by making this material available, the publisher is not advocating the use of any product described herein, nor is the publisher responsible for misuse of a product due to typographical error. Additional information on any product may be obtained from the manufacturer.

Evidence-Based Application for Your PDA

Thomson Clinical Xpert™ is a powerful medical reference developed by Thomson Healthcare for Palm® OS and Pocket PC handhelds. Designed specifically for use at the point of care, this decision-support tool puts drug, disease, and laboratory information instantly into the hands of physicians and other clinical professionals via their PDA.

Much more than a quick drug lookup, Thomson Clinical Xpert provides medical references and point of care tools you need in your daily workflow, including:

- **Drug labeling**: Search more than 4,000 trade names
- **Interaction checker**: Check up to 32 medications at one time
- **Toxicology information**: Screen 200 of the most common poisonings and drug overdoses
- **Medical calculators**: Convenient calculators: dosing, metric conversions, and more
- **News and alerts**: Get FDA announcements, clinical updates, and upcoming drug launches
- **Laboratory test information**: Identify and interpret details of more than 500 laboratory tests
- **Disease database**: Find current evidence-based treatment recommendations
- **Alternative medicine database**: Consult information on more than 300 popular herbs and dietary supplements

Thomson Clinical Xpert is available **free** to registered members of PDR.net, your medical professional web portal for drug information and much more. Go to *www.PDR.net* to put this clinical-decision support tool to work for you now.

Web-Based Clinical Resources

PDR.net, a web portal designed specifically for healthcare professionals, provides a wealth of clinical information, including full drug and disease monographs, specialty-specific resource centers, patient education, clinical news, and conference information. PDR.net gives prescribers online access to authoritative, evidence-based information they need to support or confirm diagnosis and treatment decisions, including:

- Daily feeds of specialty news, conference coverage, and monthly summaries
- FDA-approved and other manufacturer-provided product labeling for more than 4,000 brand name drugs
- Multidrug interaction checker and other tools
- Extensive disease diagnosis and treatment information
- Customizable patient education
- Professional resources

Online access is **free** for U.S.-based MDs, DOs, dentists, NPs, and PAs in full-time patient practice, as well as for medical students, residents, and other select prescribing allied health professionals. Register today at *www.PDR.net*.

Other Clinical Information Products from PDR

For complicated cases and special patient problems, there is no substitute for the in-depth data contained in *Physicians' Desk Reference*. But for those times when you need quick access to critical prescribing information, consult the **PDR® Monthly Prescribing Guide™**, the essential drug reference designed specifically for use at the point of care. Distilled from the pages of *PDR*, this digest-sized reference presents the key facts on more than 1,500 drug formulations, including therapeutic class, indications and contraindications, warnings and precautions, pregnancy rating, drug interactions and side effects, and adult and pediatric dosages. Most entries also give the *PDR* page number to turn to for further information. In addition, a full-color insert of pill images allows you to correctly identify each product. Issued monthly, the guide is regularly updated with detailed descriptions of new drugs to receive FDA approval, as well as FDA-approved revisions to existing product information. You'll also find bulletins about major new developments in the pharmaceutical industry, an overview of important new agents nearing approval, and recent clinical findings on common nutritional supplements. To learn more about this useful publication and to inquire about subscription rates, call 800-232-7379.

PDR and its major companion volumes are also found in the **PDR® Electronic Library on CD-ROM**. This Windows-compatible disc provides users with a complete database of *PDR* prescribing information, electronically searchable for instant retrieval. A standard subscription includes *PDR*'s sophisticated search software and an extensive file of chemical structures, illustrations, and full-color product photographs. Optional enhancements include the complete contents of *The Merck Manual Seventeenth Edition*, *Stedman's Medical Dictionary*, and *Stedman's Spellchecker*. For anyone who wants to run a fast double check on a proposed prescription, there's also the *PDR® Drug Interactions and Side Effects System*—sophisticated software capable of automatically screening a 20-drug regimen for conflicts, then proposing alternatives for any problematic medication. This unique decision-making tool comes free with the *PDR Electronic Library*.

For more information on these or any other members of the growing family of *PDR* products, please call, toll-free, 800-232-7379 or fax 201-722-2680.

CONTENTS

SECTION 1

INDICES

This section offers four ways to locate the product information you need:

1. Manufacturers' Index: Gives the location of each participating manufacturer's product information. If two page numbers appear, the first refers to photographs in the Product Identification Guide, the second to product information. Also listed are the addresses and telephone numbers of the company's headquarters and regional offices.

2. Product Name Index: Lists page numbers of product information alphabetically by brand name. A diamond symbol to the left of a name indicates that a photograph of the item appears in the Product Identification Guide. For these products, the first page number refers to the photograph, the second to

an entry in one of the Product Information Sections. All pharmaceuticals, equipment, and intraocular products are included.

3. Product Category Index: Lists products alphabetically by type or category, such as "Anti-Infectives" or "Hypertonic Agents." All pharmaceuticals, equipment, and intraocular products are included.

4. Active Ingredients Index: Groups products alphabetically by generic name or material, such as "Atropine Sulfate" or "Dexamethasone." Under each heading, all fully described products are listed first, followed by those with only partial descriptions. Equipment is not included.

PART I/MANUFACTURERS' INDEX

ALCON LABORATORIES, INC.   **201**
and its Affiliates
Corporate Headquarters
6201 South Freeway
Fort Worth, TX 76134
Direct Inquiries to:
Pharmaceuticals/Consumer Products:
(800) 451-3937
(Therapeutic Drugs/Lens Care)
Surgical: (800) 862-5266
(Instrumentation/Surgical Meds)
(817) 293-0450 (Main Switchboard)

ALLERGAN   **103, 218**
2525 Dupont Drive
P.O. Box 19534
Irvine, CA 92623-9534
For Medical Information, Contact:
Outside CA: (800) 433-8871
CA: (714) 246-4500
Sales and Ordering:
Outside CA: (800) 377-7790
CA: (714) 246-4500

BAUSCH & LOMB   **103, 243**
INCORPORATED
One Bausch & Lomb Place
Rochester, NY 14604
Direct Inquiries to:
Customer Service Department:
(800) 323-0000
(813) 975-7700

CORNEAL SCIENCE   **104, 259**
CORPORATION
3209-129 Gresham Lake Road
Raleigh, NC 27615
Direct Inquiries to:
(800) 325-6789
(919) 876-4444
FAX: (919) 878-5040
E-mail: techsupport@cornealscience.com
www.cornealscience.com
For Medical Emergencies Contact:
Dr. Alan Touch
(800) 325-6789
(919) 876-4444 Ext. 23

(OSI) EYETECH   **260**
140 East Hanover Avenue
Cedar Knolls, NJ 07927
(OSI) Eyetech, Inc.
Direct Inquiries to:
(973) 775-4500
Fax 1: (973) 539-9661
Fax 2: (973) 539-2665

INSPIRE PHARMACEUTICALS   **262**
4222 Emperor Boulevard
Suite 200
Durham, NC 27703
Direct Inquiries to:
(919) 941-9777
FAX: (919) 941-9797
E-mail: info@inspirepharm.com

JOHNSON & JOHNSON   **104, 263**
HEALTHCARE
Product Division of McNeil PPC, Inc.
199 Grandview Road
Skillman, NJ 08558
Direct Inquiries to:
Consumer Affairs
(888) 734-6748

KING PHARMACEUTICALS,   **105, 264**
INC.
501 Fifth Street
Bristol, TN 37620
Direct Inquiries to:
(888) 358-6436
FAX: (866) 990-0545

MEDPOINTE PHARMACEUTICALS   **267**
MedPointe Healthcare, Inc.
265 Davidson Ave., Suite 300
Somerset, NJ 08873
Direct Inquiries to:
(732) 564-2200

MERCK & CO., INC.   **105, 268**
P.O. Box 4 WP39-206
West Point, PA 19486-0004
For Medical Information Contact:
Generally:
Product and service information:
Call the Merck National Service Center,
8:00 AM to 7:00 PM (ET), Monday
through Friday:
(800) NSC-MERCK
(800) 672-6372
FAX: (800) MERCK-68
FAX: (800) 637-2568

MERCK & CO., INC.—*cont.*

Adverse Drug Experiences:
Call the Merck National Service Center,
8:00 AM to 7:00 PM (ET), Monday
through Friday:
(800) NSC-MERCK
(800) 672-6372
Pregnancy Registries
(800) 986-8999

In Emergencies:
24-hour emergency information for
healthcare professionals:
(800) NSC-MERCK
(800) 672-6372

Sales and Ordering:
For product orders and direct account
inquiries only, call the Order Management
Center, 8:00 AM to 7:00 PM (ET),
Monday through Friday:
(800) MERCK RX
(800) 637-2579

MONARCH PHARMACEUTICALS
(See KING PHARMACEUTICALS, INC.)

PHARMACIA & UPJOHN   105, 285
A division of Pfizer
235 East 42nd Street
New York, NY 10017-5755

For Medical Information, Contact:
(800) 438-1985
24 hours a day, 7 days a week

SANTEN INC.
(See VISTAKON PHARMACEUTICALS, LLC)

VISTAKON   105, 287
PHARMACEUTICALS,
LLC
7500 Centurion Parkway
Jacksonville, FL 32256
Direct Inquiries to:
(866) 427-6815

PART II/PRODUCT NAME INDEX

◆ Shown in Product Identification Guide

Italic Page Number **Indicates Brief Listing**

PART III/PRODUCT CATEGORY INDEX

PART IV/ACTIVE INGREDIENTS INDEX

Italic Page Number **Indicates Brief Listing**

SECTION 2

PHARMACEUTICALS IN OPHTHALMOLOGY

Douglas J. Rhee, MD,[1] Christopher J. Rapuano, MD,[2] and George N. Papaliodis, MD,[1] with a section on ocular toxicology by F.W. Fraunfelder, MD[3]

We are pleased to present this updated overview of pharmaceutical options in ophthalmology. This edition of the *PDR for Ophthalmic Medicines* marks the introduction of nepafenac (Nevonac) and bromfenac (Xibrom); both are topical NSAIDs. Additionally, we've included revised information on antimicrobial therapy, drug-induced ocular side effects, and off-label drug uses.

In all, this section offers 30 reference tables presenting therapeutic alternatives in all major categories of ophthalmic treatment, as well as a survey of recently identified adverse drug reactions encountered in ophthalmology. The material is divided into 14 parts as follows:

1. Mydriatics and Cycloplegics
2. Antimicrobial Therapy
3. Ocular Anti-inflammatory Agents
4. Anesthetic Agents
5. Agents for Treatment of Glaucoma
6. Medications for Dry Eye
7. Ocular Decongestants
8. Ophthalmic Irrigating Solutions
9. Hyperosmolar Agents
10. Diagnostic Agents
11. Viscoelastic Materials Used in Ophthalmology
12. Anti-Angiogenesis Treatments
13. Off-Label Drug Applications in Ophthalmology
14. Ocular Toxicology

There are a large number of excellent references related to pharmacology and treatment regimens in ophthalmology. Listed below are some of the ones we regard as particularly useful.

GENERAL REFERENCES

American Medical Association. *Drug Evaluations Annual.* Milwaukee, Wis: AMA Department of Drugs, Division of Toxicology.

Fraunfelder FT, Fraunfelder FW. *Drug-Induced Ocular Side Effects*, ed 5. Woburn, Mass: Butterworth-Heinemann; 2001.

Fraunfelder FT, Roy FH. *Current Ocular Therapy*, ed 5. Philadelphia, Pa: WB Saunders; 1999.

Kunimoto DY, Kanitkar KD, Makar M, et al. *The Wills Eye Manual, Fourth Edition, for PDA* (Palm OS, Windows CE, and Pocket PC). Philadelphia, PA: Lippincott Williams & Wilkins; 2004.

Rhee DJ, Colby KA, Rapuano CJ, Sobrin L. *Ocular Drug Guide.* New York, NY: Springer 2007.

Tasman W, Jaeger EA. *Duane's Clinical Ophthalmology on CD-ROM, 2004 Edition.* Philadelphia, PA: Lippincott Williams & Wilkins; 2004.

Vaughan D, Asbury T, Riordan-Eva P. *General Ophthalmology*, ed 15. Norwalk, Conn: Appleton & Lange; 1999.

1. Massachusetts Eye and Ear Infirmary; Boston, MA.

2. Wills Eye Hospital; Philadelphia, PA.

3. Casey Eye Institute; Portland, OR.

1. MYDRIATICS AND CYCLOPLEGICS

The autonomic drugs that produce mydriasis (pupillary dilation) and cycloplegia (paralysis of accommodation) are among the most frequently used topical medications in ophthalmic practice. The most commonly used mydriatic is the direct-acting adrenergic agent phenylephrine hydrochloride, usually in a 2.5% concentration. Phenylephrine is used alone or, more commonly, in combination with a cycloplegic agent for refraction or pupillary dilation. The 2.5% concentration is favored for most cases. There is an increased possibility of severe adverse systemic effects from the use of the 10% solution.

Anticholinergic agents have both cycloplegic and mydriatic activity. They are usually used for refraction, pupillary dilation, and relief of photosensitivity during intraocular inflammation (by minimizing movement of the inflamed iris).

It is important to remember that the effect of these medications depends on many factors, including age, race, and eye color. For example, the mydriatics and cycloplegics tend to be less effective in dark-eyed individuals than in those with blue-eyes.

When using mydriatics and cycloplegic drugs, it is important to instruct the patient to wear sunglasses and avoid driving or operating dangerous machinery.

TABLE 1

MYDRIATICS AND CYCLOPLEGICS

GENERIC NAME	TRADE NAMES	CONCENTRATION	ONSET/DURATION OF ACTION
Phenylephrine hydrochloride	AK-Dilate Mydfrin Neo-Synephrine Available generically	Soln, 2.5%, 10% Soln, 2.5% Soln, 2.5% Soln, 2.5%, 10%	30–60 min/3–5 h
Atropine sulfate	Atropine-Care Isopto Atropine Available generically	Soln, 1% Soln, 1% Soln, 1% Ointment, 1%	45–120 min/7–14 days
Cyclopentolate hydrochloride	AK-Pentolate Cyclogyl Cylate Available generically	Soln, 1% Soln, 0.5%, 1%, 2% Soln, 1% Soln, 1%	30–60 min/6–24 h
Homatropine hydrobromide	Isopto Homatropine Available generically	Soln, 2%, 5% Soln, 2%, 5%	30–60 min/3 days
Scopolamine hydrobromide	Isopto Hyoscine	Soln, 0.25%	30–60 min/4–7 days
Tropicamide	Mydriacyl Tropicacyl Available generically	Soln, 1% Soln, 0.5%, 1% Soln, 0.5%, 1%	20–40 min/4–6 h

2. ANTIMICROBIAL THERAPY

Antibiotics are routinely used in ophthalmology for both treatment and prophylaxis. They are used prophylactically in the management of foreign bodies and corneal abrasions and in preoperative and postoperative care, administered as an ophthalmic solution, ointment, or subconjunctival injection (see **Table 2**).

Many ophthalmic institutions have been using a solution of 5% povidone-iodine (Betadine) preoperatively to "sterilize" the eye, lids, and brow. Another development is the use of collagen shields (usually 12-hour) soaked in antibiotic, with or without steroid, in place of a patch and/or subconjunctival injection after surgery. While more expensive, the shields do have the advantage of being more comfortable for the patient and are less likely to cause tissue degeneration.

Also in the literature is another prophylactic measure: the addition of antibiotics to the irrigating solution. This technique is being used in several hospitals and high-volume surgicenters throughout the country. The maximum nontoxic concentrations of antibiotics are listed in **Table 3**. For prophylaxis, however, clinicians advise using half these amounts. Note that concentrations are given in micrograms per milliliter. It is critical that these medications be prepared by well trained technicians, nurses, or pharmacists.

Whether treating an external or intraocular infection, slides for gram and Giemsa stain and aerobic and anaerobic cultures should be secured prior to initiating therapy if the severity or site of infection dictates the necessity of culturing. When fungal, acanthamoebal, or atypical mycobacterial involvement is a possibility, additional stains to consider are: methenamine silver, periodic acid-Schiff (PAS), acridine orange, and calcofluor white. You can also consider using Lowenstein-Jensen culture medium. When an active or suspected superficial ocular infection is accompanied by inflammation, a variety of combination agents may be considered (see **Table 4**).

Corneal ulcers and intraocular infections require vigorous management. Most physicians and hospitals have protocols for their treatment. One such protocol for treating endophthalmitis, modified from Mandelbaum and Forster, is given in **Table 5**. Serious ocular infections are usually treated by the topical, subconjunctival, and intraocular routes of administration (see **Table 6**). Corneal ulcers are usually treated with one or more of the topical solutions listed in **Table 6**, usually given every $1/_2$ to 1 hour, in alternating doses if more than one solution is used. In severe cases, such as impending or actual perforation and scleral extension, medication is given by the topical, subconjunctival, oral, and/or intravenous route.

Fungal keratitis (keratomycosis) is relatively uncommon, but should be suspected in patients who have previously received topical steroids and/or antibiotics or have experienced ocular trauma, and in patients whose corneal ulcer does not respond to antibiotics. A recent outbreak of Fusarium keratitis in soft-contact lens wearers highlights the fact that contact lens disinfecting solutions are not 100% effective at preventing infections. Corneal scraping often permits correct clinical diagnosis. Natamycin 5% ophthalmic suspension (Natacyn) is recognized as one of the most potent broad-spectrum antifungal agents available for use in the eye. Amphotericin B 0.15% ophthalmic solution, which is extemporaneously prepared, is another commonly used antifungal agent. Topical voriconazole 1%, made from the IV solution, is gaining popularity for treating recalcitrant fungal corneal ulcers.

Endogenous fungal endophthalmitis can be seen in intravenous drug users, patients with indwelling catheters, and patients with compromised immune systems. For these infections, amphotericin B has been used subconjunctivally, intravenously, and, where indicated, intravitreally. Prior to intravitreal use, a small portion of the vitreous abscess should be aspirated for microbiologic study. In addition to amphotericin B, flucytosine has also been used to treat fungal endophthalmitis. For more on treatment of fungal infections, see **Table 7**.

There has been an increase, within the last decade, in the incidence of Acanthamoeba keratitis. This has been linked, in many cases, to use of contaminated solutions for soft-contact lenses — especially homemade saline solutions. Current therapy includes the concurrent use of polyhexamethylene biguanide compounded with Baquacil (PHMB), Neosporin, and chlorhexidine digluconate (CHX) (found in Boston Rewetting Drops).

In bacterial endophthalmitis, the use of intraocular and periocular antimicrobial therapy has significantly improved the final visual outcome. A diagnosis of bacterial endophthalmitis should be strongly suspected in a patient who is postoperative or posttraumatic, or when the intraocular inflammation is out of proportion to the situation. Ocular pain is often present before obvious inflammation. Preoperative and postoperative antibiotics may decrease the incidence of postoperative endophthalmitis.

Once endophthalmitis is suspected, prompt intervention is required. Samples of the aqueous and vitreous humors must be promptly secured and treatment quickly initiated with antimicrobials appropriate to the suspected organism(s). Fungal or anaerobic organisms should be considered in cases where inflammation occurs several weeks or more after surgery or in cases of trauma or immunosuppression.

Once the aqueous and vitreous humors have been cultured, antimicrobial agents should be directly injected into the vitreous. To prevent retinal toxicity, medications should be injected slowly into the anterior vitreous cavity, with particular caution after vitrectomy. Vitrectomy and intravitreal antibiotics should always be considered when treating endophthalmitis.

In a study by Pavan and Brinser, the use of intravenous antibiotics was found to make no difference in final visual acuity or media clarity. The authors concluded that "omission of systemic antibiotic treatment can reduce toxic effects, costs, and length of hospital stay." Despite advances in antimicrobial therapy, this premise is still supported by current publications documenting the efficacy of intravitreal antibiotics without the need for intravenous antibiotics, assuming the infection is limited to the eye.

REFERENCES

Anonymous. Results of endophthalmitis vitrectomy study. *Arch Ophthalmol.* 1995;113:1479.

Axelrod AJ, Peyman GA. Intravitreal amphotericin B treatment of experimental fungal endophthalmitis. *Am J Ophthalmol.* 1973;76:584.

Barza M. Antibacterial agents in the treatment of ocular infections. *Infect Dis Clin North Am.* 1989;3:533-551.

Baum JL. Antibiotic use in ophthalmology. In: Tasman W, Jaeger EA, eds. *Duane's Clinical Ophthalmology.* Vol. 4. Philadelphia, Pa: JB Lippincott; 1989:chap 26.

Ellis P. *Ocular Therapeutics and Pharmacology.* 7th ed. St. Louis, Mo: CV Mosby; 1985.

Forster RK. Endophthalmitis. In: Tasman W, Jaeger EA, eds. *Duane's Clinical Ophthalmology.* Vol. 4. Philadelphia, Pa: JB Lippincott; 1989:chap 24.

Gardner S. Treatment of bacterial endophthalmitis. *Ocular Therapeutics and Management.* 1991;2(1):3-4.

Lamberts DW, Potter DE, eds. *Clinical Ocular Pharmacology.* Boston, Mass: Little, Brown; 1987.

Lemp MA, Blackman HJ, Koffler BH. Therapy for bacterial and fungal infections. *Int Ophthalmol Clin.* 1980;20(3):135-145.

Pavan PR, Brinser JH. Exogenous bacterial endophthalmitis treated without systemic antibiotics. *Am J Ophthalmol.* 1987;104:121.

Peyman GA. Antibiotic administration in the treatment of bacterial endophthalmitis. II. Intravitreal injections. *Surv Ophthalmol.* 1977;21:332,339-346.

Tabbara KF, Hyndiuk RA, eds. *Infections of the Eye.* Boston, Mass: Little, Brown; 1986.

TABLE 2

COMMERCIALLY AVAILABLE OPHTHALMIC ANTIBACTERIAL AGENTS

GENERIC NAME	TRADE NAME	CONCENTRATION	
		OPHTHALMIC SOLUTION	OPHTHALMIC OINTMENT
INDIVIDUAL AGENTS			
Bacitracin	Available generically	Not available	500 units/g
Ciprofloxacin hydrochloride	Ciloxan	0.3%	0.3%
Erythromycin	Available generically	Not available	0.5%
Gatifloxacin	Zymar	0.3%	Not available
Gentamicin sulfate	Garamycin	0.3%	0.3%
	Genoptic	0.3%	Not available
	Gentak	0.3%	0.3%
	Genoptic S.O.P.	Not available	0.3%
	Available generically	0.3%	0.3%
Levofloxacin	Iquix	1.5%	Not available
	Quixin	0.5%	Not available
Moxifloxacin	Vigamox	0.5%	Not available
Ofloxacin	Ocuflox	0.3%	Not available
Sulfacetamide sodium	Bleph-10	10%	Not available
	Sulf-10 (15-mL bottle or preservative-free dropperettes)	10%	Not available
	Available generically	10%	10%
Tobramycin sulfate	AK-Tob	0.3%	Not available
	Tobrex	0.3%	0.3%
	Tobrasol	0.3%	Not available
	Available generically	0.3%	Not available
MIXTURES			
Polymyxin B/Bacitracin Zinc	AK-Poly-Bac Polysporin Polycin-B Available generically	Not available	10,000 units - 500 units/g
Polymyxin B/Neomycin/Bacitracin	Neosporin Available generically	Not available	10,000 units - 3.5 mg - 400 units/g
Polymyxin B/Neomycin/Gramicidin	Neosporin Available generically	10,000 units - 1.75 mg - 0.025 mg/mL	Not available
Polymyxin B/Oxytetracyclin	Available generically	Not available	10,000 units - 5%
Polymyxin B/Trimethoprim	Polytrim Available generically	10,000 units - 1 mg/mL	Not available

TABLE 3

ANTIBIOTICS IN INFUSION FLUID

AGENT	MAXIMUM NONTOXIC DOSE (mcg/mL)	AGENT	MAXIMUM NONTOXIC DOSE (mcg/mL)
Amikacin	10	Oxacillin	10
Ceftazidime	40	Tobramycin	10
Clindamycin	9	Vancomycin*	30
Gentamicin	8		

*Routine usage for prophylaxis is discouraged by CDC because of increased resistant organisms.
Adapted from Peyman GA, Daun M. Prophylaxis of endophthalmitis. *Ophthalmic Surg.* 1994;25:673.

TABLE 4

COMBINATION OCULAR ANTI-INFLAMMATORY AND ANTIBIOTIC AGENTS

GENERIC NAME	TRADE NAME	PREPARATION & CONCENTRATION
Dexamethasone - Neomycin - Polymyxin B	Dexasporin Maxitrol Poly-Dex Available generically	Suspension, 0.1% - 3.5 mg/mL - 10,000 units/mL
	AK-Trol Maxitrol Poly-Dex Available generically	Ointment, 0.1%-3.5 mg/g-10,000 units/mL Ointment, 0.1% - 3.5 mg/g - 10,000 units/g
Dexamethasone - Tobramycin	Tobradex Tobradex	Suspension, 0.1% - 0.3% Ointment, 0.1% - 0.3%
Fluorometholone - Sulfacetamide	FML-S	Suspension, 0.1% - 10%
Gentamicin - Prednisolone acetate	Pred-G Pred-G S.O.P.	Suspension, 0.3% - 1.0% Ointment, 0.3% - 0.6%
Hydrocortisone - Neomycin - Polymyxin B	Cortisporin Available generically	Suspension, 1% - 3.5 mg/mL - 10,000 units/mL
Hydrocortisone - Neomycin - Polymyxin B - Bacitracin	AK Spore HC Cortisporin Available generically	Ointment, 1% - 3.5 mg/g - 10,000 units/g - 400 units/g
Loteprednol etabonate - Tobramycin	Zylet	Suspension, 0.5% - 0.3%
Prednisolone acetate - Neomycin - Polymyxin B	Poly-Pred	Suspension, 0.5% - 0.35% - 10,000 units/mL
Prednisolone acetate - Sulfacetamide	Blephamide Blephamide S. O. P.	Suspension, 0.2% - 10% Ointment, 0.2% - 10%
Prednisolone sodium phosphate - Sulfacetamide	Vasocidin Available generically	Solution, 0.25% - 10% Solution, 0.25% - 10%

TABLE 5

REGIMEN FOR ENDOPHTHALMITIS

1. Diagnostic anterior chamber and vitreous aspiration; diagnostic vitrectomy when liquid vitreous fails to aspirate or in cases of suspected fungal endophthalmitis.

2. Initial therapy (in operating room after diagnostic technique).

A. Intraocular: gentamicin 100 mcg or amikacin 400 mcg and vancomycin 1000 mcg or ceftazidime 2000 mcg

B. Subconjunctival: gentamicin 40 mg and triamcinolone acetonide (Kenalog) 40 mg*

C. Topical: gentamicin 9.1 or 13.4 mg/mL and cefazolin 50 mg/mL and prednisolone acetate 1%; alternatively; a 3rd or 4th generation fluoroquinolone (along with prednisolone acetate 1%)

D. Systemic: cefazolin (Ancef or Kefzol) 1000 mg every 6 to 8 hours or Imipenen/Cilastatin 500 mg IV q 6 hours. (Ceftriaxone has good penetration of the blood-ocular barrier and may be used as an alternative.) The use of systemic antibiotics is controversial; many practitioners do not employ them.

3. If cultures are positive for virulent bacteria, consider repeating the above intraocular injections at the bedside on the second and fourth postoperative days. Continue topical treatment every half hour, subconjunctival treatment daily, and systemic ther-apy. Consider therapeutic vitrectomy with repeat intraocular antibiotics.

4. If cultures are negative after 48 hours, do not repeat intraocular antibiotics. Consider tapering topical, subconjunctival, and systemic antibiotic therapy while continuing topical and subconjunctival corticosteroids.

5. If endophthalmitis presents as a *delayed inflammation* in which a fungal etiology is considered, the vitreous sample should be obtained by a vitreous instrument using membrane filters; intraocular amphotericin B (Fungizone) at a dosage of 5 mcg should be considered.

6. If endophthalmitis presents as a delayed inflammation or chronic indolent infection, a *Propionibacterium acnes* infection should be considered.

Source: Mandelbaum S, Forster RK.
Anonymous. Results of endophthalmitis vitrectomy study. *Arch Ophthalmol.* 1995;113:1479.

*Subconjunctival corticosteroids should be deferred 48 to 72 hours to await culture growth and confirmation if a fungal etiology is suspected or the inflammation is delayed.

TABLE 6

CONCENTRATIONS AND DOSAGE OF PRINCIPAL ANTIBIOTIC AGENTS

DRUG NAME*	TOPICAL	SUBCONJUNCTIVAL	INTRAVITREAL	INTRAVENOUS[†]
Amikacin sulfate	10 mg/mL	25 mg	400 mcg	15 mg/kg daily in 2–3 doses
Ampicillin sodium	50 mg/mL	50–150 mg	5 mg	4–12 g daily in 4 doses
Bacitracin zinc	10,000 units/mL	5000 units	. . .	. . .
Cefazolin sodium	50 mg/mL	100 mg	2250 mcg	2–4 g daily in 3–4 doses
Ceftazidime	50 mg/mL	100 mg	2000 mcg	1 g daily in 2–3 doses
Ceftriaxone	50 mg/mL	. . .	. . .	1–4 g daily in 1–2 doses
Ciprofloxacin	0.3%	. . .	. . .	400 mg IV q 8 hours
Clindamycin	50 mg/mL	15–50 mg	1000 mcg	900–1800 mg daily in 2–3 doses
Colistimethate sodium	10 mg/mL	15–25 mg	100 mcg	2.5–5 mg/kg daily in 2–4 doses
Erythromycin	50 mg/mL	100 mg	500 mcg	. . .
Gentamicin sulfate	8–15 mg/mL	10–20 mg	100–200 mcg	3–5 mg/kg daily in 2–3 doses
Imipenem/Cilastatin sodium	5 mg/mL	. . .	. . .	2 g daily in 3–4 doses
Kanamycin sulfate	30–50 mg/mL	30 mg	500 mcg	. . .
Levofloxacin	1.5%	0.5%	. . .	500 mg IV q 24 hours
Neomycin sulfate	5–8 mg/mL	125–250 mg	. . .	. . .
Penicillin G	100,000 units/mL	0.5–1.0 million units	300 units	12–24 million units daily in 4–6 doses
Piperacillin	12.5 mg/mL	100 mg	. . .	. . .
Polymyxin B sulfate	10,000 units/mL	100,000 units	. . .	. . .
Ticarcillin disodium	6 mg/mL	100 mg	. . .	200–300 mg/kg daily 3 x in 4–6 doses
Tobramycin sulfate	8–15 mg/mL	10–20 mg	100–200 mcg	3–5 mg/kg daily in 2–3 doses
Vancomycin hydrochloride‡	20–25 mg/mL	25 mg	1000 mcg	15–30 mg/kg daily in 1–2 doses

*Most penicillins and cephalosporins are physically incompatible when combined in the same bottle with aminoglycosides such as amikacin, gentamicin, or tobramycin. †Adult doses. ‡Usage discouraged by CDC because of increased resistant organisms.

TABLE 7

ANTIFUNGAL AGENTS

GENERIC (TRADE) NAME	ROUTE	DOSAGE	SPECTRUM
Amphotericin B (Fungizone)	Topical	0.1–0.5% solution (most commonly 0.15%); dilute with water for injection or dextrose 5% in water	*Blastomyces (Fungizone), Candida, Coccidioides, Histoplasma*
	Subconjunctival	0.8–1.0 mg	
	Intravitreal	5 mcg	
	Intravenous	*	
Caspofungin (Cancidas)	Intravenous	50 mg daily	*Candida, Aspergillus*
Clotrimazole	Oral	One troche 5 times a day	*Candida*
Eraxis (Anidulafungin)	Intravenous	100 mg daily	*Candida*
Fluconazole (Diflucan)	Oral	150 mg single dose 200 mg on day 1, then 100 mg daily in divided doses 400 mg on day 1, then 200 mg daily in divided doses	*Candida, Cryptococcus*
	Intravenous	200-400 mg IV daily*	
Flucytosine (Ancobon)	Oral	50–150 mg/kg daily in 4 divided doses*	*Candida, Cryptococcus*
Griseofulvin	Oral	500 mg daily	*Tinea*
Gris-PEG (Griseofulvin ultramicrosize)	Oral	375 mg daily 750 mg daily (divided doses)	*Tinea*
Itraconazole (Sporanox)	Oral	200–400 mg daily*	*Blastomyces, Histoplasma, Aspergillus, Onychomyces*
	Intravenous	200 mg IV twice a day for 4 doses, then 200 mg IV daily for 14 days*	
Ketoconazole (Nizoral)	Oral	200–400 mg daily*	*Candida, Cryptococcus, Histoplasma*
Natamycin (Natacyn)	Topical	5% suspension	*Candida, Aspergillus, Cephalosporium, Fusarium, Penicillium*
Posaconazole (Noxafil)	Oral	200 mg three times a day 100mg (2.5mL) twice a day on day 1, then 100mg daily for 13 days	*Candida, Aspergillus*
Terbinafine (Lamisil)	Oral	250 mg daily	*Tinea*
Voriconazole (Vfend)	Topical	1% (made from IV solution); dosing ranges from hourly to bid as determined by the clinician.	*Aspergillus, Blastomyces, Candida, Cryptococcus, Fusarium, Histoplasma, Penicillium, Scedosporium*
	Oral	200 mg twice a day	
	Intravenous	3-6 mg/kg every 12 hours*	

*Because of potential side effects and toxicity, the practitioner should consult the main *PDR* for possible dosage adjustments and warnings.

TABLE 8

ANTIVIRAL AGENTS

GENERIC (TRADE) NAME	TOPICAL CONC.	INTRAVIT. DOSE	SYSTEMIC DOSAGE*
Trifluridine (Viroptic) Available generically	1.0% (oph. solution)	. . .	. . .
Acyclovir sodium (Zovirax) Available generically	. . .	. . .	Oral–Herpes simplex keratitis, acute infection: 400 mg 5 times daily for 7–14 days; prophylactic dose: 400 mg 2 times daily. Oral–Herpes zoster ophthalmicus: 600–800 mg 5 times daily for 7-10 days; IV therapy[†]
Cidofovir (Vistide)	. . .	. . .	IV–Induction: 5 mg/kg constant infusion over 1 hour administered once weekly for 2 consecutive weeks. Maintenance: 5mg/kg constant infusion over 1 hour administered once every 2 weeks
Famciclovir (Famvir)	. . .	. . .	Oral–Herpes zoster ophthalmicus: 500 mg 3 times daily for 7 days
Foscarnet sodium (Foscavir)	. . .	. . .	IV–by controlled infusion only, either by central vein or by peripheral vein-Induction: 60 mg/kg (adjusted for renal function) given over 1 h every 8 h for 14–21 days. Maintenance: 90–120 mg/kg given over 2 hours once daily
Ganciclovir sodium (Cytovene)	. . .	200 mcg	IV–Induction: 5 mg/kg every 12 h for 14–21 days Maintenance: 5 mg/kg daily for 7 days or 6 mg once daily for 5 days/week. Oral– After IV induction: 1000 mg 3 times daily with food or 500 mg 6 times daily every 3 h
Ganciclovir sodium (Vitrasert)	. . .	4.5 mg	Sterile intravitreal insert designed to release the drug over a 5- to 8-month period
Valacyclovir (Valtrex)	. . .	. . .	Oral–Herpes zoster ophthalmicus: 1 gram 3 times daily for 7 days
Valganciclovir (Valcyte)	. . .	. . .	Oral–CMV retinaitis: 900 mg every 12 hours for 21 days then daily

*Because of potential side effects and toxicity, the practitioner should consult the main *PDR* for possible dosage adjustments and warnings.
[†]IV therapy should be considered if the patient is immunocompromised.

3. OCULAR ANTI-INFLAMMATORY AGENTS

A wide variety of medications are available for therapy. They are listed in **Table 9**. Corticosteroids are the most commonly used. Many are available in combination with antibiotics and/or other medications.

At one time, it was felt that corticosteroids were contraindicated in infectious disease states. However, it is now appreciated that steroids, when used in conjunction with appropriate antimicrobial, antifungal, or antiviral agents, may help prevent more serious ocular damage.

TABLE 9

TOPICAL ANTI-INFLAMMATORY AGENTS

NAME AND DOSAGE FORM	TRADE NAME	CONCENTRATION
Dexamethasone Sodium Phosphate Ophthalmic Solution or Ointment	Maxidex Ocu-Dex	0.1% 0.1%, 0.5%
Fluorometholone Ophthalmic Ointment	FML S.O.P.	0.1%
Fluorometholone Ophthalmic Suspension	Fluor-Op FML FML Forte Available generically	0.1% 0.1% 0.25% 0.1%
Fluorometholone Acetate Ophthalmic Suspension	Flarex	0.1%
Loteprednol Etabonate Ophthalmic Suspension	Alrex Lotemax	0.2% 0.5%
Medrysone Ophthalmic Suspension	HMS	1%
Prednisolone Acetate Ophthalmic Suspension	Pred Mild Econopred Plus Pred Forte Available generically	0.12% 1% 1% 1%
Prednisolone Sodium Phosphate Ophthalmic Solution	Inflamase Mild AK-Pred Inflamase Forte Available generically	0.125% 1% 1% 0.125%, 1%
Rimexolone Ophthalmic Suspension	Vexol	1%
NONSTEROIDAL ANTI-INFLAMMATORY DRUGS		
Bromfenac Ophthalmic	Xibrom	0.09%
Diclofenac Sodium Ophthalmic Solution	Voltaren	0.1%
Flurbiprofen Sodium Ophthalmic Solution	Ocufen Available generically	0.03% 0.03%
Ketorolac Tromethamine Ophthalmic Solution	Acular LS Acular Acular PF Available generically	0.4% 0.5% 0.5% 0.5%
Nepafenac Ophthalmic	Nevanac	0.1%

Steroids may be administered by four different routes in the treatment of ocular inflammation. **Table 10** lists the preferred route in various conditions.

Topical corticosteroids can elevate intraocular pressure and, in susceptible individuals, can induce glaucoma. Some corticosteroids, such as fluorometholone acetate, medrysone, and loteprednol cause less elevation of intraocular pressure than others. Corticosteroids, particularly topically administered corticosteroids, may also cause cataract formation. However, long-term systemic use can also accelerate cataract formation.

In addition to topical, subtenons, and singular intravitreal dosing, sustained release dosing of fluocinolone acetonide 0.59 mg (Retisent) is also available.

There are also five nonsteroidal anti-inflammatory drugs (NSAIDs) available. They are: bromfenac (Xibrom), diclofenac (Voltaren); flurbiprofen (Ocufen); ketorolac (Acular) and nepafenac (Nevanac). Flurbiprofen is indicated solely for inhibition of intraoperative miosis. Diclofenac has an official indication for the postoperative prophylaxis and treatment of ocular inflammation. Ketorolac is indicated for the treatment of postoperative inflammation and for relief of ocular itching due to seasonal allergic conjunctivitis. It has also shown some success in alleviating the pain associated with keratotomy, although unapproved for this use. Both diclofenac and ketorolac have also been used successfully to prevent and treat cystoid macular edema. NSAIDs cause little, if any, rise in intraocular pressure. However, in rare instances, topical NSAIDs have been associated with corneal melts and perforations, especially in older patients with ocular surface disease such as dry eyes.

TABLE 10

USUAL ROUTE OF STEROID ADMINISTRATION IN OCULAR INFLAMMATION

CONDITION	ROUTE
Anterior uveitis	Topical and/or periocular
Blepharitis	Topical
Conjunctivitis	Topical
Cranial arteritis	Systemic
Endophthalmitis	Systemic-periocular, and/or intravitreal
Episcleritis	Topical
Keratitis	Topical
Optic neuritis	Systemic or periocular
Posterior uveitis	Systemic and/or periocular, and/or intravitreal
Scleritis	Topical and/or systemic
Sympathetic ophthalmia	Systemic and topical

Other useful agents include mast-cell inhibitors, antihistamines, low-concentration steroids, and decongestants to treat vernal conjunctivitis or allergic keratoconjunctivitis. Tetracycline, taken orally, in doses of 250 mg 4 times daily for 4 weeks, then 250 mg once daily, is useful in treating ocular rosacea. Alternatively, doxycycline or minocycline, taken orally, in doses of 100 mg twice daily for 1 to 2 weeks, then 40-100 mg once daily or in divided doses may be used.

Agents useful in treatment of seasonal allergic conjunctivitis are listed in **Table 11.**

TABLE 11

AGENTS FOR RELIEF OF SEASONAL ALLERGIC CONJUNCTIVITIS

GENERIC NAME	TRADE NAME	CLASS	TYPICAL DAILY DOSE
Azelastine HCl	Astelin, Optivar	H_1-Antagonist/Mast-cell inhibitor	2
Cromolyn sodium	Crolom Available generically	Mast-cell inhibitor	4-6
Emedastine difumarate	Emadine	H_1-Antagonist	4
Epinastine HCl	Elestat	H_1- and H_2-antagonist/ Mast-cell inhibitor	2
Ketorolac tromethamine	Acular, Acular LS, Acular PF	NSAID	4
Ketotifen fumarate	Alaway, Zaditor (OTC)	H_1-Antagonist/Mast-cell inhibitor	2
Levocabastine HCl	Livostin	H_1-Antagonist	4
Lodoxamide tromethamine	Alomide	Mast-cell inhibitor	4
Loteprednol etabonate	Alrex Lotemax	Corticosteroid	4
Naphazoline/antazoline	Vasocon-A (OTC)	Antihistamine/decongestant	4
Naphazoline/pheniramine	Naphcon-A (OTC) Opcon-A (OTC) Visine-A (OTC)	Antihistamine/decongestant	4
Nedocromil sodium	Alocril	H_1-Antagonist/Mast-cell inhibitor	2
Olopatadine HCl 0.1%	Patanol	H_1-Antagonist/Mast-cell inhibitor	2
Olopatadine HCl 0.2%	Pataday	H_1-Antagonist/Mast-cell inhibitor	1
Pemirolast potassium	Alamast	Mast-cell inhibitor	4

4. ANESTHETIC AGENTS

A. Topical anesthetics

The agents listed in **Table 12** permit the clinician to perform ocular procedures such as tonometry, removal of foreign bodies from the surface of the eye, and lacrimal canalicular manipulation and irrigation. Cocaine, the prototype topical anesthetic, is a natural compound; the others are synthetic.

Cocaine is rarely used as an anesthetic agent because it causes damage to the corneal epithelium, produces pupillary dilation, and may affect intraocular pressure. However, it is considered useful when removal of the corneal epithelium is desired, as in epithelial debridement for dendritic keratitis.

The table lists available agents and concentrations. Most begin working within a minute and continue acting for 10 to 20 minutes. A transient, superficial punctate keratitis may develop rapidly after instillation of the agent.

B. Regional anesthetics

The actions, benefits, and drawbacks of the most common regional anesthetic agents used in ophthalmic surgery are summarized in **Table 13**.

TABLE 12

TOPICAL ANESTHETIC AGENTS

USP OR NF NAME	TRADE NAME	CONCENTRATION
Cocaine hydrochloride*	. . .	1%–4%
Proparacaine hydrochloride	Alcaine	0.5%
	Ocu-Caine	0.5%
	Ophthetic	0.5%
	Paracaine	0.5%
	Available generically	0.5%
Tetracaine hydrochloride	Pontocaine	0.5%, 1%, 2%
	Available generically	0.5%

*Extemporaneous formulation.

TABLE 13

REGIONAL ANESTHETICS*

USP OR NF NAME	CONCENTRATION/ MAXIMUM DOSE	ONSET OF ACTION	DURATION OF ACTION	MAJOR ADVANTAGES/ DISADVANTAGES
Bupivacaine[†,‡]	0.25%–0.75%	5–11 min	480–720 min (with epinephrine)	
Etidocaine[†]	1%	3 min	300–600 min	
Lidocaine[†]	1%–2%/500 mg	4–6 min	40–60 min 120 min (with epinephrine)	Spreads readily without hyaluronidase
Mepivacaine[†]	1%–2%/500 mg	3–5 min	120 min	Duration of action greater without epinephrine[2]
Prilocaine[†]	1%–2%/600 mg	3–4 min	90–120 min (with epinephrine)	As effective as lidocaine
Procaine[§]	1%–4%/500 mg	7–8 min	30–45 min 60 min (with epinephrine)	Short duration. Poor absorption from mucous membranes
Tetracaine[§]	0.25%	5–9 min	120–140 min (with epinephrine)	

*Retrobulbar injection has been reported to cause apnea.
[†]Amide type compound.
[‡]A mixture of bupivacaine, lidocaine, and epinephrine has been shown to be effective in retinal detachment surgery under local anesthesia.[1]
[§]Ester type compound.

REFERENCES

1. Holekamp TLR, Arribas NP, Boniuk I. Bupivacaine anesthesia in retinal detachment surgery. *Arch Ophthalmol.* 1979;97:109.
2. Everett WG, Vey EK, Finlay JW. Duration of oculomotor akinesia of injectable anesthetics. *Trans Am Acad Ophthalmol.* 1961;65:308.

5. AGENTS FOR TREATMENT OF GLAUCOMA

A. α_2 Selective agonists — see Table 14
There are two medications in this class: apraclonidine and brimonidine. Apraclonidine is available as a single-dose applicator of a 1% solution for suppression of the acute intraocular pressure spikes that occur after laser treatments. A 0.5% concentration is also available, supplied in a multiple-dose bottle for use with other glaucoma medications to control pressure in patients who are not responding adequately to maximally tolerated glaucoma therapy. The medication is generally useful only for short-term therapy, since it has been associated with tachyphylaxis within 3 months in up to 48% of patients. Brimonidine, the second agent in this class, is 23 to 32 times more selective for alpha$_2$ versus alpha$_1$ adrenoreceptors than is apraclonidine. This allows the medication to be used on a chronic basis with reduced risk of tachyphylaxis. Brimonidine ophthalmic solution is available in concentrations of 0.2% (generic), 0.15% (Alphagan-P), and 0.1% (Alphagan-P).

B. β-Adrenergic blocking agents — see Table 15
These medications work by blocking β-adrenergic receptor sites and decreasing aqueous production, thereby reducing intraocular pressure. Because β-adrenergic receptors occur in a number of organ systems, systemic side effects of these drugs may include slowed heart rate, decreased blood pressure, and exacerbation of intrinsic bronchial asthma and emphysema. These agents can also enhance the effects of a number of systemic medications including β-blockers, digitalis alkaloids, and reserpine. Since betaxolol is a cardioselective β-blocker, it has significantly less effect on the respiratory system and can be used in some patients with respiratory illnesses.

C. Carbonic anhydrase inhibitors — see Table 16
Used both topically and systemically, these drugs decrease the formation and secretion of aqueous humor. The systemic forms are usually used to supplement various topical agents (but not topical CAIs). Use of the systemic agents is limited by their side effects, which include paresthesias, anorexia, gas-trointestinal disturbances, headaches, altered taste and smell, sodium and potassium depletion, ureteral colic, a predisposition to form renal calculi, and, rarely, bone marrow suppression. The most commonly reported adverse effects of the topical solution are superficial punctate keratitis and ocular allergic reactions. Less frequently reported are blurred vision, tearing, ocular dryness, and photophobia. Infrequent are headache, nausea, asthenia, and fatigue. Rarely, skin rashes, urolithiasis, and iridocyclitis may occur.

Carbonic anhydrase inhibitors have a sulfonamide moiety and should be avoided in patients with known drug allergies to sulfonamides. In addition to hypersensitivity mediated allergic reactions, systemic CAIs have been associated with bilateral acute angle-closure glaucoma and acute myopia.

D. Hyperosmotic agents — see Table 17
These medications decrease intraocular pressure by creating an osmotic gradient between the blood and intraocular fluid, causing fluid to move out of the aqueous and vitreous humors into the bloodstream. They are used for acute situations and are not to be used chronically. These agents are employed to decrease pressure in an attack of acute-closure glaucoma, and to give a "soft" eye during surgery. Increased intravascular osmolarity increases the intravascular fluid volume and has the potential to increase cardiovascular stress. Therefore, these agents should be used with caution in patients with a history of cardiac disease.

E. Miotics — see Table 18
Parasympathomimetic agents (miotics) are used primarily as topical therapy for glaucoma. A secondary use is the control of accommodative esotropia. This class of agents mimics the effect of acetylcholine on parasympathomimetic postganglionic nerve endings within the eye. The class is subdivided into direct-acting (cholinergic) agents and indirect-acting (anticholinesterase) agents, based on their respective abilities to bind acetylcholine receptors and inhibit the enzymatic hydrolysis of acetylcholine. Table 18 lists the parasympathomimetics approved for topical use in the United States. In addition, two agents are available for intraocular use: Miochol-E, a 1% solution of acetylcholine, and Miostat or Carbastat, a 0.01% solution of carbachol.

F. Prostaglandins — see Table 19
A single evening dose of latanoprost, travoprost, or bimatoprost has each been shown to be more effective in reducing intraocular pressure than timolol 0.5% administered twice daily. Ocular side effects—hyperemia, itching, foreign-body sensation, and stinging—appear to be minimal, and systemic side effects have not been observed. An increase in pigmentation in the iris occurs in approximately 10% of patients; the rate is higher in eyes with mixed-color irises and lower in blue or brown irises. Changes in periocular skin pigmentation have also been noted.

G. Sympathomimetics — see Table 20
These medications work by improving aqueous outflow and, to a lesser extent, improving uveoscleral output. The prodrug dipivefrin causes fewer systemic side effects than epinephrine and can sometimes be used in patients who have developed a sensitivity to epinephrine.

H. Combination Agents — see Table 21
Another option for the treatment of glaucoma is the brand Cosopt (Merck), which is a combination of the β-adrenergic blocker timolol with the carbonic anhydrase inhibitor dorzolamide. Cosopt is the only combination agent available in the United States.

Other combination agents may be available in some countries. These include: Combigan by Allergan (timolol 0.5% with brimonidine 0.2%), Duotrav by Alcon (timolol 0.5% with travoprost 0.004%), Gantfort by Allergan (timolol 0.5% with bimatoprost 0.03%), and Xalacom by Pfizer (timolol 0.5% and latanoprost 0.005%).

REFERENCES
Fiscella RG, Winarko T. Glaucoma—new therapeutic options. *U.S. Pharmacist*, December 1996.

Rhee DJ, Colby KA, Rapuano CJ, Sorbin L. Ophthalmic Drug Guide, New York, NY: Springer. 2007.

TABLE 14

α_2 SELECTIVE AGONISTS

GENERIC NAME	TRADE NAME	CONCENTRATION	SIZES (mL)
Apraclonidine	Iopidine	0.5% 1.0%	5, 10 single-use container
Brimonidine	Alphagan P Available generically	0.1%, 0.15% 0.15%, 0.2%	5, 10, 15 5, 10, 15

TABLE 15

β-ADRENERGIC BLOCKING AGENTS

GENERIC NAME	TRADE NAME	CONCENTRATION	SIZES (mL)
Betaxolol hydrochloride	Betoptic-S Available generically	0.25% 0.5%	2.5, 5, 10, 15 5, 10, 15
Carteolol hydrochloride	Available generically	1%	5, 10, 15
Levobunolol hydrochloride	Betagan Available generically	0.25%, 0.5% 0.25%, 0.5%	2, 5, 10, 15 5, 10, 15
Metipranolol	OptiPranolol Available generically	0.3% 0.3%	5, 10 5, 10
Timolol	Betimol	0.25%, 0.5%	5, 10, 15
Timolol maleate	Timoptic Available generically	0.25%, 0.5% 0.25%, 0.5%	2.5, 5, 10, 15 5, 10, 15
Timolol maleate (gel)	Timoptic - XE Available generically	0.25%, 0.5% 0.25%, 0.5%	5 2.5, 5

TABLE 16

CARBONIC ANHYDRASE INHIBITORS

USP OR NF NAME	TRADE NAME	PREPARATION	ONSET/DURATION OF ACTION
Acetazolamide	Diamox	500 mg (extended-release) capsules	. . ./18-24 h
	Available generically	125, 250 mg tablets	2 h/8-12 h
Brinzolamide	Azopt	1% ophthalmic suspension	. . .
Dorzolamide HCl	Trusopt	2% ophthalmic solution	. . .
Methazolamide	Available generically	25, 50 mg tablets	2-4 h/10–18 h

TABLE 17

HYPEROSMOTIC AGENTS

USP OR NF NAME	TRADE NAME	PREPARATION	DOSE	ROUTE	ONSET/DURATION OF ACTION
Glycerin	Osmoglyn	50%	1–1.5 g/kg	Oral	. . .
Mannitol*	Osmitrol	5%–20%	0.5–2 g/kg	IV	30–60 min/4–6 h
Urea	Ureaphil	Powder (4 g) for reconstitution to 30% soln	0.5–2 g/kg	IV	30–45 min/5–6 h

TABLE 18

MIOTICS

GENERIC NAME	TRADE NAME	STRENGTHS	SIZES
CHOLINERGIC AGENTS			
Carbachol	Isopto Carbachol	1.5%, 3%	15, 30 mL
	Miostat	0.01%	1.5 mL x 12
Pilocarpine hydrochloride	Isopto Carpine	0.25%, 1%, 2%, 4%	15 & 30 mL
	Pilopine-HS gel	4%	3.5 g
	Available generically	0.5%, 1%, 2%, 3%, 4%, 6%	15 mL

TABLE 19

PROSTAGLANDINS

GENERIC NAME	TRADE NAME	CONCENTRATION	SIZES (mL)
Bimatoprost	Lumigan	0.03%	2.5, 5, 7.5
Latanoprost	Xalatan	0.005%	2.5
Travoprost	Travatan	0.004%	2.5, 5

TABLE 20

SYMPATHOMIMETICS

GENERIC NAME	TRADE NAME	CONCENTRATION	SIZES (mL)
Dipivefrin hydrochloride	Propine	0.1%	5, 10, 15
	Available generically	0.1%	5, 10, 15
Epinephrine hydrochloride	Epifrin	0.5%, 1%, 2%	5, 10, 15

TABLE 21

COMBINATION AGENT (AVAILABLE IN THE U.S.)

GENERIC NAME	TRADE NAME	CONCENTRATION	SIZES (mL)
Dorzolamide HCl and timolol maleate	Cosopt	2% dorzolamide/0.5% timolol	5, 10

*Do not confuse with mannitol hexanitrate, an antianginal agent.

6. MEDICATIONS FOR DRY EYE

Dry eye refers to a deficiency in either the lipid, aqueous or mucin components of the precorneal tear film. The most commonly encountered aqueous-deficient dry eye in the United States is keratoconjunctivitis sicca, while mucin-deficient dry eyes may be seen in cases of hypovitaminosis A, Stevens-Johnson syndrome, ocular pemphigoid, extensive trachoma, and chemical burns. Dry eye is treated with artificial tear preparations (see **Table 22**), prescription medication (see **Table 23**) and ophthalmic lubricants (see **Table 24**). The lubricants form an occlusive film over the ocular surface and protect the eye from drying. Administered as a nighttime medication, they are useful both for dry eye and in cases of recurrent corneal erosion. Topical cyclosporin A 0.05% is very helpful in many patients with mild-to-severe dry eyes. Punctal occlusion can also be helpful in some patients with dry eyes.

TABLE 22

ARTIFICIAL TEAR PREPARATIONS

MAJOR COMPONENT(S)	CONCENTRATION	TRADE NAME	PRESERVATIVE/EDTA*
Carboxymethylcellulose	0.25% 0.5% 1% 0.25%	GenTeal Gel Refresh Plus Refresh Tears Refresh Liquigel TheraTears	Sodium perborate None Purite Purite Sodium perborate
Carboxymethylcellulose, Glycerin	0.5%, 0.9%	Optive	Purite
Glycerin	1.0%	Computer Eye Drops	Benzalkonium chloride, EDTA
Glycerin, polysorbate 80	1%, 1%	Refresh Endura	None
Glycerin, Propylene glycol	0.3%, 1.0%	Moisture Eyes	Benzalkonium chloride
Hydroxypropyl cellulose	5 mg/insert	Lacrisert (biodegradable insert)	None
Hydroxypropyl methylcellulose (Hypromellose)	0.2% 0.3% 0.5%	GenTeal Mild GenTeal Moderate GenTeal Severe GenTeal Gel GenTeal PF Tearisol	Sodium perborate Sodium perborate Sodium perborate Sodium perborate None Benzalkonium chloride, EDTA
Hydroxypropyl methylcellulose, dextran 70	0.3%, 0.1%	Tears Renewed	Benzalkonium chloride, EDTA
Hydroxypropyl methylcellulose, glycerin, dextran 70	0.3%, 0.2%, 0.1%	Tears Naturale Forte Tears Naturale Free	Polyquaternium-1 None
Hydroxypropyl methylcellulose, glycerin, PEG-400	0.2%, 0.2%, 1%	Visine Tears Visine Pure Tears	Benzalkonium chloride None
Hypromellose, dextran 70	0.8%, 0.1%	Moisture Eyes	None
Hypromellose, glycerin		Clear Eyes CLR Visine for Contacts	Sorbic acid, EDTA Potassium sorbate, EDTA
Hypromellose/Glycerin Polyethylene glycol 400	0.36%, 0.2%, 1% 0.2%, 0.2%, 1%	Visine Tears Lasting Relief Visine Pure Tears	None
Methylcellulose	1%	Murocel	Methylparabens, propylparabens
Mineral oil, white petrolatum	15%, 85%	GenTeal PM	None
Polysorbate 80	1%	VIVA Lubricating	None
Polysorbate 80, hypromellose, glycerin, zinc sulfate	1%, 0.3%, 0.125%, 0.25%	VIVA Ultratears Lubricating + MR	None
Polyvinyl alcohol	1.4%	AKWA Tears	Benzalkonium chloride, EDTA
Polyvinyl alcohol, PEG-400	1%, 1%	HypoTears	Benzalkonium chloride
Polyvinyl alcohol, povidone	0.5% , 0.6%	Murine Tears	Benzalkonium chloride
Proplylene alcohol, povidone, Tetrahydrozoline HCl	0.5%, 0.6%, 0.05%	Murine Tears Plus	Benzalkonium chloride
Propylene glycol	0.95%	Moisture Eyes Preservative Free	None
Propylene glycol, PEG-400	0.3%, 0.4%	Systane, Systane Preservative Free	Polyquaternium-1, also available as preservative free
Restoryl (neutral oils)	Not available	Soothe	Polyhexamethylene biguanide

EDTA = ethylenediaminetetraacetic acid.

TABLE 23

PRESCRIPTION MEDICINE FOR DRY EYE SYNDROME

MAJOR COMPONENT	CONCENTRATION	DOSE	TRADE NAME	PRESERVATIVE
Cyclosporine	0.05%	q 12h	Restasis	None

TABLE 24

OPHTHALMIC LUBRICANTS

TRADE NAME	COMPOSITION OF STERILE OINTMENT
AKWA Tears Ointment	White petrolatum, liquid lanolin, and mineral oil
HypoTears Ointment Tears Renewed	White petrolatum and light mineral oil
Lacri-Lube S.O.P.	White petrolatum, mineral oil, chlorobutanol, and lanolin alcohols
Refresh P.M.	42.5% mineral oil, 57.3% white petrolatum, and lanolin alcohols

7. OCULAR DECONGESTANTS

These topically applied adrenergic medications are commonly used to whiten the eye. Those containing naphazoline and tetrahydrozoline are more stable than those with phenylephrine. Usual dosage is 1 or 2 drops no more than 4 times a day (see **Table 25**).

TABLE 25

OCULAR DECONGESTANTS

DRUG	TRADE NAME	ADDITIONAL COMPONENTS
Naphazoline hydrochloride	AK-Con (0.1%)	Benzalkonium chloride, edetate disodium
	Albalon (0.1%)	Benzalkonium chloride, edetate disodium
	All Clear (0.012%)	Benzalkonium chloride, edetate disodium, PEG-300, polyethylene glycol
	All Clear AR (0.03%)	Benzalkonium chloride, edetate disodium, hydroxypropyl methylcellulose 0.5%
	Clear Eyes (0.012%)	Benzalkonium chloride, edetate disodium
	Available generically	Benzalkonium chloride, EDTA[†]
Oxymetazoline hydrochloride	Visine L.R. (0.025%)	Benzalkonium chloride, edetate disodium
Phenylephrine hydrochloride	AK-Nefrin (0.12%) Available generically	Benzalkonium chloride, edetate disodium
Tetrahydrozoline hydrochloride	Murine Tears Plus (0.05%)	Benzalkonium chloride, edetate disodium, polyvinyl alcohol, povidone
	Visine (0.05%)	Benzalkonium chloride, edetate disodium
	Visine Advanced Relief (0.05%)	Benzalkonium chloride, edetate disodium, PEG-400, povidone, dextran 70
	Available generically	Benzalkonium chloride, edetate disodium, PEG-400, povidone, dextran 70
DECONGESTANT/ASTRINGENT COMBINATIONS		
Naphazoline hydrochloride plus antazoline phosphate	Vasocon-A	Benzalkonium chloride, edetate disodium
Naphazoline hydrochloride plus pheniramine maleate	Visine-A Naphcon-A	Benzalkonium chloride, edetate disodium Benzalkonium chloride, edetate disodium
Naphazoline hydrochloride plus zinc sulfate	Clear Eyes ACR (0.125%) (allergy/cold relief)	Benzalkonium chloride, edetate disodium, glycerin
Tetrahydrozoline plus zinc sulfate	Visine A.C.	Benzalkonium chloride, edetate disodium
DECONGESTANT/LUBRICANT		
Naphazoline hydrochloride, Polysorbate 80	VIVA Lubricating Redness Relief	Citric acid, edetate disodium, sodium chloride

[†]EDTA = ethylenediaminetetraacetic acid.

8. OPHTHALMIC IRRIGATING SOLUTIONS

Listed in **Table 26** are sterile isotonic solutions for general ophthalmic use. They are all over-the-counter products. There are also intraocular irrigating solutions available for use during surgical procedures.

They include prescription medications such as Bausch & Lomb's Balanced Salt Solution, Alcon's BSS and BSS Plus, and Iolab's Iocare Balanced Salt Solution.

TABLE 26

OPHTHALMIC IRRIGATING SOLUTIONS

TRADE NAME	COMPONENTS	ADDITIONAL COMPONENTS
Collyrium Fresh Eyes	Boric acid and sodium borate	Benzalkonium chloride
Dacriose	Sodium and potassium chlorides, and sodium phosphate	Benzalkonium chloride, edetate disodium
Eye Wash Solution	Boric acid, sodium borate, and sodium chloride	EDTA*, sorbic acid

*EDTA = ethylenediaminetetraacetic acid.

9. HYPEROSMOLAR AGENTS

Hyperosmolar (hypertonic) agents are used to reduce corneal edema. They act through osmotic attraction of water through the semipermeable corneal epithelium.

TABLE 27

HYPEROSMOLAR AGENTS

GENERIC NAME	TRADE NAME	CONCENTRATION
Sodium chloride	Muro-128	2% or 5% (solution), 5% (ointment)
	Available generically	5% (solution and ointment)

10. DIAGNOSTIC AGENTS

Some of the more common diagnostic agents and tests used in ophthalmologic practice are listed below.

A. Examination of the Conjunctiva, Cornea, and Lacrimal Apparatus

Fluorescein, applied primarily as a 2% alkaline solution, and with impregnated paper strips, is used to examine the integrity of the conjunctival and corneal epithelia. Defects in the corneal epithelium will appear bright green in ordinary light and bright yellow when a cobalt blue filter is used in the light path. Similar lesions of the conjunctiva appear bright orange-yellow in ordinary illumination.

Fluorescein has also come into wide use in the fitting of rigid contact lenses, though it cannot be used for soft lenses, which absorb the dye. Proper fit is determined by examining the pattern of fluorescein beneath the contact lens.

In addition, fluorescein is used in performing applanation tonometry. Also, one test of lacrimal apparatus patency (Jones test) uses 1 drop of 1% fluorescein instilled into the conjunctival sac. If the dye appears in the nose, drainage is normal.

Rose bengal, available as 1% solution or in impregnated strips, is particularly useful for demonstrating abnormal conjunctival or corneal epithelium. Devitalized cells stain bright red, while normal cells show no change. *Lissamine green,* available as 1% solution or in impregnated strips, also stains abnormal conjunctival and corneal cells. It is less irritating to the eye than rose bengal. The abnormal epithelial cells that present in dry eye disorders are effectively revealed by these stains.

The *Schirmer* test is a valuable method of assessing tear production. It employs prepared strips of filter paper 5 by 30 mm in size. The strips are inserted into the topically anesthetized conjunctival sac at the junction of the middle and outer third of the lower lid, with approximately 25 mm of paper exposed. After 5 minutes, the strip is removed and the amount of moistening measured. The normal range is 10 to 25 mm. If inadequate production of tears is found on the initial test, a Schirmer II test can be performed by repeating the procedure while stimulating the nasal mucosa. A number of variations of the Schirmer test can be found in textbooks and journals.

B. Examination of Acquired Ptosis or Extraocular Muscle Palsy

To confirm myasthenia gravis as the cause of ptosis or muscle palsy, an intravenous injection of 2 mg of *edrophonium chloride* is administered, followed 45 seconds later by an additional 8 mg if there is no response to the first dose. (In case of a severe reaction to the edrophonium, immediately give atropine sulfate, 0.6 mg intravenously.) Alternatively, a non-invasive, low-risk test, such as the "ice test" may be used. The ice test has approximately a 0.94 sensitivity for ocular myasthenia and 0.82 sensitivity for generalized disease. The ice test also has a 0.97 specificity for ocular myasthenia and 0.96 specificity for generalized disease.

C. Examination of the Retina and Choroid

Sodium fluorescein solution, in concentrations of 5%, 10%, and 25%, is injected intravenously to study the retinal and choroidal circulation. It has been used primarily in examination of lesions at the posterior pole of the eye, but anterior segment fluorescein angiography (wherein the vessels of the iris, sclera, and conjunctiva are studied) is also a useful clinical tool.

Intravascular fluorescein is normally prevented from entering the retina by the intact retinal vascular endothelium (blood-retinal barrier) and the intact retinal pigment epithelium. Defects in either the retinal vessels or the pigment epithelium will allow leakage of fluorescein, which can then be studied by either direct observation or photography. For good results, appropriate filters are needed to excite the fluorescein and exclude unwanted wavelengths. The peak frequencies for excitation lie between 485 and 500 nm and, for emission, between 520 and 530 nm.

Fluorescein has proved to be a safe diagnostic agent, the most common side effects being nausea and vomiting. However, occasional allergic and vagal reactions do occur, so oxygen and emergency equipment should be readily available when angiography is performed. Patients should also be warned that the dye will temporarily stain their skin and urine; in the average patient this lasts no more than a day.

Indocyanine green (IC-Green) has been used in recent years, either alone or with fluorescein, to obtain better frames of choroid neovascularization.

D. Examination of Abnormal Pupillary Responses

Methacholine, as a 2.5% solution instilled into the conjunctival sac, will cause the tonic pupil (Adie's pupil) to contract, but will leave a normal pupil unchanged. A similar pupillary response is seen following instillation of 2.5% methacholine in patients with familial dysautonomia (Riley-Day syndrome).

Table 28 shows the effects of several drugs on miosis due to interruption of the sympathetic nervous system (Horner's syndrome). The effect depends on the location of the lesion in the sympathetic chain.

TABLE 28

HORNER'S SYNDROME

TOPICAL DROP (CENTRAL)	NEURON III (POST-GANGLIONIC)	NEURON II (PRE-GANGLIONIC)	NEURON I
Cocaine 2%–10%	–	–	+/–
Epinephrine (Adrenalin) 1:1000	+++	+	–
Phenylephrine 1%	+++	+	+/–

Pilocarpine may be used to determine whether a fixed dilated pupil is due to an atropine-like drug or interruption of the pupil's parasympathetic innervation.[3] If an atropine-like drug is involved, the pupil will not react to pilocarpine. If dilation is due to interruption of the parasympathetic innervation (compression by aneurysm, Adie's tonic pupil) instillation of pilo- carpine will cause the pupil to constrict.

REFERENCES

Benatar M. A systemic review of diagnostic studies in myasthenia gravis. *Neuromus Dis.* 2000;16:459-467.

Hecht SD. Evaluation of the lacrimal drainage system. *Ophthalmology.* 1978;85:1250.

Thompson HS, Mensher JH. Adrenergic mydriasis in Horner's syndrome: hydroxyampheta mine test for diagnosis of post-ganglionic defects. *Am J Ophthalmol.* 1971;72:472.

Thompson HS, Newsome DA, Lowenfeld IE. The fixed dilated pupil. Sudden iridoplegia or mydriatic drops; a simple diagnostic test. *Arch Ophthalmol.* 1971;86:12.

11. VISCOELASTIC MATERIALS USED IN OPHTHALMOLOGY

Viscoelastic substances are used in ophthalmic surgery to maintain the anterior chamber, hydraulically dissect tissues, act as a vitreous substitute/tamponade, and prevent mechanical damage to tissue, especially the corneal endothelium. The individual characteristics of the various viscoelastic materials are the result of the chain length and intra- and interchain molecular interactions of the compounds comprising the viscoelastic substance. All viscoelastic materials have the potential to produce a large postoperative increase in pressure if they are not adequately removed from the anterior chamber following surgery.

AMVISC (Bausch and Lomb) – Composed of sodium hyaluronate 1.2% in physiologic saline. The viscosity is 40,000 cSt (@25°C, 1/sec shear rate), and molecular weight is ≥2,000,000 daltons. Its shelf life is estimated at 2 years.

AMVISC PLUS (Bausch and Lomb) – Composed of sodium hyaluronate 1.6% in physiologic saline. The viscosity is 55,000 cSt (@25°C, 1/sec shear rate), and molecular weight is approximately 1,500,000 daltons. The greater viscosity is obtained by increasing total concentration and using sodium hyaluronate of lower molecular weight. Its shelf life is estimated at 1 year.

BIOLON (Akorn) – Composed of sodium hyaluronate 1%. The viscosity is 215,000 cps, and the molecular weight is approximately 3,000,000 daltons. The product does not require refrigeration and its shelf life is estimated to be approximately 2 years.

DUOVISC (Alcon) – Package contains two separate syringes. One syringe containing Provisc; the other containing Viscoat. Please see individual descriptions below for details of each.

HEALON (Advanced Medical Optics) – Composed of sodium hyaluronate 1% in physiologic saline. The viscosity is 200,000 (@ 0/sec shear rate), and the molecular weight is approximately 4,000,000 daltons.

HEALON GV (Advanced Medical Optics) – Composed of sodium hyaluronate 1.4% in physiologic saline. The viscosity is 2,000,000 (@ 0/sec shear rate), and the molecular weight is approximately 5,000,000 daltons. In the presence of high positive vitreous pressure, Healon GV has 3 times more resistance to pressure than does Healon.

HEALON 5 (Advanced Medical Optics) – Composed of sodium hyaluronate 2.3%. The viscosity is 7,000,000 cP (@ 25°C, 1/sec shear rate), and the molecular weight is 4,000,000 daltons.

OCUCOAT (Storz – Bausch and Lomb) – Composed of hydroxypropylmethylcellulose 2% in balance salt solution (BSS). The viscosity is 4,000 cSt (@ 37°C measured on Cannon-Fenske Viscometer), and the molecular weight is approximately 80,000 daltons. Occucoat is termed a viscoadherent rather than a viscoelastic because of its coating ability, which is related to its contact angle and low surface tension.

PROVISC (Alcon) – Composed of sodium hyaluronate 1% in physiologic saline. The viscosity is 39,000 cps (@ 25°C, 2/sec shear rate) and the molecular weight is approximately 1,900,000 daltons. Clinical studies demonstrate that ProVisc functions in a similar fashion to Healon.

VISCOAT (Alcon) – Composed of a 1:3 mixture of chondroitin sulfate 4% (CS) and sodium hyaluronate 3% (SH) in physiologic saline. The viscosity is 40,000 cps (@ 25°C, 2/sec shear rate), and the molecular weight is 22,500 daltons for CS and 500,000 daltons for SH.

VITRAX (Allergan) – Composed of sodium hyaluronate 3% in balanced salt solution (BSS). The viscosity is 30,000 cps (@ 2/sec shear rate) and the molecular weight is 500,000 daltons. It is highly concentrated to produce a significantly viscous material. It does not require refrigeration and has a shelf life of 18 months.

12. ANTI-ANGIOGENESIS TREATMENTS

These medications are used for the treatment of wet age-related macular degeneration.

TABLE 29

ANTI-ANGIOGENESIS TREATMENTS

GENERIC NAME	TRADE NAME	DOSAGE	FDA-APPROVED INDICATION
Verteporfin for injection	Visudyne	6 mg/m^2 intravenously over 10 min at 3 mL/min.*	Treatment of predominantely classic subfoveal CNV due to AMD, pathologic myopia, or presumed ocular histoplasmosis
Pegaptanib sodium	Macugen	0.3 mg intravitreal q 6 weeks	Treatment of wet AMD (all subtypes, including predominantly classic, minimally classic, and occult)
Ranibizumab	Lucentis	0.3 mg or 0.5 mg intravitreal q month	Treatment of wet AMD (all subtypes, including predominantly classic, minimally classic, and occult)

*Initiate photoactivation with laser light therapy with nonthermal diode laser 15 minutes after starting intravenous infusion. Re-evaluate every 3 months and repeat if CNV leakage is detected on fluorescein angiography.

AMD = age-related macular degeneration; CNV = choroidal neovascularization.

REFERENCE
Gragoudas ES, et al. Pegaptanib for neovascular age-related macular degeneration. *N Engl J Med*. 2004;351:2805.

13. OFF-LABEL DRUG APPLICATIONS IN OPHTHALMOLOGY

A. Acetylcysteine
This agent is used to treat corneal conditions such as alkali burns, corneal melts, and keratoconjunctivitis sicca. It is thought to improve healing by inhibiting the action of collagenase, which may contribute to delay in healing. The drug is available generically or under the trade name Mucomyst in 10% and 20% solutions. Though none of the commercially available solutions are approved for use in ophthalmology, they have been administered as frequently as hourly in acute cases, and up to 4 times a day in maintenance therapy, usually in the 10% concentration.

B. Alteplase (tissue plasminogen activator)
This thrombolytic agent, available under the trade name Activase, is used to treat fibrin formation in postvitrectomy patients. Though initial studies were

based on intraocular injections of 25 mcg, more recent work has shown the drug to be effective in doses of as little as 3 to 6 mcg. Because by-products of alteplase activity may mediate endothelial cell toxicity, the lower doses are preferred. This agent has also been used for submacular hemorrage, but this use is controversial.

C. Antimetabolites

5-Fluorouracil (5-FU). This drug inhibits fibroblast proliferation and diminishes scarring after glaucoma filtering surgery. Initial recommendations of the 5-FU study group called for subconjunctival injections of 5 mg twice daily for 7 days postoperatively and once daily for the next 7 days (total 21 injections). Other physicians achieve success with five injections over 15 days. Many physicians are using an intraoperative application of 50 mg/mL solution soaked into a murocell sponge lasting for 3 to 5 minutes, with a body of literature supporting its effectiveness (see references listed at the end of this section). Use of this drug is associated with a number of complications, including conjunctival wound leak, corneal epithelial defects, hypotony associated with permanently reduced vision acuity, serious corneal infections in eyes with preexistent corneal epithelial edema, and increased susceptibility to late-onset bleb infections. The drug should be considered only when there is a high risk of surgical failure.

Mitomycin. This potent chemotherapeutic agent, available under the trade name Mutamycin, is being used in glaucoma filtering surgery for the same purpose and on the same type of patients as 5-FU. It is applied once during surgery on a small piece of Gelfilm or Weck cell sponge in a concentration of 0.2 mg/mL (0.02%) to 0.4 mg/mL (0.04%). Reported side effects are similar to those of 5-FU. However, some serious side effects may go unreported, since there is a possibility of delayed reactions 6 to 24 months after surgery. Mitomycin has also been administered in a concentrated solution of 0.2 mg/mL (0.02%) to 0.4 mg/mL (0.04%) 2 to 4 times a day — and more recently as a one-time application in the operating room — to prevent recurrence after pterygium surgery and reduce scarring after corneal surgery, especially excimer laser surgery. Serious side effects associated with this therapy include corneal melts and scleral ulceration and calcification.

Physicians should bear in mind the possibility of major side effects from all antineoplastic agents and carefully weigh the risks and benefits of their use. Remember, too, that these agents should always be handled and discarded in accordance with OSHA, AMA, ASHP, and/or hospital policies regarding the safe use of antineoplastics.

D. Cyclosporine

This potent immunosuppressant has a high degree of selectivity for T lymphocytes. Available under the trade name Sandimmune, it has been used in a 0.5–2% topical solution as prophylaxis against rejection in high-risk, penetrating keratoplasty and for treating severe vernal conjunctivitis resistant to conventional therapy, ligneous conjunctivitis unrespon-

sive to other topical therapy, and noninfectious peripheral ulcerative keratitis associated with systemic autoimmune disorders.

E. Doxycycline and Minocycline

These derivatives of tetracycline are used for the treatment of ocular rosacea meibomianitis, and certain conditions involving corneal melting. The usual dose is 100 mg PO 1-2 times per day for 6 to 12 weeks, although lower doses (eg 40-50 mg/day) are thought to provide an anti-inflammatory effect. They have the same side effects, contraindications, and interactions as tetracycline, although doxycycline may be taken with food.

F. Edetate disodium

This chelating agent plays a role in treating band keratopathy. After removal of the corneal epithelium, it is used to remove calcium from Bowman's membrane.

REFERENCES

Dietze PJ, Feldman RM, Gross RL. Intraoperative application of 5-fluorouracil during trabeculectomy. *Ophthalmic Surg Lasers.* 1992;23(10):662.

Dunn J, Seamone S, Ostler H. Development of scleral ulceration and calcification after pterygium excision and mitomycin therapy. *Am J Ophthalmol.* 1991;112:343.

Feldman RM, Dietze PJ, Gross RL, et al. Intraoperative 5 fluorouracil administration in trabeculectomy. *J Glaucoma.* 1994;3:302.

Frucht-Perry J, et al. The effect of doxycycline on ocular rosacea. *Am J Ophthalmol.* 1989;170(4):434.

Jaffe G, Abrams G, et al. Tissue plasminogen activator for post vitrectomy fibrin formation. *Ophthalmology.* 1990;97:189.

Goldenfeld M, Krupin T, Ruderman JM, et al. 5-Fluorouracil in initial trabeculectomy. A prospective, randomized, multicenter study. *Ophthalmology.* 1994;101(6):1024.

Lanigan L, Sturmer J, Baez KA, Hitchings RA, Khaw PT. Single intraoperative applications of 5-fluorouracil during filtration surgery: early results. *Br J Ophthalmol.* 1994;78(1):33.

Lish A, Camras C, Podos S. Effect of apraclonidine on intraocular pressure in glaucoma patients receiving maximally tolerated medications. *Glaucoma.* 1992;1:19.

McDermott M, Edelhauser H, et al. Tissue plasminogen activator and corneal endothelium. *Am J Ophthalmol.* 1989;108:91-92.

Mora JS, Nguyen N, Iwach AG, et al. Trabeculectomy with intraoperative sponge 5-fluorouracil. *Ophthalmology.* 1996;103(6):963. Review.

Perry HD, Donnenfeld ED. Medications for dry eye syndrome: a drug-therapy review. *Manag Care.* 2003;12(suppl 12):26.

Pflugfelder SC. Antiinflammatory therapy for dry eye. *Am J Ophthalmol.* 2004;137:337.

Quarterman MJ, et al. Signs, symptoms, and tear studies before and after treatment with doxycycline. *Arch Dermatol.* 1997;133:89.

Rothman RF, Liebmann JM, Ritch R. Low-dose 5-fluorouracil trabeculectomy as initial surgery in uncomplicated glaucoma: long-term followup. *Ophthalmology.* 2000;107(6):1184.

Rubinfeld R, Pfister R, et al. Serious complications of topical mitomycin-C after pterygium surgery. *Ophthalmology.* 1992;99:1647.

Sall K, Stevenson OD, Nundorf TK, Reis BL. Two multicenter, randomized studies of the efficacy and safety of cyclosporine ophthalmic emulsion in moderate to severe dry eye disease. CsA Phase 3 Study Group. *Ophthalmology.* 2000;107:631. Erratum in: *Ophthalmology.* 2000;107:1220.

Smith MF, Sherwood MB, Doyle JW, Khaw PT. Results of intraoperative 5-fluorouracil supplementation on trabeculectomy for open-angle glaucoma. *Am J Ophthalmol.* 1992;114(6):737.

Stevenson D, Tauber J, Reis BL. Efficacy and safety of cyclosporine A ophthalmic emulsion in the treatment of moderate-to-severe dry eye disease: a dose-ranging, randomized trial. The Cyclosporin A Phase 2 Study Group. *Ophthalmology.* 2000;107:967.

Three-year follow-up of the Fluorouracil Filtering Surgery Study. *Am J Ophthalmol.* 1993;115(1):82.

Williams D, Benett S, et al. Low-dose intraocular tissue plasminogen activator for treatment of postvitrectomy firbrin formations. *Am J Opthalmol.* 1990;109:606.

14. OCULAR TOXICOLOGY — F. W. FRAUNFELDER, MD

The table on the following pages lists recently reported ocular side effects of drugs as they relate to the eye. The list is not intended to be comprehensive but should provide clinicians with an overview of some of the more clinically relevant side effects that have been reported. For more extensive information, please consult our book *Clinical Ocular Toxicology* or our website at www.eyedrugregistry.com.

Toxicology data are cataloged by the National Registry of Drug-Induced Ocular Side Effects. To report a suspected adverse drug response, or to obtain references for the information listed in the table, please contact:

F.W. Fraunfelder, MD, Director, National Registry of Drug-Induced Ocular Side Effects
Casey Eye Institute
Oregon Health & Science University
3375 SW Terwilliger Blvd.
Portland, OR 97239-4197
Phone: (503) 494-4318
Fax: (503) 418-2284
E-mail: eyedrug@ohsu.edu
Website: www.eyedrugregistry.com

REFERENCES

Fraunfelder FT, Fraunfelder FW. *Drug-Induced Ocular Side Effects*, ed 5. Woburn, Mass: Butterworth-Heinemann; 2001.

Fraunfelder FT, Fraunfelder FW, Edwards R: Ocular side effects possibly associated with isotretinoin usage. *Am J Ophthalmol*. 2001;132(3): 299-305.

Fraunfelder FW. Corneal toxicity from topical ocular and systemic medications. *Cornea*. 2006 Dec;25(10):1133-8.

Fraunfelder FW. Ocular side effects associated with bisphosphonates. *Drugs of Today*. 2003;39(11):829-835.

Fraunfelder FW. Ocular side effects associated with COX-2 inhibitors. *Arch Ophthalmol*. 2006 Feb; 124(2):277-9.

Fraunfelder FW. Twice-yearly exams not necessary for patients taking quetiapine. *Am J Ophthalmol*. 2004;138(5):870-871.

Fraunfelder FW. Visual side effects associated with erectile dysfunction agents. *Am J Ophthalmol*. 2005 Oct; 140(4):723-4.

Fraunfelder FW, Fraunfelder FT: Topiramate associated acute, bilateral, secondary angle-closure glaucoma. *Ophthalmol*. 2004;111(1):109-111.

Fraunfelder FW, Fraunfelder FT: Oculogyric crisis in patients taking cetirizine. *Am J Ophthalmol*. 2004;137(2):355-57.

Fraunfelder FW, Fraunfelder FT: Scleritis associated with pamidronate disodium use. *Am J Ophthalmol*. 2003;135(2):219-222.

Fraunfelder FW, Fraunfelder FT, Corbett JJ: Isotretinoin-associated intracranial hypertension. *Ophthalmology*. 2004;111(6):1248-1250.

Fraunfelder FW, Harrison D. Peripheral ulcerative keratitis-like findings associated with filgrastim. *Cornea*. 2007 Apr;26(3):368-9.

Fraunfelder FW, Pomeranz H, Egan RA. Nonarteritic ischemic optic neuropathy and sildenafil. *Arch Ophthalmol*. 2006 May; 124(5): 733-4.

Fraunfelder FW, Rich LF: Possible adverse effects of drugs used in refractive surgery. *J Cataract Refractive Surg*. 2003;29(1):170-175.

Wheeler D, Fraunfelder FW: Ocular motility dysfunction associated with chemotherapeutic agents. *J Am Assoc Pediatr Ophthalmol Strabismus*. 2004;8(1):15-17.

TABLE 30

ADVERSE DRUG EFFECTS

GENERIC NAME	PRINCIPAL GENERAL USE	POSSIBLE ADVERSE EFFECTS
I. MEDICATION BY INJECTION		
Adrenal Corticosteroids		
Depo-steroids	Allergic disorders Anti-inflammatory disorders	If injected into a blood vessel, eg, the tonsillar fossa, may cause unilateral or bilateral retinal arterial occlusions due to emboli of depo-steroid. Permanent bilateral blindness may ensue.
Triamcinolone	Allergic disorders Anti-inflammatory disorders	Fatty atrophy in area of injection, ie, enophthalmus if given retrobulbar or, if given in periocular skin, some deformity can occur in area due to loss of fat. 50% chance of an IOP elevation.
Alpha-blocker		
Tamsulosin	Benign prostatic hyperplasia	Intraoperative floppy iris syndrome
Antifungals		
Amphotericin B	Aspergillosis, blastomycosis, candidiasis, coccidioidomycosis, histoplasmosis	Ischemic necrosis after subconjunctival injection Subconjunctival nodule, yellow discoloration
Antineoplastics		
Carmustine	Brain tumors Multiple myeloma	Optic neuritis Retinal vascular disorders
Cisplatin	Metastatic testicular or ovarian tumors. Advanced bladder carcinoma	Cortical blindness Papilledema, retrobulbar or optic neuritis
Fluorouracil	Carcinoma of the colon, rectum, breast, stomach, and pancreas	Ocular irritation with tearing, conjunctival hyperemia, canalicular fibrosis, ocular motility dysfunction
Ophthalmic Dyes		
Fluorescein	Ocular diagnostic tests	Nausea, vomiting, urticaria, rhinorrhea, dizziness, hypotension, pharyngoedema, anaphylactic reaction

GENERIC NAME	PRINCIPAL GENERAL USE	POSSIBLE ADVERSE EFFECTS
Parasympathomimetics		
Acetylcholine	Produces prompt, short-term miosis	Hypotension and bradycardia with intraocular injection

II. ORAL

GENERIC NAME	PRINCIPAL GENERAL USE	POSSIBLE ADVERSE EFFECTS
Anthelmintics		
Levamisol hydrochloride	Connective tissue disorders Ascaris infestation	Patients with Sjögren's syndrome and possibly keratitis sicca have marked increase in systemic side effects, including pruritus and muscle weakness
Antiarrhythmics		
Amiodarone hydrochloride	Cardiac abnormalities Ventricular arrhythmias	Keratopathy Lens opacities, optic neuropathy, color vision defects Discoloration of conjunctiva and eyelids
Propranolol	Cardiovascular abnormalities Certain hypertensive states	May precipitate latent myotonia May mask hyperthyroidism; when taken off drug, thyroid stare and exophthalmos may occur
Antibiotics and Antituberculars		
Chloramphenicol Ethambutol hydrochloride Rifampin	Typhoid fever Pulmonary tuberculosis Asymptomatic carriers of meningococcus Many gram-negative and gram-positive cocci, including *Neisseria* and *Haemophilus influenzae* Pulmonary tuberculosis	Aplastic anemia Optic neuropathy Conjunctival hyperemia Exudative conjunctivitis Increased lacrimation
Minocycline	Useful against gram-negative and gram-positive bacteria Members of lymphogranuloma-psittacosis group *Mycoplasma* Acne rosacea	Pseudotumor cerebri and papilledema as early as 3 days after onset of medication in infants and in young adults Transient myopia Permanent pigmentation of sclera
Antihistamines		
Cetirizine	Treatment of perennial allergic rhinitis, chronic urticaria, and allergic rhinitis	Oculogyric crisis (primarily in children)
Antihypertensives		
Sodium nitroprusside	Provides controlled hypertension during anesthesia Management of severe hypertension	Contraindicated in Leber's hereditary optic atrophy and tobacco amblyopia
Antileprotics		
Clofazimine	Dermatologic diseases—psoriasis, pyoderma gangrenosum Leprosy	Conjunctival, corneal, and macular pigmentation
Antimalarials and Anti-inflammatories		
Hydroxychloroquine	Malaria Lupus erythematosus Rheumatoid arthritis	Disturbance of accommodation Corneal changes Bull's-eye maculopathy—central, pericentral, or paracentral scotomas
Antineoplastics		
Busulfan	Chronic myelogenous leukemia	Cataracts Decreased lacrimation
Tamoxifen	Metastatic breast carcinoma	Corneal opacities Refractile retinal deposits Posterior subcapsular cataracts Decreased color perception
Bisphosphonates	Osteoporosis Hypercalcemia of malignancy	Scleritis, uveitis, conjunctivitis, episcleritis (reversible)
Imatinib mesylate	Treatment of chronic myelogenous leukemia and gastrointestinal stromal tumors	Periorbital edema, epiphora, conjunctivitis
Antipsychotics		
Lithium carbonate	Manic phase of manic/depressive psychosis	Exophthalmos, oculogyric crisis, myoclonus
Seroquel	Schizophrenia	Cataracts unlikely

GENERIC NAME	PRINCIPAL GENERAL USE	POSSIBLE ADVERSE EFFECTS
Antiseizure Topiramate	Refractory epilepsy	Acute angle-closure glaucoma, myopia, uveal effusion
Antispasmodics Baclofen	Muscle spasms in multiple sclerosis and disorders associated with increased muscular tone	Blurred vision Hallucinations
Carbonic Anhydrase Inhibitors Acetazolamide Methazolamide	Glaucoma	Aggravation of metabolic acidosis, primarily in known CO_2-retaining diseases such as emphysema and bronchiectasis, and in patients with poor vital capacity Aplastic anemia, various blood disorders Decreased libido Impotency
Chelating Agents Penicillamine	Cystinuria Heavy metal antagonist—iron, lead, copper, mercury poisoning Wilson's disease	Facial or ocular myasthenia, including extraocular muscle paralysis, ptosis, and diplopia Ocular pemphigoid Optic neuritis and color-vision problems
Erectile Dysfunction Agents Sildenafil Tadalafil Vardenafil	Erectile dysfunction	Transitory changes in color perception, blurred vision, changes in light perception, electroretinography (ERG) changes, conjunctival hyperemia, ocular pain, photophobia, subconjunctival hemorrhages, optic neuropathy possible
Hormonal Agents Oral contraceptives	Amenorrhea Dysfunctional uterine bleeding Dysmenorrhea Hypogonadism Oral contraception Premenstrual tension	Contraindicated in patients with preexisting retinal vascular diseases Decrease in color vision with chronic use Macular edema
Hydantoins Phenytoin	Chronic epilepsy	Optic nerve hypoplasia in infants with epileptic mothers on the drug; ocular teratogenic effects, including strabismus, ptosis, hypertelorism, epicanthus
Nonsteroidal Anti-inflammatory Drugs COX-2 inhibitors (celecoxib, rofecoxib, valdecoxib) Ibuprofen Naproxen Sulindac	Rheumatoid arthritis Osteoarthritis Rheumatoid arthritis Osteoarthritis Rheumatoid arthritis Osteoarthritis Ankylosing spondylitis Rheumatoid arthritis Osteoarthritis Ankylosing spondylitis	Blurred vision Irritative conjunctivitis Decreased color vision Optic neuritis, Visual field defects Corneal opacity Periorbital edema Keratitis Stevens-Johnson syndrome
Psychedelics Marijuana	Cerebral sedative or narcotic	Conjunctival hyperemia; decreased lacrimation; decreased intraocular pressure; dyschromatopsia with chronic long-term use
Sedatives and Hypnotics Ethanol	Antiseptic Used as a beverage	Fetal alcohol syndrome: offspring of alcoholic mothers may have epicanthus, small palpebral fissures, and microphthalmia
Synthetic Retinoids Isotretinoin	Severe recalcitrant nodular acne	Permanent night blindness, color vision defects, keratitis sicca. **Note:** All retinoids, in rare instances, can cause intracranial hypertension.

GENERIC NAME	PRINCIPAL GENERAL USE	POSSIBLE ADVERSE EFFECTS
III. TOPICAL		
Anticholinergics		
Cyclopentolate hydrochloride	Used as a cycloplegic and mydriatic	Central nervous system toxicity, including slurred speech, ataxia, hallucinations, hyperactivity, seizures, syncope, and paralytic ileus
Tropicamide	Used as a cycloplegic and mydriatic	Cyanosis, muscle rigidity, nausea, pallor, vomiting, vasomotor collapse
Parasympathomimetics or Anticholinesterases		
Echothiophate iodide	Glaucoma	Retinal detachments primarily in eyes with peripheral retinal or retinal-vitreal disease. (Patients need to be warned of this possible effect when first placed on this medication.)
Pilocarpine		Miotic upper respiratory infection—rhinorrhea, sensation of chest constriction, cough, conjunctival hyperemia; seen primarily in young children on anticholinesterase agents
Prostaglandins		
Latanoprost	Open-angle glaucoma	Flu-like syndrome; increased pigmentation of iris, eyelid skin, eyelid and eyelash; eyelashes—increased number, growth, and curling; iritis
Sulfonamides		
Carbonic anhydrase inhibitors	Open-angle glaucoma and ocular hypertension	Ciliary body and uveal effusion causing acute myopia and bilateral angle closure glaucoma
Sympathomimetics		
Dipivefrin	Open-angle glaucoma	Follicular blepharoconjunctivitis, keratitis
Epinephrine	Used as a bronchodilator	Cicatricial pemphigoid
	Open-angle glaucoma	Stains soft-contact lenses black
	Used as a vasoconstrictor to prolong anesthetic action	Hypertension, headache
10% Phenylephrine	Used as a mydriatic and vasoconstrictor	Cardiac arrhythmias and cardiac arrests with pledget form or subconjunctival injection, possible myocardial infarcts, systemic hypertension
Betaxolol	Open-angle glaucoma	Cardiac syncope, bradycardia, light-headedness, fatigue, congestive heart failure; in diabetics—hyperglycemia; in myasthenia gravis—severe dysarthria
Levobunolol hydrochloride		
Timolol		

SUTURE MATERIALS

Although sutureless cataract surgery is diminishing the need for certain sutures, there is still no other discipline that requires as many specialized needles and suture materials as ophthalmic surgery. To meet this need, manufacturers offer the ophthalmologist a comprehensive array of precisely manufactured reverse-cutting and spatula needles swaged to suture materials of collagen (plain and chromic), silk (black and white braided), virgin silk (black and white twisted), Nylon, Dacron, and synthetics.

Suture material intended for use in ophthalmic surgery can be either absorbable or nonabsorbable. Following is a list of various suture materials available with a brief description of each.

Absorbable

The absorption of sutures occurs in two distinct phases. After implantation, the suture's tensile strength diminishes during the early postoperative period. When most of the strength is lost, the remaining suture mass begins to decrease in what may be termed the second phase of absorption. The mass-loss phase then proceeds until the entire suture has been absorbed.

Plain Catgut—Prepared from the submucosal or mucosal layers of sheep or beef intestine, respectively, this material consists primarily of collagen—a fibrous protein—which is absorbed by the body. The material is chemically purified to minimize tissue reaction. Available in sizes 4–0 through 6–0.

Chromic Catgut—same as plain catgut except that it is treated with chromium salts to delay the absorption time. Available in sizes 4–0 through 7–0.

Plain Collagen—prepared from bovine deep flexor tendon. The tendon is purified and converted to a uniform suspension of collagen fibril. This fibrillar suspension is then extruded into suture strands and chemically treated to accurately control absorption rate. Available in sizes 4–0 through 7–0.

TABLE 1

COMPARISON OF OPHTHALMIC SUTURE MATERIALS

SUTURE MATERIAL	RELATIVE TENSILE STRENGTH*	RELATIVE HOLDING DURATION†	RELATIVE TISSUE REACTION‡	EASE OF HANDLING	SPECIAL KNOT REQUIRED	BEHAVIOR OF EXPOSED ENDS	AVAILABLE SIZES§
ABSORBABLE							
Surgical gut or collagen							
Plain	6	1 week	4+	Fair	No	Stiff	4–0 to 7–0
Chromic	6	<2 weeks	3+	Fair	No	Stiff	4–0 to 8–0
SYNTHETIC ABSORBABLE							
Polyglactin 910							
Braided	9	2 weeks	2+	Good	Yes	Stiff	4–0 to 9–0
Monofilament	9	2 weeks	2+	Good	Yes	Stiff	9–0 to 10–0
Polyglycolic acid	9	2 weeks	2+	Good	Yes	Stiff	4–0 to 10–0
NONABSORBABLE							
Silk							
Virgin	7	2 months	3+	Excellent	No	Softest	8–0 to 9–0
Braided	8	2 months	3+	Good	No	Soft	4–0 to 9–0
Polyamide (Nylon)	9	6 months	1+	Fair	Yes	Stiff, sharp	8–0 to 11–0
Polypropylene	10	>12 months	1+	Fair	Yes	Stiff, sharp	4–0 to 6–0 9–0 to 10–0

*The higher the number, the greater the relative tensile strength. Strength varies with size of material; estimates apply mainly to size 8–0 sutures.

† Holding duration will vary with location and size of suture, health of patient, medications employed, etc. The time given in this table is an average of the time at which about 30% of tensile strength is lost.

‡ 1+ indicates least inflammatory response, 4+ greatest.

§ With needles appropriate for ophthalmic use. Sizes available will vary from time to time.

Adapted from Spaeth GL. *Ophthalmic Surgery, Principles and Practice.* Philadelphia, Pa: WB Saunders; 1982:64.

Chromic Collagen—prepared in the same way as plain collagen except that chromium salts are added during the chemical treatment to further delay absorption. Available in sizes 4–0 through 8–0.

Synthetic Absorbable Sutures—Products include Vicryl (Polyglactin 910, a copolymer of lactide and glycolide) and Dexon (polyglycolic acid). These materials offer high tensile strength and minimal tissue reaction during the critical postoperative healing period, followed by predictable absorption. Coated Vicryl sutures are also available. Manufactured in size 4–0 through 10–0 (coated 4–0 through 8–0).

Nonabsorbable

Virgin Silk—twisted with the individual silk filaments still embedded in their natural sericin coating, providing a smooth, uniform suture in very fine sizes. The suture is offered in black or white, permitting optimum contrast with tissues. Available in sizes 8–0 and 9–0.

Black Braided Silk Suture—braided under controlled conditions to maximize strength and assure resistance to breaking while knots are tied. Gums and other impurities are removed, resulting in a suture that remains tightly braided, with virtually no loose filaments and minimal tendency to broom. Available in sizes 4–0 through 9–0.

Monofilament Nylon Sutures (Ethilon, Dermalon, and Supramid)—These sutures offer high tensile strength and minimal tissue reaction. Nylon has been reported to lose tensile strength postoperatively at a rate of approximately 15% per year. Available in sizes 8–0 through 11–0.

Polypropylene Suture (Prolene)—a monofilament suture with high tensile strength and minimal tissue reaction. The material is not degraded or weakened by tissue enzymes. Available in sizes 4-0 to 6-0 and 9-0 to 10-0.

Polyester Fiber Sutures—Products include Mersilene and Ti Cron. They exhibit minimal tissue reaction and are braided by a special method for tightness, uniformity, and a smooth surface that minimizes trauma. Available in sizes 4–0 through 6–0.

A variety of physical characteristics of different sutures have been published. In addition, the United States Pharmacopeia has established specifications for various suture materials. Some of the useful parameters measured have been: (1) tensile strength, (2) elasticity, (3) suture diameters, and (4) weight per unit length. Data are summarized in **Tables 1** through **3**.

TABLE 2

ELASTICITY OF SELECTED SUTURES

SUTURE MATERIAL	ELONGATION OF STANDARD 30.5-cm SEGMENT	INCREASE IN LENGTH	WEIGHT AT BREAKING POINT
6–0 plain gut	4.7 cm	15.4%	264 g
6–0 chromic gut	4.3 cm	14.1%	257 g
6–0 Mersilene	1.9 cm	6.3%	254 g
6–0 braided silk	1.2 cm	3.9%	237 g
7–0 chromic gut	3.6 cm	1.8%	118 g
7–0 braided silk	0.9 cm	3.0%	126 g
8–0 virgin silk	0.8 cm	2.6%	53 g
10–0 Nylon	8.7 cm	28.5%	23 g

From Middleton DG, McCulloch C. *Adv Ophthalmol.* 1970;22:35.

TABLE 3

WEIGHT OF SELECTED SUTURE MATERIAL

SUTURE MATERIAL	WEIGHT/LENGTH (mg/cm)
6–0 plain gut (wet)	0.170
6–0 chromic gut (wet)	0.176
6–0 Mersilene	0.116
6–0 braided silk	0.165
7–0 chromic gut (wet)	0.062
7–0 braided silk	0.065
8–0 virgin silk	0.025
10–0 Nylon	0.007

OPHTHALMIC LENSES

1. COMPARISON AND CONVERSION TABLES

TABLE 1

RELATIVE MAGNIFICATION PRODUCED BY CONTACT AND SPECTACLE LENSES
The percentage increase (or decrease) in the size of the retinal image afforded by contact lenses in comparison with orthodox spectacles fitted at 12 mm from the cornea.

SPECTACLE REFRACTION	EQUIVALENT POWER OF CONTACT LENS SYSTEM	PERCENTAGE INCREASE AFFORDED BY CONTACT LENS	SPECTACLE REFRACTION	EQUIVALENT POWER OF CONTACT LENS SYSTEM	PERCENTAGE INCREASE AFFORDED BY CONTACT LENS	SPECTACLE REFRACTION	EQUIVALENT POWER OF CONTACT LENS SYSTEM	PERCENTAGE INCREASE AFFORDED BY CONTACT LENS
−20	−15.73	27.2	−8	−7.07	12.9	+6	+6.10	−4.7
−18	−14.41	24.8	−6	−5.42	10.5	+8	+8.29	−7.4
−16	−13.06	22.5	−4	−3.69	7.8	+10	+10.62	−10.3
−14	−11.65	20.1	−2	−1.88	5.4	+12	+13.07	−13.8
−12	−10.19	17.8	+2	+1.96	1.2	+14	+15.64	−17.3
−10	−8.66	15.3	+4	+3.99	−1.7			

Bennet AG. *Optics of Contact Lenses,* ed 4. London: Hatton Press; 1966.

TABLE 2

INDEX OF REFRACTION OF LENS MATERIAL

	CROWN GLASS	1.6-INDEX CROWNLITE GLASS	HILITE GLASS	8-INDEX GLASS	CR−39 PLASTIC	HIRI PLASTIC	1.6-INDEX PLASTIC	POLY− CARBONATE THIN−LITE PLASTIC
INDEX OF REFRACTION The higher the number, the thinner the material	1.523	1.601	1.701	1.805	1.498	1.56	1.6	1.586
SPECIFIC GRAVITY The higher the number, the heavier the material	2.5	2.67	2.99	3.37	1.32	1.216	1.34	1.20
DISPERSION The higher the number, the less chromatic aberration (Abbe value)	59	42.24	31	25	58	38	37	31
PERSONALITY	Temperable, coatable, ease in handling, vast availability	Chemically temperable, ease in handling, limited availability	Chemically temperable, fairly easy to handle, SV and multifocals; vacuum coatings cause lens to become highly sensitive to scratching	SV, difficult to temper, highly reflective so A/R coatings recommended, but have same problems as hilite; mfrs suggest having patient sign liability waiver when ground thin. Multifocal available in laminate.	Strong, tintable, coatable, ease in handling, vast availability	SV and bifocal, tints well before SRC, edges well, must be SRC, extremely brittle	SV only, tints well before SRC, edges well, must be SRC	SV and multifocal, strongest lens material available, limited tintability, must be SPC, no fast fabrication, special edging equipment needed, a must for children and athletes

SV = single-vision lenses. A/R = antireflective. SRC = scratch-resistant coating. SPC = scratch-proof coating.

TABLE 3

CORNEAL RADIUS EQUIVALENCE DIOPTERS/MILLIMETERS

DIOPTERS	mm	DIOPTERS	mm	DIOPTERS	mm	DIOPTERS	mm	DIOPTERS	mm	DIOPTERS	mm	DIOPTERS	mm	DIOPTERS	mm
20.00	16.875	36.00	9.375	39.00	8.653	42.00	8.035	45.00	7.500	48.00	7.031	51.00	6.617	54.00	6.250
22.00	15.340	36.12	9.343	39.12	8.627	42.12	8.012	45.12	7.480	48.12	7.013	51.12	6.602	54.12	6.236
24.00	14.062	36.25	9.310	39.25	8.598	42.25	7.988	45.25	7.458	48.25	6.994	51.25	6.585	54.25	6.221
26.00	12.980	36.37	9.279	39.37	8.572	42.37	7.965	45.37	7.438	48.37	6.977	51.37	6.569	54.37	6.207
27.00	12.500	36.50	9.246	39.50	8.544	42.50	7.941	45.50	7.417	48.50	6.958	51.50	6.553	54.50	6.192
28.00	12.053	36.62	9.216	39.62	8.518	42.62	7.918	45.62	7.398	48.62	6.941	51.62	6.538	54.62	6.179
29.00	11.638	36.75	9.183	39.75	8.490	42.75	7.894	45.75	7.377	48.75	6.923	51.75	6.521	54.75	6.164
29.50	11.441	36.87	9.153	39.87	8.465	42.87	7.872	45.87	7.357	48.87	6.906	51.87	6.506	54.87	6.150
30.00	11.250	37.00	9.121	40.00	8.437	43.00	7.848	46.00	7.336	49.00	6.887	52.00	6.490	55.00	6.136
30.50	11.065	37.12	9.092	40.12	8.412	43.12	7.826	46.12	7.317	49.12	6.870	52.12	6.475	55.12	6.123
31.00	10.887	37.25	9.060	40.25	8.385	43.25	7.803	46.25	7.297	49.25	6.852	52.25	6.459	55.25	6.108
31.50	10.714	37.37	9.031	40.37	8.360	43.37	7.781	46.37	7.278	49.37	6.836	52.37	6.444	55.37	6.095
32.00	10.547	37.50	9.000	40.50	8.333	43.50	7.758	46.50	7.258	49.50	6.818	52.50	6.428	55.50	6.081
32.50	10.385	37.62	8.971	40.62	8.308	43.62	7.737	46.62	7.239	49.62	6.801	52.62	6.413	55.62	6.068
33.00	10.227	37.75	8.940	40.75	8.282	43.75	7.714	46.75	7.219	49.75	6.783	52.75	6.398	55.75	6.054
33.50	10.075	37.87	8.912	40.87	8.257	43.87	7.693	46.87	7.200	49.87	6.767	52.87	6.383	55.87	6.041
34.00	9.926	38.00	8.881	41.00	8.231	44.00	7.670	47.00	7.180	50.00	6.750	53.00	6.367	56.00	6.027
34.25	9.854	38.12	8.853	41.12	8.207	44.12	7.649	47.12	7.162	50.12	6.733	53.12	6.353	56.50	5.973
34.50	9.783	38.25	8.823	41.25	8.181	44.25	7.627	47.25	7.142	50.25	6.716	53.25	6.338	57.00	5.921
34.75	9.712	38.37	8.795	41.37	8.158	44.37	7.606	47.37	7.124	50.37	6.700	53.37	6.323	57.50	5.869
35.00	9.643	38.50	8.766	41.50	8.132	44.50	7.584	47.50	7.105	50.50	6.683	53.50	6.308	58.00	5.819
35.25	9.574	38.62	8.738	41.62	8.109	44.62	7.563	47.62	7.087	50.62	6.667	53.62	6.294	58.50	5.769
35.50	9.507	38.75	8.708	41.75	8.083	44.75	7.541	47.75	7.068	50.75	6.650	53.75	6.279	59.00	5.720
35.75	9.440	38.87	8.682	41.87	8.060	44.87	7.521	47.87	7.050	50.87	6.634	53.87	6.265	60.00	5.625

TABLE 4

VERTEX DISTANCE CONVERSION SCALE (mm)

SPECTACLE LENS	PLUS LENSES								MINUS LENSES							
POWER	8	9	10	11	12	13	14	15	8	9	10	11	12	13	14	15
4.00	4.12	4.12	4.12	4.12	4.25	4.25	4.25	4.25	3.87	3.87	3.87	3.87	3.87	3.75	3.75	3.75
4.50	4.62	4.75	4.75	4.75	4.75	4.75	4.75	4.87	4.37	4.37	4.25	4.25	4.25	4.25	4.25	4.25
5.00	5.25	5.25	5.25	5.25	5.25	5.37	5.37	5.37	4.75	4.75	4.75	4.75	4.75	4.75	4.62	4.62
5.50	5.75	5.75	5.75	5.87	5.87	5.87	6.00	6.00	5.25	5.25	5.25	5.12	5.12	5.12	5.12	5.12
6.00	6.25	6.37	6.37	6.37	6.50	6.50	6.50	6.62	5.75	5.62	5.62	5.62	5.62	5.50	5.50	5.50
6.50	6.87	6.87	7.00	7.00	7.00	7.12	7.12	7.25	6.12	6.12	6.12	6.00	6.00	6.00	6.00	5.87
7.00	7.37	7.50	7.50	7.62	7.62	7.75	7.75	7.75	6.62	6.62	6.50	6.50	6.50	6.37	6.37	6.37
7.50	8.00	8.00	8.12	8.12	8.25	8.25	8.37	8.50	7.12	7.00	7.00	6.87	6.87	6.87	6.75	6.75
8.00	8.50	8.62	8.75	8.75	8.87	8.87	9.00	9.12	7.50	7.50	7.37	7.37	7.25	7.25	7.25	7.25
8.50	9.12	9.25	9.25	9.37	9.50	9.50	9.62	9.75	8.00	7.87	7.87	7.75	7.75	7.62	7.62	7.50
9.00	9.75	9.75	9.87	10.00	10.12	10.25	10.37	10.37	8.37	8.37	8.25	8.25	8.12	8.00	8.00	8.00
9.50	10.25	10.37	10.50	10.62	10.75	10.87	11.00	11.12	8.87	8.75	8.62	8.62	8.50	8.50	8.37	8.37
10.00	10.87	11.00	11.12	11.25	11.37	11.50	11.62	11.75	9.25	9.12	9.12	9.00	8.87	8.87	8.75	8.75
10.50	11.50	11.62	11.75	11.87	12.00	12.12	12.25	12.50	9.62	9.62	9.50	9.37	9.37	9.25	9.12	9.12
11.00	12.00	12.25	12.37	12.50	12.75	12.87	13.00	13.12	10.12	10.00	9.87	9.75	9.75	9.62	9.50	9.50
11.50	12.62	12.87	13.00	13.12	13.37	13.50	13.75	13.87	10.50	10.37	10.37	10.25	10.12	10.00	9.87	9.87
12.00	13.25	13.50	13.62	13.87	14.00	14.25	14.50	14.62	11.00	10.87	10.75	10.62	10.50	10.37	10.25	10.12
12.50	13.87	14.12	14.25	14.50	14.75	15.00	15.25	15.37	11.37	11.25	11.12	11.00	10.87	10.75	10.62	10.50
13.00	14.50	14.75	15.00	15.25	15.50	15.62	16.00	16.12	11.75	11.62	11.50	11.37	11.25	11.12	11.00	10.87
13.50	15.12	15.37	15.62	15.87	16.12	16.37	16.62	16.87	12.25	12.00	11.87	11.75	11.62	11.50	11.37	11.25
14.00	15.75	16.00	16.25	16.50	16.75	17.12	17.50	17.75	12.62	12.50	12.25	12.12	12.00	11.87	11.75	11.50
14.50	16.50	16.75	17.00	17.25	17.50	17.87	18.25	18.50	13.00	12.75	12.62	12.50	12.37	12.25	12.00	11.87
15.00	17.00	17.37	17.75	18.00	18.25	18.62	19.00	19.37	13.37	13.25	13.00	12.87	12.75	12.50	12.37	12.25
15.50	17.75	18.00	18.25	18.75	19.00	19.37	19.75	20.25	13.75	13.62	13.50	13.25	13.00	12.87	12.75	12.62
16.00	18.25	18.75	19.00	19.37	19.75	20.25	20.50	21.00	14.25	14.00	13.75	13.62	13.50	13.25	13.00	12.87
16.50	19.00	19.37	19.75	20.25	20.50	21.00	21.50	21.87	14.50	14.37	14.12	14.00	13.75	13.62	13.50	13.25
17.00	19.75	20.25	20.50	21.00	21.50	22.00	22.25	22.87	15.00	14.75	14.50	14.25	14.12	14.00	13.75	13.50
17.50	20.50	20.75	21.25	21.75	22.25	22.75	23.25	23.75	15.37	15.12	14.87	14.75	14.50	14.25	14.00	13.87
18.00	21.00	21.50	22.00	22.50	23.00	23.50	24.00	24.62	15.75	15.50	15.25	15.00	14.75	14.62	14.37	14.12
18.50	21.75	22.25	22.75	23.25	23.75	24.50	25.00	25.62	16.12	15.87	15.62	15.37	15.12	14.87	14.75	14.50
19.00	22.50	23.00	23.50	24.00	24.75	25.25	26.00	26.50	16.50	16.25	16.00	15.75	15.50	15.25	15.00	14.75

TABLE 5

MJK SPHEROCYLINDRICAL VERTEX CHART

VERTEX DISTANCE = 13.00 mm					SPHERE INCREMENT = 0.125 DIOPTER						CYLINDER INCREMENT = 0.25 DIOPTER		
SR	SRV	−0.25	−0.50	−0.75	−1.00	−1.25	−1.50	−1.75	−2.00	−2.25	−2.50	−2.75	−3.00
−3.00	−2.87	−0.25	−0.50	−0.75	−1.00	−1.25	−1.25	−1.50	−1.75	−2.00	−2.25	−2.50	−2.75
−3.25	−3.12	−0.25	−0.50	−0.75	−1.00	−1.25	−1.25	−1.50	−1.75	−2.00	−2.25	−2.50	−2.75
−3.50	−3.37	−0.25	−0.50	−0.75	−1.00	−1.25	−1.25	−1.50	−1.75	−2.00	−2.25	−2.50	−2.75
−3.75	−3.62	−0.25	−0.50	−0.75	−1.00	−1.00	−1.25	−1.50	−1.75	−2.00	−2.25	−2.50	−2.75
−4.00	−3.75	−0.25	−0.50	−0.75	−1.00	−1.00	−1.25	−1.50	−1.75	−2.00	−2.25	−2.50	−2.50
−4.25	−4.00	−0.25	−0.50	−0.75	−1.00	−1.00	−1.25	−1.50	−1.75	−2.00	−2.25	−2.50	−2.50
−4.50	−4.25	−0.25	−0.50	−0.75	−1.00	−1.00	−1.25	−1.50	−1.75	−2.00	−2.25	−2.25	−2.50
−4.75	−4.50	−0.25	−0.50	−0.75	−1.00	−1.00	−1.25	−1.50	−1.75	−2.00	−2.25	−2.25	−2.50
−5.00	−4.75	−0.25	−0.50	−0.75	−0.75	−1.00	−1.25	−1.50	−1.75	−2.00	−2.25	−2.25	−2.50
−5.25	−4.87	−0.25	−0.50	−0.75	−0.75	−1.00	−1.25	−1.50	−1.75	−2.00	−2.25	−2.25	−2.50
−5.50	−5.12	−0.25	−0.50	−0.75	−0.75	−1.00	−1.25	−1.50	−1.75	−2.00	−2.00	−2.25	−2.50
−5.75	−5.37	−0.25	−0.50	−0.75	−0.75	−1.00	−1.25	−1.50	−1.75	−2.00	−2.00	−2.25	−2.50
−6.00	−5.62	−0.25	−0.50	−0.75	−0.75	−1.00	−1.25	−1.50	−1.75	−2.00	−2.00	−2.25	−2.50
−6.25	−5.75	−0.25	−0.50	−0.75	−0.75	−1.00	−1.25	−1.50	−1.75	−1.75	−2.00	−2.25	−2.50
−6.50	−6.00	−0.25	−0.50	−0.75	−0.75	−1.00	−1.25	−1.50	−1.75	−1.75	−2.00	−2.25	−2.50
−6.75	−6.25	−0.25	−0.50	−0.75	−0.75	−1.00	−1.25	−1.50	−1.75	−1.75	−2.00	−2.25	−2.50
−7.00	−6.37	−0.25	−0.50	−0.50	−0.75	−1.00	−1.25	−1.50	−1.75	−1.75	−2.00	−2.25	−2.50
−7.25	−6.62	−0.25	−0.50	−0.50	−0.75	−1.00	−1.25	−1.50	−1.75	−1.75	−2.00	−2.25	−2.50
−7.50	−6.87	−0.25	−0.50	−0.50	−0.75	−1.00	−1.25	−1.50	−1.50	−1.75	−2.00	−2.25	−2.50
−7.75	−7.00	−0.25	−0.50	−0.50	−0.75	−1.00	−1.25	−1.50	−1.50	−1.75	−2.00	−2.25	−2.50
−8.00	−7.25	−0.25	−0.50	−0.50	−0.75	−1.00	−1.25	−1.50	−1.50	−1.75	−2.00	−2.25	−2.50
−8.25	−7.50	−0.25	−0.50	−0.50	−0.75	−1.00	−1.25	−1.50	−1.50	−1.75	−2.00	−2.25	−2.25
−8.50	−7.62	−0.25	−0.50	−0.50	−0.75	−1.00	−1.25	−1.50	−1.50	−1.75	−2.00	−2.25	−2.25
−8.75	−7.87	−0.25	−0.50	−0.50	−0.75	−1.00	−1.25	−1.50	−1.50	−1.75	−2.00	−2.25	−2.25
−9.00	−8.00	−0.25	−0.50	−0.50	−0.75	−1.00	−1.25	−1.25	−1.50	−1.75	−2.00	−2.25	−2.25
−9.25	−8.25	−0.25	−0.50	−0.50	−0.75	−1.00	−1.25	−1.25	−1.50	−1.75	−2.00	−2.00	−2.25
−9.50	−8.50	−0.25	−0.50	−0.50	−0.75	−1.00	−1.25	−1.25	−1.50	−1.75	−2.00	−2.00	−2.25
−9.75	−8.62	−0.25	−0.50	−0.50	−0.75	−1.00	−1.25	−1.25	−1.50	−1.75	−2.00	−2.00	−2.25
−10.00	−8.87	−0.25	−0.50	−0.50	−0.75	−1.00	−1.25	−1.25	−1.50	−1.75	−2.00	−2.00	−2.25
−10.25	−9.00	−0.25	−0.50	−0.50	−0.75	−1.00	−1.25	−1.25	−1.50	−1.75	−2.00	−2.00	−2.25
−10.50	−9.25	−0.25	−0.50	−0.50	−0.75	−1.00	−1.25	−1.25	−1.50	−1.75	−2.00	−2.00	−2.25
−10.75	−9.37	−0.25	−0.50	−0.50	−0.75	−1.00	−1.25	−1.25	−1.50	−1.75	−2.25	−2.00	−2.25
+4.00	+4.25	−0.25	−0.50	−0.75	−1.00	−1.25	−1.75	−2.00	−2.25	−2.50	−2.75	−3.00	−3.25
+4.25	+4.50	−0.25	−0.50	−0.75	−1.00	−1.50	−1.75	−2.00	−2.25	−2.50	−2.75	−3.00	−3.25
+4.50	+4.75	−0.25	−0.50	−0.75	−1.00	−1.50	−1.75	−2.00	−2.25	−2.50	−2.75	−3.00	−3.25
+4.75	+5.12	−0.25	−0.50	−0.75	−1.00	−1.50	−1.75	−2.00	−2.25	−2.50	−2.75	−3.00	−3.25
+5.00	+5.37	−0.25	−0.50	−0.75	−1.00	−1.50	−1.75	−2.00	−2.25	−2.50	−2.75	−3.00	−3.25
+5.25	+5.62	−0.25	−0.50	−0.75	−1.00	−1.50	−1.75	−2.00	−2.25	−2.50	−2.75	−3.00	−3.25
+5.50	+5.87	−0.25	−0.50	−0.75	−1.00	−1.50	−1.75	−2.00	−2.25	−2.50	−2.75	−3.00	−3.25
+5.75	+6.25	−0.25	−0.50	−0.75	−1.00	−1.50	−1.75	−2.00	−2.25	−2.50	−2.75	−3.00	−3.25
+6.00	+6.50	−0.25	−0.50	−0.75	−1.00	−1.50	−1.75	−2.00	−2.25	−2.50	−2.75	−3.00	−3.50
+6.25	+6.75	−0.25	−0.50	−1.00	−1.00	−1.50	−1.75	−2.00	−2.25	−2.50	−2.75	−3.25	−3.50
+6.50	+7.12	−0.25	−0.50	−1.00	−1.00	−1.50	−1.75	−2.00	−2.25	−2.50	−3.00	−3.25	−3.50
+6.75	+7.37	−0.25	−0.50	−1.00	−1.00	−1.50	−1.75	−2.00	−2.25	−2.50	−3.00	−3.25	−3.50
+7.00	+7.75	−0.25	−0.50	−1.00	−1.00	−1.50	−1.75	−2.00	−2.25	−2.75	−3.00	−3.25	−3.50
+7.25	+8.00	−0.25	−0.50	−1.00	−1.00	−1.50	−1.75	−2.00	−2.25	−2.75	−3.00	−3.25	−3.50
+7.50	+8.25	−0.25	−0.50	−1.00	−1.00	−1.50	−1.75	−2.00	−2.50	−2.75	−3.00	−3.25	−3.50
+7.75	+8.62	−0.25	−0.50	−1.00	−1.00	−1.50	−1.75	−2.00	−2.50	−2.75	−3.00	−3.25	−3.50
+8.00	+8.87	−0.25	−0.50	−1.00	−1.00	−1.50	−1.75	−2.25	−2.50	−2.75	−3.00	−3.25	−3.50
+8.25	+9.25	−0.25	−0.50	−1.00	−1.00	−1.50	−1.75	−2.25	−2.50	−2.75	−3.00	−3.25	−3.50
+8.50	+9.25	−0.25	−0.75	−1.00	−1.25	−1.50	−1.75	−2.25	−2.50	−2.75	−3.00	−3.25	−3.75
+8.75	+9.87	−0.25	−0.75	−1.00	−1.25	−1.50	−1.75	−2.25	−2.50	−2.75	−3.00	−3.25	−3.75
+9.00	+10.25	−0.25	−0.75	−1.00	−1.25	−1.50	−2.00	−2.25	−2.50	−2.75	−3.00	−3.50	−3.75
+9.25	+10.50	−0.25	−0.75	−1.00	−1.25	−1.50	−2.00	−2.25	−2.50	−2.75	−3.00	−3.50	−3.75
+9.50	+10.87	−0.25	−0.75	−1.00	−1.25	−1.50	−2.00	−2.25	−2.50	−2.75	−3.25	−3.50	−3.75
+9.75	+11.12	−0.25	−0.75	−1.00	−1.25	−1.50	−2.00	−2.25	−2.50	−2.75	−3.25	−3.50	−3.75
+10.00	+11.50	−0.25	−0.75	−1.00	−1.25	−1.50	−2.00	−2.25	−2.50	−3.00	−3.25	−3.50	−3.75
+10.25	+11.87	−0.25	−0.75	−1.00	−1.25	−1.75	−2.00	−2.25	−2.50	−3.00	−3.25	−3.50	−3.75
+10.50	+12.12	−0.25	−0.75	−1.00	−1.25	−1.75	−2.00	−2.25	−2.50	−3.00	−3.25	−3.50	−3.75
+10.75	+12.50	−0.25	−0.75	−1.00	−1.25	−1.75	−2.00	−2.25	−2.50	−3.00	−3.25	−3.50	−4.00
+11.00	+12.87	−0.25	−0.75	−1.00	−1.25	−1.75	−2.00	−2.25	−2.75	−3.00	−3.25	−3.50	−4.00
+11.25	+13.12	−0.25	−0.75	−1.00	−1.25	−1.75	−2.00	−2.25	−2.75	−3.00	−3.25	−3.50	−4.00
+11.50	+13.50	−0.25	−0.75	−1.00	−1.25	−1.75	−2.00	−2.25	−2.75	−3.00	−3.25	−3.75	−4.00
+11.75	+13.87	−0.25	−0.75	−1.00	−1.25	−1.75	−2.00	−2.25	−2.75	−3.00	−3.25	−3.75	−4.00

Example: Spectacle refraction (SR) at 13 mm = −5.75 − 2.50 × 180.
Matching up −5.75 (see highlighted boxes) on the left, gives effective spherical power (SRV) of −5.37.
Following values to the right and reading in the −2.50 cylinder column gives a cylinder value of −2.00.

Corneal plane refraction = −5.37 − 2.00 × 180.

Legend: In this chart of spherocylindrical corneal plane refractions, the spherical value is calculated and rounded off to the nearest 0.125 diopter, while the cylinder value is rounded off to the nearest 0.25 diopter.

2. SOFT-CONTACT LENSES MANUFACTURER DIRECTORY

This section provides a convenient list of the companies that manufacture soft-contact lenses, together with the information needed if you have further inquiries.

ACCU LENS, INC.
5353 West Colfax Avenue
Denver, CO 80214
Phone: (303) 232-6244
Toll-free: (800) 525-2470
Fax: 303-235-0472
Website: www.acculens.com

ACUITY ONE, LLC.
7642 East Gray Road, Suite 103
Scottsdale, AZ 85260
Phone: (480) 607-2998
Toll-free: (877) 228-4891
Fax: (877) 607-2871
E-mail: info@acuityone.com
Website: acuityone.com

ALDEN OPTICAL LABORATORIES, INC.
13295 Broadway
Alden, NY 14004
Phone: (716) 937-9181
Toll-free: (800) 253-3669
Fax: (800) 899-5612
E-mail: info@aldenoptical.com
Website: www.aldenoptical.com

BAUSCH & LOMB
1400 North Goodman Street
Rochester, NY 14603
Phone: (585) 338-6000
Toll-free: (800) 553-5340
Fax: (585) 338-6896
Website: www.bausch.com

BLANCHARD CONTACT LENS
8025 S. Willow St.
Manchester, NH 03103
Toll-free: (800) 367-4009
Fax: (603) 627-3280
E-mail: blanchardlabs@prodigy.net
Website: www.blanchardlab.com

CIBA VISION CORPORATION
11460 Johns Creek Parkway
Duluth, GA 30097
Phone: (678) 415-3937
Toll-free: (800) 241-5999
Fax: (800) 845-8842
Website: www.cibavision.com

CONTINENTAL SOFT LENS, INC.
P.O. Box 621029
Littleton, CO 80162
Phone: (303) 795-2130
Toll-free: (800) 637-3845
Fax: (303) 795-6984

COOPERVISION, INC.
370 Woodcliff Drive, Suite 200
Fairport, NY 14450
Phone: (585) 385-6810
Toll-free: (800) 341-2020
Fax: (888) 385-3217
E-mail: info@coopervision.com
Website: www.coopervision.com

CUSTOM COLOR CONTACTS
55 West 49th Street
New York, NY 10020
Phone: (212) 765-4444
Toll-free: (800) 598-2020
Fax: (212) 765-4459
E-mail: info@customcontacts.com
Website: www.customcontacts.com

EXTREME H2O/ HYDROGEL VISION CORP.
7575 Commerce Court
Sarasota, FL 34243
Toll-free: (877) 336-2482
Fax: (888) 612-6379
E-mail: customercare@extreme-h2o.com
Website: www.extreme-h2o.com

IDEAL OPTICS, INC.
2255 Cumberland Parkway
Building 500
Atlanta, GA 30339
Phone: (770) 432-0048
Toll-free: (800) 554-7353
Fax: (770) 434-8291

KONTUR KONTACT LENS CO.
642 Alfred Nobel Dr.
Hercules, CA 94547
Phone: (510) 964-9760
Toll-free: 800-227-1320
Fax: (800) 650-6525
E-mail: kontur55@aol.com

LENS DYNAMICS, INC.
14998 West 6th Avenue, Suite 830
Golden, CO 80401
Phone: (303) 237-6927
Toll-free: (800) 228-2691
Fax: (800) 661-6707
    (303) 274-6707
E-mail: vaske@lensdynamics.com
Website: www.lensdynamics.com

METRO OPTICS, INC.
P.O. Box 81189
Austin, TX 78708
Phone: (512) 251-2382
Toll-free: (800) 223-1858
Fax: (512) 251-6554
E-mail: info@metro-optics.com
Website: www.metro-optics.com

OCU-EASE OPTICAL PRODUCTS, INC.
920 San Pablo Avenue
Pinole, CA 94564
Toll-free: (800) 521-8984
Fax: (800) 628-3273
E-mail: custom@ocuease.com
Website: www.ocuease.com

PC OPTICAL PRODUCTS, INC.
801 12th Avenue North
Minneapolis, MN 55411
Toll-free: (800) 433-4885
Fax: (800) 895-8235

PERMEABLE CONTACT LENSES OF NJ/LIFESTYLE COMPANY, INC.
1800 Rt. 34 North
Suite 401
Wall, NJ 07719
Toll-free: (877) 787-5367
Fax: (732) 972-9205
E-mail: lenses@lifestylecompany.com
Website: www.purilens.com

PRECISION VISION, LTD.
1490 S. Yampa Way
Aurora, CO 80017
Phone: (303) 743-0494
Toll-free: (800) 843-5367
Fax: (303) 632-8216
E-mail: info@precisionvision.com
Website: www.precisionvision.com

PREFERRED OPTICS, INC.
393 North Sessions Street
Marietta, GA 30060
Phone: (770) 426-4015
Toll-free: (800) 253-0351
Fax: (770) 424-4341

SODERBERG CONTACT LENS
230 Eva Street
Saint Paul, MN 55107
Phone: (651) 291-1400
Toll-free: (866) 566-0387
Fax: (800) 838-2972
E-mail: info@soderberginc.com
Website: www.soseyes.com

TRU-FORM OPTICS
400 S Industrial Boulevard,
Euless, TX 76040-4246
Phone: (817) 267-9261
Toll-free: (800) 792-1095
Fax: (817) 354-8319
E-mail: info@tfoptics.com
Website: www.tfoptics.com

UNILENS CORPORATION, USA
10431 72nd Street North
Largo, FL 33777
Phone: (727) 544-2531
Toll-free: (800) 446-2020
Fax: (727) 545-1883
    (800) 808-8264
E-mail: unilens@aol.com *or*
    information@unilens.com
Website: www.unilens.com

UNITED CONTACT LENS, INC.
917 134th Street Southwest, Suite A-4
Everett, WA 98204
Phone: (425) 743-7343
Toll-free: (800) 446-1666
Fax: (425) 743-8795
Website: www.unitedcontactlens.com

VALLEY CONTAX
200 South Mill Street
Springfield, OR 97477
Phone: (541) 744-9393
Toll-free: (800) 547-8815
Fax: (541) 744-9399
E-mail: contax@valleycontax.com
Website: www.valleycontax.com

VISTAKON
7500 Centurion Parkway, Suite 100
Mail Stop D-CREL
Jacksonville, FL 32256
Phone: (904) 443-1000
Toll-free: (800) 843-2020
Fax: (800) 456-2733
Website: www.acuvue.com

WESTCON CONTACT LENS COMPANY, INC.
611 Eisenhauer Street
Grand Junction, CO 81505
Phone: (970) 245-3845
Toll-free: (800) 346-4303
Fax: (970) 245-4516
    (800) 715-3388
E-mail: westcon@westconlens.com
Website: www.westconlens.com

X-CEL CONTACTS/ A WALMAN COMPANY
2775 Premiere Parkway, Suite 600
Duluth, GA 30097
(See website for more office locations.)
Phone: (770) 622-9235
Toll-free: (800) 241-9312
Fax: (800) 622-8989
Website: www.walman.com

SECTION 5

VISION STANDARDS AND LOW-VISION AIDS

1. VISION STANDARDS

TABLE 1

VISION STANDARDS FOR PILOTS

	WITHOUT RX[1]	REQUIRING RX[1] CORRECTED TO	NEAR VISION WITH/ WITHOUT RX	PHORIAS[2]	FIELDS	COLOR	PATHOLOGY
1st class	20/20	20/100 to 20/20	20/40 (J_3)	6 D eso/exo 1 Δ hyper	Normal	Normal	4
2nd class	20/20	20/100 to 20/20	20/40 (J_3)	6 D eso/exo 1 Δ hyper	Normal	3	5
3rd class	20/50	To 20/30	20/60 (J_6)	. . .	. . .	3	5

1. Each eye.
2. If exceeded, further evaluation required to determine bifoveal fixation and adequate vergence phoria relationship.
3. Able to distinguish aviation signal red, aviation signal green, and white.
4. No acute or chronic pathologic condition of either eye of adnexa that might interfere with its proper function, might progress to that degree, or be aggravated by flying.
5. No serious pathology.
Note: By amendment regulations (12/21/76) correction may be by spectacles or contact lenses.

TABLE 2

VISION STANDARDS FOR ADMISSION TO SERVICE ACADEMIES

US Coast Guard Academy	Minimum uncorrected 20/200 each eye; correctable to 20/20 each eye; refractive error not more than ±5.50 D any meridian; astigmatism not over 3.00 D; anisometropia not exceeding 3.50 D; full visual fields; normal color vision; no chronic, disfiguring, disabling, ocular pathology.
US Merchant Marine Academy	Minimum uncorrected 20/100 each eye; correctable to 20/20 each eye; refractive error as for Coast Guard Academy; color vision normal by Farnsworth lantern test or pseudoisochromatic plates; certain pathologies may disqualify.
US Naval Academy	Uncorrected vision 20/20 each eye; limited waivers if correctable to 20/20 each eye and to refraction standards, Coast Guard Academy; color vision normal–no waivers; no chronic, disfiguring, disabling ocular pathology.
US Military Academy	Distance vision correctable to 20/20 each eye; refractive error as for Coast Guard Academy; able to distinguish vivid red and green; ET less than 15 prism diopters; XT less than 10 prism diopters; hypertropia less than 2 prism diopters; certain pathologies may disqualify.
US Air Force Academy	*Pilot:* Uncorrected vision 20/20 or better each eye, far and near; refractive error hyperopia no greater than +1.75 D and nearsightedness less than plano in any one meridian; the astigmatic error must not exceed 0.75 D. *Navigator:* Uncorrected vision 20/70 or better correctable with ordinary glasses to 20/20 each eye; near acuity 20/20 or better each eye, uncorrected; hyperopia not greater than +3.00 D and myopia not greater than −1.50 D any meridian; astigmatism not to exceed 2.00 D. *Commission:* Distance acuity correctable 20/40 one eye and 20/70 other, or 20/30 one eye and 20/100 other; near acuity correctable to 20/20 (J_1) one eye and 20/30 (J_2) in other; refractive error of equivalent sphere not more than ±8.00 D; no chronic, disfiguring, disabling ocular pathology.

Based on information as of May 17, 1983, Medical Examination Review Board, Department of Defense.

TABLE 3

VISION STANDARDS FOR COMMERCIAL DRIVERS

	VISUAL ACUITY BINOC	VISUAL FIELD (degrees) MONOC	BINOC	COLOR	OTHER	RETEST
Alabama	20/40	No	No	ND	No	No
Alaska	20/40	No	No	No	No	Periodic
Arizona	20/40	70/35	No	PD	No	Periodic
Arkansas	20/50	105	NS	No	NS	NS
California	20/40	No	No	No	NS	Periodic
Colorado	20/40	No	No	No	ST	Periodic
Connecticut	20/40	100	140	No	ST	No
Delaware	20/40	No	No	No	No	Periodic
Florida	20/70	No	130	No	No	Periodic
Georgia	20/60	140, 140	140	No	No	Periodic
Hawaii	20/40	70, 70	140	No	ST, EC	Periodic
Idaho	20/40	NS	NS	NS	NS	Periodic
Illinois	20/40	105	140	NS	NS	Periodic
Indiana	20/40	70	120	No	NS	Periodic
Iowa	20/40	No	140	PD	NS	Periodic
Kansas	20/40	55	110	No	NS	Periodic
Kentucky	20/45, PV	80	120	No	No	No
Louisiana	20/40	No	No	No	No	Periodic
Maine	20/40	NS	140	No	NS	No
Maryland	20/40	NS	140	PD	No	Periodic
Massachusetts	20/40	90,90	120	Yes	No	Periodic
Michigan	20/40	70, 70	140	No	NS	Periodic
Minnesota	20/40	NS	105	No	NS	Periodic
Mississippi	20/40	70(T)/35(N)	140	No	ST	No
Missouri	20/40	55, 55	No	No	No	Periodic
Montana	20/40	No	No	No	ST	Periodic
Nebraska	20/40	No	140	PD	No	Periodic
Nevada	20/40	No	140	NS	No	Periodic
New Hampshire	20/40	No	No	No	NS	Periodic
New Jersey	20/50	70, 70	No	No	No	NS
New Mexico	20/40	NS	120(T)/30(N)	No	NS	Periodic
New York	20/40	NS	140	No	NS	Periodic
North Carolina	20/50	No	60	No	No	Periodic
North Dakota	20/40	70, 70	105	No	No	Periodic
Ohio	20/40	70, 70	No	Yes	No	Periodic
Oklahoma	20/60	No	70	No	No	No
Oregon	20/40	No	110	No	No	No
Pennsylvania	20/40	No	120	No	No	No
Rhode Island	20/40	NS	NS	Yes	No	Periodic
South Carolina	20/40	NS	140	NS	NS	Periodic
South Dakota	20/40	No	No	No	No	Periodic
Tennessee	20/40	No	No	PD	No	No
Texas	20/50	No	No	ND	No	Periodic
Utah	20/40	NS	120(H)/20(V)	No	ST	Periodic
Vermont	20/40	60,60	No	No	NS	No
Virginia	20/40	100, 100	100	No	NS	Periodic
Washington	20/40	No	110	ND,PD	No	Periodic
West Virginia	20/40	No	No	No	No	No
Wisconsin	20/40	70, 70	140	PD	No	Periodic
Wyoming	20/40	No	120	No	No	Periodic

Note: Visual acuity is expressed in Snellen notation; visual field is given in degrees along the horizontal meridian.
Key: EC = eye coordination; H = horizontal; N = nasal field; ND = new driver; No = no standard; NS = standard not specified; PD = professional driver; PV = default to private vehicle standard; ST = stereopsis (absence of); T = with telescope; V = vertical.

Sources: US Dept of Transportation. *Visual Disorders and Commercial Drivers.* Washington, DC: Federal Highway Administration, Office of Motor Carriers; Nov 1991. US Dept of Transportation publication FHWA-MC-92-003, HCS-10/1-92(200)E.

Wang CC, Kosinski CJ, Schwartzberg JG, et al. *Physician's Guide to Assessing and Counseling Older Drivers.* Washington, DC: National Highway Traffic Safety Administration; 2003.

2. LOW-VISION AIDS

Under federal regulation, a patient is considered legally blind when the best vision attained in the better eye is 20/200 or less, or when, whatever the acuity achieved, the field of vision of the better eye is 20° or less. While most states have adopted these standards, individual variations may exist at the local level.

Patients whose vision is reduced or inadequate for their visual tasks — those whose best corrected vision ranges from 20/50 downward toward the 20/200 level — can frequently be aided by the same techniques and devices used for the legally blind and visually rehabilitated. These modalities include rehabilitation training programs and optical and nonoptical aids. They often can help restore independence and mobility, allowing the patient to remain productive.

For those patients considered partially sighted rather than partially blind, increased vision is obtained by magnification or approximation. For distance, this may be accomplished by telescopic devices. Although difficult to use while moving about, these instruments may be quite effective for distinguishing a street sign or the number of a house or bus. They are also useful aids in the theater or classroom and at sporting events.

Telescopic devices can be obtained in magnifications of 2.2, 2.5, 3.0, 3.5, 4.0, 6.0, 8.0, and 10× from suppliers such as Designs for Vision, Keeler, Nikon, Selsi, Walters, and Zeiss. Some are fixed focus; others may be refocused for viewing closer material. Telescopes fitted with reading cap lenses permit reading at greater distances than high-plus aids. A familiar example of this system is the surgical loupe.

Because the field diminishes as the power increases, the magnification of telescopic devices should be kept to the minimum needed to secure desired acuity. Differences in design and construction of these devices may cause slight variations in the fields produced at a given magnification. A representative sample may be drawn from the devices produced by Designs for Vision:

MAGNIFICATION	FIELD AT 20 FEET
2.2 standard	12°
2.2 wide angle	17°
3.0 standard	8°
3.0 wide angle	12°
4.0 standard	6°

Near vision can be augmented by higher adds, high-plus "Micro" lenses (American Optical, Lucerne Optical), binocular loupes, and handheld or stand magnifiers. The higher plus values permit approximation to increase the angle subtended with little or no demand on accommodation. The add to obtain J_5 can be estimated by the inverse of the best distance vision obtained. For example, if best distance vision is 20/200, the add is 200/20, or 10 D.

Greater detail can be obtained through increased add power or supplementary magnifiers. If the patient will not read at extremely close range, lower adds may be used in combination with magnifiers. Required magnification at desired working distance can also be provided by a telemicroscope system modified with a reading cap or objective lens, as in a surgical loupe.

When binocular function is present, prism base-in may be required in the near prescription (about 1 prism diopter per diopter of add). Plastic-lens, half-eye spectacles of 6, 8, or 10 D with incorporated prism are available from American Optical and Lucerne Optical. Handheld magnifiers ranging from 23 to 83 are available from Bausch & Lomb, Coburn, Coil, Eschenbach, McLeod, and Selsi. Once again, the higher powers have reduced fields of view. Patients with physical infirmities can use stand magnifiers that rest on the material and remain in focus as they are moved across the page.

Nonoptical aids include reading masks, large-print publications, heavily ruled stationery, check-writing guides, large playing cards, and easy-to-thread needles. Also available are fixed-power opaque projection magnifiers (Nesbit Co) and closed-circuit television devices with variable magnification.

Television permits a greater range of magnification and can, when polarity is reversed, provide a white-on-black image instead of the usual black-on-white. This effect, for many, is an additional aid. Products are available from Telesensory Systems and Visualtek. Advances in electronics have also made possible talking clocks, calculators, computers, and word processors whose "voices" open the way to gainful employment for the visually impaired.

For those with clouded vision, absorptive lenses provide glare protection and can help improve acuity. Neutral gray lenses with 5–15% transmission are specifically recommended for achromatopes, who may also require the protection of wide side-shield frames. Albinotic patients are aided by brown tints with 75% transmission indoors and 25% outdoors. Retinitis pigmentosa patients generally require daytime outdoor protection with the darker sunglass tints. Many are aided in night vision by the Kalichrome lenses (Bausch & Lomb) and the Hazemaster line (American Optical).

For more information on optical aids and other resources for the visually impaired, contact:

American Council of the Blind
Phone: 800-424-8666, 202-467-5081
Website: www.acb.org

American Foundation for the Blind
Phone: 800-232-5463, 212-502-7600
Website: www.afb.org

Library of Congress, National Library Service for the Blind and Physically Handicapped
Phone: 800-424-8567, 202-707-5100
Website: www.loc.gov/nls

PRODUCT IDENTIFICATION GUIDE

To aid in quick identification, manufacturers participating in this section have furnished full-color photographs of selected ophthalmic products. Capsules and tablets are shown in actual size. Tubes, bottles, boxes, and other types of packaging appear in reduced size to fit available space.

For more information on any of the products in this section, please turn to the Pharmaceutical and Equipment Product Information Section, or check directly with the manufacturer. The page number of each product's text entry appears above its photograph.

While every effort has been made to guarantee faithful reproduction of the products in this section, changes in size, color, and design are always a possibility. Be sure to confirm a product's identity with the manufacturer or your pharmacist.

MANUFACTURERS INDEX

PRODUCT INDEX

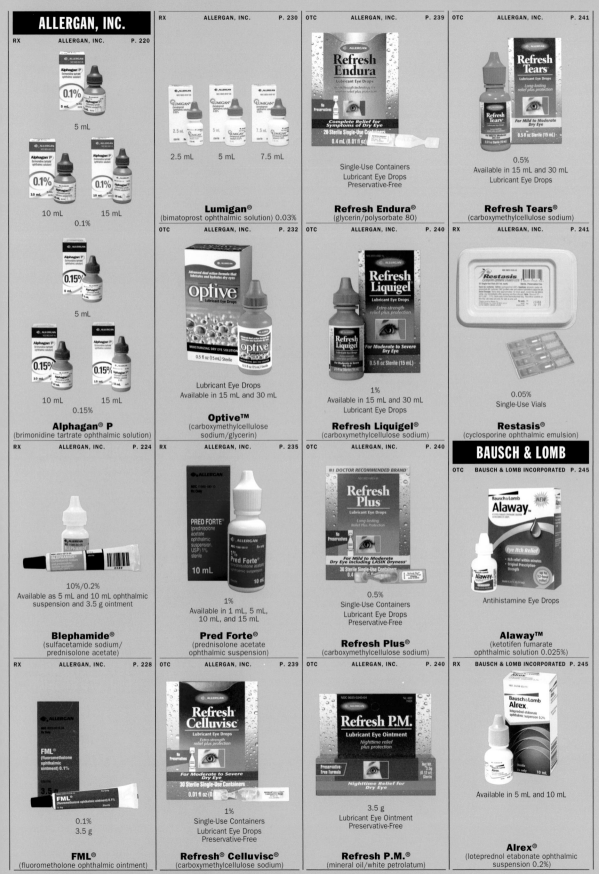

ALLERGAN, INC.

RX ALLERGAN, INC. P. 220

5 mL

10 mL   15 mL
0.1%

5 mL

10 mL   15 mL
0.15%

Alphagan® P
(brimonidine tartrate ophthalmic solution)

RX ALLERGAN, INC. P. 224

10%/0.2%
Available as 5 mL and 10 mL ophthalmic
suspension and 3.5 g ointment

Blephamide®
(sulfacetamide sodium/
prednisolone acetate)

RX ALLERGAN, INC. P. 228

0.1%
3.5 g

FML®
(fluorometholone ophthalmic ointment)

RX ALLERGAN, INC. P. 230

2.5 mL   5 mL   7.5 mL

Lumigan®
(bimatoprost ophthalmic solution) 0.03%

OTC ALLERGAN, INC. P. 232

Lubricant Eye Drops
Available in 15 mL and 30 mL

Optive™
(carboxymethylcellulose
sodium/glycerin)

RX ALLERGAN, INC. P. 235

1%
Available in 1 mL, 5 mL,
10 mL, and 15 mL

Pred Forte®
(prednisolone acetate
ophthalmic suspension)

OTC ALLERGAN, INC. P. 239

1%
Single-Use Containers
Lubricant Eye Drops
Preservative-Free

Refresh® Celluvisc®
(carboxymethylcellulose sodium)

OTC ALLERGAN, INC. P. 239

Single-Use Containers
Lubricant Eye Drops
Preservative-Free

Refresh Endura®
(glycerin/polysorbate 80)

OTC ALLERGAN, INC. P. 240

1%
Available in 15 mL and 30 mL
Lubricant Eye Drops

Refresh Liquigel®
(carboxymethylcellulose sodium)

OTC ALLERGAN, INC. P. 240

0.5%
Single-Use Containers
Lubricant Eye Drops
Preservative-Free

Refresh Plus®
(carboxymethylcellulose sodium)

OTC ALLERGAN, INC. P. 240

3.5 g
Lubricant Eye Ointment
Preservative-Free

Refresh P.M.®
(mineral oil/white petrolatum)

OTC ALLERGAN, INC. P. 241

0.5%
Available in 15 mL and 30 mL
Lubricant Eye Drops

Refresh Tears®
(carboxymethylcellulose sodium)

RX ALLERGAN, INC. P. 241

0.05%
Single-Use Vials

Restasis®
(cyclosporine ophthalmic emulsion)

BAUSCH & LOMB

OTC BAUSCH & LOMB INCORPORATED P. 245

Antihistamine Eye Drops

Alaway™
(ketotifen fumarate
ophthalmic solution 0.025%)

RX BAUSCH & LOMB INCORPORATED P. 245

Available in 5 mL and 10 mL

Alrex®
(loteprednol etabonate ophthalmic
suspension 0.2%)

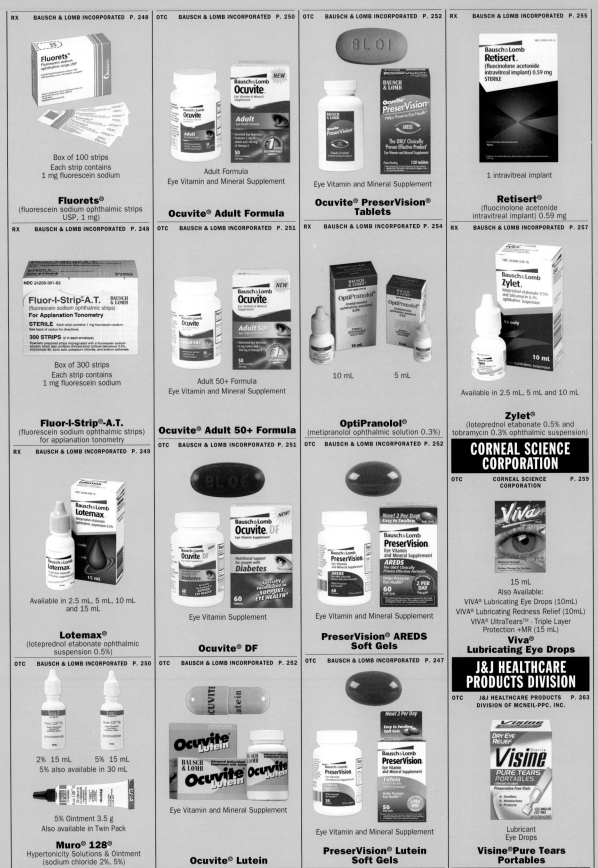

RX   BAUSCH & LOMB INCORPORATED   P. 248

Box of 100 strips
Each strip contains
1 mg fluorescein sodium

Fluorets®
(fluorescein sodium ophthalmic strips
USP, 1 mg)

RX   BAUSCH & LOMB INCORPORATED   P. 248

Box of 300 strips
Each strip contains
1 mg fluorescein sodium

Fluor-I-Strip®-A.T.
(fluorescein sodium ophthalmic strips)
for applanation tonometry

RX   BAUSCH & LOMB INCORPORATED   P. 249

Available in 2.5 mL, 5 mL, 10 mL
and 15 mL

Lotemax®
(loteprednol etabonate ophthalmic
suspension 0.5%)

OTC   BAUSCH & LOMB INCORPORATED   P. 250

2%   15 mL   5%   15 mL
5% also available in 30 mL

5% Ointment 3.5 g
Also available in Twin Pack

Muro® 128®
Hypertonicity Solutions & Ointment
(sodium chloride 2%, 5%)

OTC   BAUSCH & LOMB INCORPORATED   P. 250

Adult Formula
Eye Vitamin and Mineral Supplement

Ocuvite® Adult Formula

OTC   BAUSCH & LOMB INCORPORATED   P. 251

Adult 50+ Formula
Eye Vitamin and Mineral Supplement

Ocuvite® Adult 50+ Formula

OTC   BAUSCH & LOMB INCORPORATED   P. 251

Eye Vitamin Supplement

Ocuvite® DF

OTC   BAUSCH & LOMB INCORPORATED   P. 252

Eye Vitamin and Mineral Supplement

Ocuvite® Lutein

OTC   BAUSCH & LOMB INCORPORATED   P. 252

Eye Vitamin and Mineral Supplement

**Ocuvite® PreserVision®
Tablets**

RX   BAUSCH & LOMB INCORPORATED   P. 254

10 mL   5 mL

OptiPranolol®
(metipranolol ophthalmic solution 0.3%)

OTC   BAUSCH & LOMB INCORPORATED   P. 252

Eye Vitamin and Mineral Supplement

**PreserVision® AREDS
Soft Gels**

OTC   BAUSCH & LOMB INCORPORATED   P. 247

Eye Vitamin and Mineral Supplement

**PreserVision® Lutein
Soft Gels**

RX   BAUSCH & LOMB INCORPORATED   P. 255

1 intravitreal implant

Retisert®
(fluocinolone acetonide
intravitreal implant) 0.59 mg

RX   BAUSCH & LOMB INCORPORATED   P. 257

Available in 2.5 mL, 5 mL and 10 mL

Zylet®
(loteprednol etabonate 0.5% and
tobramycin 0.3% ophthalmic suspension)

CORNEAL SCIENCE CORPORATION

OTC   CORNEAL SCIENCE   P. 259
CORPORATION

15 mL
Also Available:
VIVA® Lubricating Eye Drops (10mL)
VIVA® Lubricating Redness Relief (10mL)
VIVA® UltraTears™ - Triple Layer
Protection +MR (15 mL)
**Viva®
Lubricating Eye Drops**

J&J HEALTHCARE PRODUCTS DIVISION

OTC   J&J HEALTHCARE PRODUCTS   P. 263
DIVISION OF MCNEIL-PPC, INC.

Lubricant
Eye Drops
**Visine®Pure Tears
Portables**

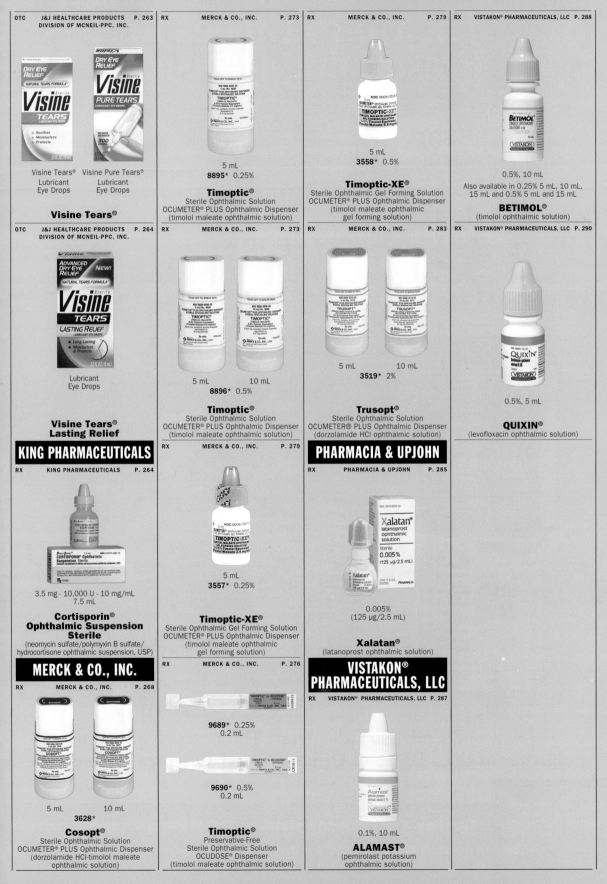

OTC   J&J HEALTHCARE PRODUCTS   P. 263
DIVISION OF MCNEIL-PPC, INC.

Visine Tears®
Lubricant
Eye Drops

Visine Pure Tears®
Lubricant
Eye Drops

Visine Tears®

OTC   J&J HEALTHCARE PRODUCTS   P. 264
DIVISION OF MCNEIL-PPC, INC.

Lubricant
Eye Drops

Visine Tears®
Lasting Relief

KING PHARMACEUTICALS

RX   KING PHARMACEUTICALS   P. 264

3.5 mg - 10,000 U - 10 mg/mL
7.5 mL

Cortisporin®
Ophthalmic Suspension
Sterile
(neomycin sulfate/polymyxin B sulfate/
hydrocortisone ophthalmic suspension, USP)

MERCK & CO., INC.

RX   MERCK & CO., INC.   P. 268

5 mL   10 mL

3628*

Cosopt®
Sterile Ophthalmic Solution
OCUMETER® PLUS Ophthalmic Dispenser
(dorzolamide HCl-timolol maleate
ophthalmic solution)

RX   MERCK & CO., INC.   P. 273

5 mL
8895* 0.25%

Timoptic®
Sterile Ophthalmic Solution
OCUMETER® PLUS Ophthalmic Dispenser
(timolol maleate ophthalmic solution)

RX   MERCK & CO., INC.   P. 273

5 mL   10 mL
8896* 0.5%

Timoptic®
Sterile Ophthalmic Solution
OCUMETER® PLUS Ophthalmic Dispenser
(timolol maleate ophthalmic solution)

RX   MERCK & CO., INC.   P. 279

5 mL
3557* 0.25%

Timoptic-XE®
Sterile Ophthalmic Gel Forming Solution
OCUMETER® PLUS Ophthalmic Dispenser
(timolol maleate ophthalmic
gel forming solution)

RX   MERCK & CO., INC.   P. 276

9689* 0.25%
0.2 mL

9690* 0.5%
0.2 mL

Timoptic®
Preservative-Free
Sterile Ophthalmic Solution
OCUDOSE® Dispenser
(timolol maleate ophthalmic solution)

RX   MERCK & CO., INC.   P. 279

5 mL
3558* 0.5%

Timoptic-XE®
Sterile Ophthalmic Gel Forming Solution
OCUMETER® PLUS Ophthalmic Dispenser
(timolol maleate ophthalmic
gel forming solution)

RX   MERCK & CO., INC.   P. 283

5 mL   10 mL
3519* 2%

Trusopt®
Sterile Ophthalmic Solution
OCUMETER® PLUS Ophthalmic Dispenser
(dorzolamide HCl ophthalmic solution)

PHARMACIA & UPJOHN

RX   PHARMACIA & UPJOHN   P. 285

0.005%
(125 µg/2.5 mL)

Xalatan®
(latanoprost ophthalmic solution)

VISTAKON®
PHARMACEUTICALS, LLC

RX   VISTAKON® PHARMACEUTICALS, LLC   P. 287

0.1%, 10 mL

ALAMAST®
(pemirolast potassium
ophthalmic solution)

RX   VISTAKON® PHARMACEUTICALS, LLC   P. 288

0.5%, 10 mL
Also available in 0.25% 5 mL, 10 mL,
15 mL and 0.5% 5 mL and 15 mL

BETIMOL®
(timolol ophthalmic solution)

RX   VISTAKON® PHARMACEUTICALS, LLC   P. 290

0.5%, 5 mL

QUIXIN®
(levofloxacin ophthalmic solution)

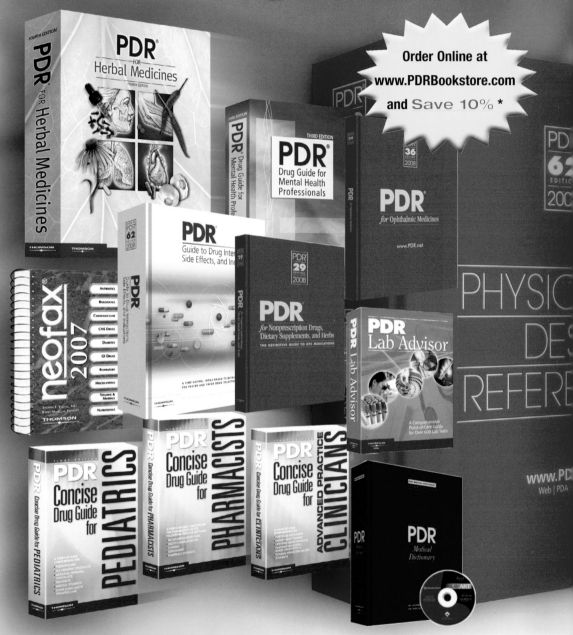

PRODUCT INFORMATION ON PHARMACEUTICALS AND EQUIPMENT

This book is made possible through the courtesy of the manufacturers whose products appear in this and the following section. The information concerning each pharmaceutical product has been prepared by the manufacturer, and edited and approved by the manufacturer's medical department, medical director, or medical counsel.

For those products that have official package circulars, the descriptions in *Physicians' Desk Reference For Ophthalmic Medicines* must be in full compliance with Food and Drug Administration regulations pertaining to the labeling of prescription drugs. For more information, please turn to the Foreword. In presenting the following material, the publisher is not necessarily advocating the use of any product listed.

Alcon Laboratories, Inc.
and its affiliates
CORPORATE HEADQUARTERS
6201 SOUTH FREEWAY
FORT WORTH, TX 76134

Address Inquiries to:
Pharmaceuticals/Consumer
Products   800-451-3937
(Therapeutic Drugs/Lens Care)
Surgical   800-862-5266
(Instrumentation/Surgical Meds)
(817) 293-0450 (Main Switchboard)

AZOPT®   ℞
(brinzolamide ophthalmic suspension) 1%

Description: AZOPT® (brinzolamide ophthalmic suspension) 1% contains a carbonic anhydrase inhibitor formulated for multidose topical ophthalmic use. Brinzolamide is described chemically as: (R)-(+)-4-Ethylamino-2-(3-methoxypropyl)-3,4-dihydro-2H-thieno [3,2-e]-1,2-thiazine-6-sulfonamide-1,1-dioxide. Its empirical formula is $C_{12}H_{21}N_3O_5S_3$.
Brinzolamide has a molecular weight of 383.5 and a melting point of about 131°C. It is a white powder, which is insoluble in water, very soluble in methanol and soluble in ethanol.
AZOPT® (brinzolamide ophthalmic suspension) 1% is supplied as a sterile, aqueous suspension of brinzolamide which has been formulated to be readily suspended and slow settling, following shaking. It has a pH of approximately 7.5 and an osmolality of 300 mOsm/kg. Each mL of AZOPT® (brinzolamide ophthalmic suspension) 1% contains 10 mg brinzolamide. Inactive ingredients are mannitol, carbomer 974P, tyloxapol, edetate disodium, sodium chloride, hydrochloric acid and/or sodium hydroxide (to adjust pH), and purified water. Benzalkonium chloride 0.01% is added as a preservative.
Clinical Pharmacology: Carbonic anhydrase (CA) is an enzyme found in many tissues of the body including the eye. It catalyzes the reversible reaction involving the hydration of carbon dioxide and the dehydration of carbonic acid. In humans, carbonic anhydrase exists as a number of isoenzymes, the most active being carbonic anhydrase II (CA-II), found primarily in red blood cells (RBCs), but also in other tissues. Inhibition of carbonic anhydrase in the ciliary processes of the eye decreases aqueous humor secretion, presumably by slowing the formation of bicarbonate ions with subsequent reduction in sodium and fluid transport.
The result is a reduction in intraocular pressure (IOP).
AZOPT® (brinzolamide ophthalmic suspension) 1% contains brinzolamide, an inhibitor of carbonic anhydrase II (CA-II). Following topical ocular administration, brinzolamide inhibits aqueous humor formation and reduces elevated intraocular pressure. Elevated intraocular pressure is a major risk factor in the pathogenesis of optic nerve damage and glaucomatous visual field loss.
Following topical ocular administration, brinzolamide is absorbed into the systemic circulation. Due to its affinity for CA-II, brinzolamide distributes extensively into the RBCs and exhibits a long half-life in whole blood (approximately 111 days). In humans, the metabolite N-desethyl brinzolamide is formed, which also binds to CA and accumulates in RBCs. This metabolite binds mainly to CA-I in the presence of brinzolamide. In plasma, both parent brinzolamide and N-desethyl brinzolamide concentrations are low and generally below assay quantitation limits (<10 ng/mL). Binding to plasma proteins is approximately 60%. Brinzolamide is eliminated predominantly in the urine as unchanged drug. N-Desethyl brinzolamide is also found in the urine along with lower concentrations of the N-desmethoxypropyl and O-desmethyl metabolites.
An oral pharmacokinetic study was conducted in which healthy volunteers received 1 mg capsules of brinzolamide twice per day for up to 32 weeks. This regimen approximates the amount of drug delivered by topical ocular administration of AZOPT® (brinzolamide ophthalmic suspension) 1% dosed to both eyes three times per day and simulates systemic drug and metabolite concentrations similar to those achieved with long-term topical dosing. RBC CA activity was measured to assess the degree of systemic CA inhibition. Brinzolamide saturation of RBC CA-II was achieved within 4 weeks (RBC concentrations of approximately 20 µM). N-Desethyl brinzolamide accumulated in RBCs to steady-state within 20–28 weeks reaching concentrations ranging from 6–30 µM. The inhibition of CA-II activity at steady- state was approximately 70–75%, which is below the degree of inhibition expected to have a pharmacological effect on renal function or respiration in healthy subjects. In two, three-month clinical studies, AZOPT® (brinzolamide ophthalmic suspension) 1% dosed three times per day (TID) in patients with elevated intraocular pressure (IOP), produced significant reductions in IOPs (4–5 mmHg). These IOP reductions are equivalent to the reductions observed with TRUSOPT* (dorzolamide hydrochloride ophthalmic solution) 2% dosed TID in the same studies.
In two clinical studies in patients with elevated intraocular pressure, AZOPT® (brinzolamide ophthalmic suspension) 1% was associated with less stinging and burning upon instillation than TRUSOPT* 2%.
Indications and Usage: AZOPT® (brinzolamide ophthalmic suspension) 1% is indicated in the treatment of elevated intraocular pressure in patients with ocular hypertension or open-angle glaucoma.
Contraindications: AZOPT® (brinzolamide ophthalmic suspension) 1% is contraindicated in patients who are hypersensitive to any component of this product.
Warnings: AZOPT® (brinzolamide ophthalmic suspension) 1% is a sulfonamide and although administered topically it is absorbed systemically. Therefore, the same types of adverse reactions that are attributable to sulfonamides may occur with topical administration of AZOPT® (brinzolamide ophthalmic suspension) 1%. Fatalities have occurred, although rarely, due to severe reactions to sulfonamides including Stevens-Johnson syndrome, toxic epidermal necrolysis, fulminant hepatic necrosis, agranulocytosis, aplastic anemia, and other blood dyscrasias. Sensitization may recur when a sulfonamide is re-administered irrespective of the route of administration. If signs of serious reactions or hypersensitivity occur, discontinue the use of this preparation.
Precautions
General:
Carbonic anhydrase activity has been observed in both the cytoplasm and around the plasma membranes of the corneal endothelium. The effect of continued administration of AZOPT® (brinzolamide ophthalmic suspension) 1% on the corneal endothelium has not been fully evaluated. The management of patients with acute angle-closure glaucoma requires therapeutic interventions in addition to ocular hypotensive agents. AZOPT® (brinzolamide ophthalmic suspension) 1% has not been studied in patients with acute angle-closure glaucoma.
AZOPT® (brinzolamide ophthalmic suspension) 1% has not been studied in patients with severe renal impairment (CrCl <30 mL/min). Because AZOPT® (brinzolamide ophthalmic suspension) 1% and its metabolite are excreted predominantly by the kidney, AZOPT® (brinzolamide ophthalmic suspension) 1% is not recommended in such patients.
AZOPT® (brinzolamide ophthalmic suspension) 1% has not been studied in patients with hepatic impairment and should be used with caution in such patients.
There is a potential for an additive effect on the known systemic effects of carbonic anhydrase inhibition in patients receiving an oral carbonic anhydrase inhibitor and AZOPT®

Continued on next page

Azopt—Cont.

(brinzolamide ophthalmic suspension) 1%. The concomitant administration of AZOPT® (brinzolamide ophthalmic suspension) 1% and oral carbonic anhydrase inhibitors is not recommended.

Information For Patients:
AZOPT® (brinzolamide ophthalmic suspension) 1% is a sulfonamide and although administered topically, it is absorbed systemically; therefore, the same types of adverse reactions attributable to sulfonamides may occur with topical administration. Patients should be advised that if serious or unusual ocular or systemic reactions or signs of hypersensitivity occur, they should discontinue the use of the product and consult their physician (see **Warnings**).

Vision may be temporarily blurred following dosing with AZOPT® (brinzolamide ophthalmic suspension) 1%. Care should be exercised in operating machinery or driving a motor vehicle.

Patients should be instructed to avoid allowing the tip of the dispensing container to contact the eye or surrounding structures or other surfaces, since the product can become contaminated by common bacteria known to cause ocular infections. Serious damage to the eye and subsequent loss of vision may result from using contaminated solutions.

Patients should also be advised that if they have ocular surgery or develop an intercurrent ocular condition (e.g., trauma or infection), they should immediately seek their physician's advice concerning the continued use of the present multidose container.

If more than one topical ophthalmic drug is being used, the drugs should be administered at least ten minutes apart. The preservative in AZOPT® (brinzolamide ophthalmic suspension) 1%, benzalkonium chloride, may be absorbed by soft contact lenses. Contact lenses should be removed during instillation of AZOPT® (brinzolamide ophthalmic suspension) 1%, but may be reinserted 15 minutes after instillation.

Drug Interactions:
AZOPT® (brinzolamide ophthalmic suspension) 1% contains a carbonic anhydrase inhibitor. Acid-base and electrolyte alterations were not reported in the clinical trials with brinzolamide. However, in patients treated with oral carbonic anhydrase inhibitors, rare instances of drug interactions have occurred with high-dose salicylate therapy. Therefore, the potential for such drug interactions should be considered in patients receiving AZOPT® (brinzolamide ophthalmic suspension) 1%.

Carcinogenesis, Mutagenesis, Impairment of Fertility:
Carcinogenicity data on brinzolamide are not available. The following tests for mutagenic potential were negative: (1) *in vivo* mouse micronucleus assay; (2) *in vivo* sister chromatid exchange assay; and (3) Ames *E. coli* test. The *in vitro* mouse lymphoma forward mutation assay was negative in the absence of activation, but positive in the presence of microsomal activation.

In reproduction studies of brinzolamide in rats, there were no adverse effects on the fertility or reproductive capacity of males or females at doses up to 18 mg/kg/day (375 times the recommended human ophthalmic dose).

Pregnancy:
Teratogenic Effects: Pregnancy Category C.
Developmental toxicity studies with brinzolamide in rabbits at oral doses of 1, 3, and 6 mg/kg/day (20, 62, and 125 times the recommended human ophthalmic dose) produced maternal toxicity at 6 mg/kg/day and a significant increase in the number of fetal variations, such as accessory skull bones,

which was only slightly higher than the historic value at 1 and 6 mg/kg. In rats, statistically decreased body weights of fetuses from dams receiving oral doses of 18 mg/kg/day (375 times the recommended human ophthalmic dose) during gestation were proportional to the reduced maternal weight gain, with no statistically significant effects on organ or tissue development. Increases in unossified sternebrae, reduced ossification of the skull, and unossified hyoid that occurred at 6 and 18 mg/kg were not statistically significant. No treatment-related malformations were seen. Following oral administration of 14C-brinzolamide to pregnant rats, radioactivity was found to cross the placenta and was present in the fetal tissues and blood.

There are no adequate and well-controlled studies in pregnant women. AZOPT® (brinzolamide ophthalmic suspension) 1% should be used during pregnancy only if the potential benefit justifies the potential risk to the fetus.

Nursing Mothers:
In a study of brinzolamide in lactating rats, decreases in body weight gain in offspring at an oral dose of 15 mg/kg/day (312 times the recommended human ophthalmic dose) were seen during lactation. No other effects were observed. However, following oral administration of 14C-brinzolamide to lactating rats, radioactivity was found in milk at concentrations below those in the blood and plasma.

It is not known whether this drug is excreted in human milk. Because many drugs are excreted in human milk and because of the potential for serious adverse reactions in nursing infants from AZOPT® (brinzolamide ophthalmic suspension) 1%, a decision should be made whether to discontinue nursing or to discontinue the drug, taking into account the importance of the drug to the mother.

Pediatric Use:
Safety and effectiveness in pediatric patients have not been established.

Geriatric Use: No overall differences in safety or effectiveness have been observed between elderly and younger patients.

Adverse Reactions:
In clinical studies of AZOPT® (brinzolamide ophthalmic suspension) 1%, the most frequently reported adverse events associated with AZOPT® (brinzolamide ophthalmic suspension) 1% were blurred vision and bitter, sour or unusual taste. These events occurred in approximately 5–10% of patients. Blepharitis, dermatitis, dry eye, foreign body sensation, headache, hyperemia, ocular discharge, ocular discomfort, ocular keratitis, ocular pain, ocular pruritus and rhinitis were reported at an incidence of 1–5%.

The following adverse reactions were reported at an incidence below 1%: allergic reactions, alopecia, chest pain, conjunctivitis, diarrhea, diplopia, dizziness, dry mouth, dyspnea, dyspepsia, eye fatigue, hypertonia, keratoconjunctivitis, keratopathy, kidney pain, lid margin crusting or sticky sensation, nausea, pharyngitis, tearing and urticaria.

Overdosage: Although no human data are available, electrolyte imbalance, development of an acidotic state, and possible nervous system effects may occur following oral administration of an overdose. Serum electrolyte levels (particularly potassium) and blood pH levels should be monitored.

Dosage and Administration: Shake well before use. The recommended dose is 1 drop of AZOPT® (brinzolamide ophthalmic suspension) 1% in the affected eye(s) three times daily. AZOPT® (brinzolamide ophthalmic suspension) 1% may be used concomitantly with other topical ophthalmic drug products to lower intraocular pressure.

If more than one topical ophthalmic drug is being used, the drugs should be administered at least ten minutes apart.

How Supplied: AZOPT® (brinzolamide ophthalmic suspension) 1% is supplied in plastic DROP-TAINER® dispensers with a controlled dispensing-tip as follows:

NDC 0065-0275-24	2.5 mL
NDC 0065-0275-05	5 mL
NDC 0065-0275-10	10 mL
NDC 0065-0275-15	15 mL

Storage: Store AZOPT® (brinzolamide ophthalmic suspension) 1% at 4–30°C (39–86°F).

℞ Only

U.S. Patent Numbers: 5,240,923; 5,378,703; 5,461,081; 6,071,904.

*TRUSOPT is a registered trademark of Merck & Co., Inc.

BETADINE® 5% ℞
Sterile Ophthalmic Prep Solution
[bē'tă-dīne]
(povidone-iodine ophthalmic solution)
(0.5% available iodine)

Description: Povidone-Iodine is a broad-spectrum microbicide with the chemical formulas: 2-pyrrolidinone, 1-ethenyl-, homopolymer, compound with iodine; 1-vinyl-2-pyrrolidinone polymer, compound with iodine.
BETADINE® 5% Sterile Ophthalmic Prep Solution contains 5% povidone-iodine (0.5% available iodine) as a sterile dark brown solution stabilized by glycerin. Inactive Ingredients: citric acid, glycerin, nonoxynol-9, sodium chloride, sodium hydroxide, and dibasic sodium phosphate.

Clinical Pharmacology: A placebo-controlled study in 38 normal volunteers yielded data for 36 subjects who showed a mean $\log_{10}$ reduction of 3.05 $\log_{10}$ units in total aerobes at 10 minutes following prepping the skin with BETADINE 5% Sterile Ophthalmic Prep Solution compared with reduction of 1.58 $\log_{10}$ units after prepping with vehicle free of the iodine complex. This placebo-controlled study indicates a mean $\log_{10}$ reduction by the iodine complex compared with the control solution of 1.47 $\log_{10}$ units at 10 minutes and 1.79 $\log_{10}$ units at 45 minutes. The base-line mean aerobic bacterial count was 7,586 organisms per square cm.

Indications and Usage: BETADINE 5% Sterile Ophthalmic Prep Solution for the eye is indicated for prepping of the periocular region (lids, brow, and cheek) and irrigation of the ocular surface (cornea, conjunctiva, and palpebral fornices).

Contraindications: Do not use on individuals known to be sensitive to iodine, or other components of this product.

Warnings: FOR EXTERNAL USE ONLY. NOT FOR INTRAOCULAR INJECTION OR IRRIGATION.

Precautions:
General: No studies are available in patients with thyroid disorders; therefore, caution is advised in using BETADINE 5% Sterile Ophthalmic Prep Solution in these patients due to the possibility of iodine absorption.

Carcinogenesis, Mutagenesis, Impairment of Fertility: No long term studies in animals have been performed to evaluate the carcinogenic or mutagenic potential of povidone-iodine. One report of the mutagenic potential of povidone-iodine indicated that it was positive in a modification of the Ames S. **typhimurium** model, but these results could not be reproduced by another researcher. Another test using mouse lymphoma and Balb/3T3 cells showed that povidone-iodine has no significant mutagenic or transformation capabilities.

Other data indicated that it does not produce mutagenic effects in mice or hamsters according to the dominant lethal test, micronucleus test, and chromosome analysis.

Pregnancy Category C: Animal reproduction studies have not been conducted with BETADINE® 5% Sterile Ophthalmic Prep Solution. It is also not known whether BETADINE 5% Sterile Ophthalmic Prep Solution can cause fetal harm when administered to a pregnant woman or can affect reproductive capacity. BETADINE 5% Sterile Ophthalmic Prep Solution should only be used on a pregnant woman if clearly needed.

Nursing Mothers: Because of the potential for serious adverse reactions in nursing infants from BETADINE 5% Sterile Ophthalmic Prep Solution, a decision should be made to discontinue nursing or discontinue the drug, taking into account the importance of the drug to the mother.

Pediatric Use: Safety and effectiveness in pediatric patients have not been established.

Geriatric Use: No overall differences in safety or effectiveness have been observed between elderly and younger patients.

Adverse Reactions: Local sensitivity has been exhibited by some individuals to povidone-iodine ophthalmic solution.

Dosage and Administration: While the inner surface and contents of the immediate container (i.e. bottle) are sterile, the outer surface of the bottle is not sterile. The use of the bottle in a sterile field should be avoided.
BETADINE 5% Sterile Ophthalmic Prep Solution is used as follows:

1. Make sure container is intact before use. To open, COMPLETELY TWIST OFF TAB, do not pull off. Gently squeeze entire contents of bottle into a sterile prep cup.
2. Saturate sterile cotton-tipped applicator to prep lashes and lid margins using one or more applicators per lid; repeat once.
3. Saturate sterile prep sponge or other suitable material to prep lids, brow and cheek in a circular ever-expanding fashion until the entire field is covered; repeat prep three (3) times.
4. While separating the lids, irrigate the cornea, conjunctiva and palpebral fornices with BETADINE 5% Sterile Ophthalmic Prep Solution using a sterile bulb syringe.
5. After the BETADINE 5% Sterile Ophthalmic Prep Solution has been left in contact for two minutes, sterile saline solution in a bulb syringe should be used to flush the residual prep solution from the cornea, conjunctiva, and the palpebral fornices.

How Supplied: BETADINE 5% Sterile Ophthalmic Prep Solution is packaged under sterile conditions and supplied in 1 fl.oz. (30 mL) form sealed blue HDPE bottles (NDC #0065 0411 30). Twenty-four (24) bottles are packed in each shipper.
Store at 15-25°C (59-77°F).
℞ Only
Single use only
    BETADINE® is a registered trademark of The Purdue Frederick Company.

BETOPTIC S®   ℞
(betaxolol HCl)
0.25% as base
Sterile Ophthalmic Suspension

Description: BETOPTIC S® Ophthalmic Suspension 0.25% contains betaxolol hydrochloride, a cardioselective beta-adrenergic receptor blocking agent, in a sterile resin suspension formulation. Betaxolol hydrochloride is a white, crystalline powder, with a molecular weight of 343.89.
Empirical Formula: $C_{18}H_{29}NO_3 \cdot HCl$

Chemical Name:
$(\pm)$ - 1 - [p - [2 - (cyclopropylmethoxy) ethyl] phenoxy] - 3 - (isopropylamino) - 2 - propanol hydrochloride.
Each mL of BETOPTIC S® Ophthalmic Suspension contains: **Active:** betaxolol HCl 2.8 mg equivalent to 2.5 mg of betaxolol base. **Preservative:** benzalkonium chloride 0.01%. **Inactive:** Mannitol, Poly(Styrene-Divinyl Benzene) sulfonic acid, Carbomer 934P, edetate disodium, hydrochloric acid or sodium hydroxide (to adjust pH) and purified water.

Clinical Pharmacology: Betaxolol HCl, a cardioselective (beta-1-adrenergic) receptor blocking agent, does not have significant membrane-stabilizing (local anesthetic) activity and is devoid of intrinsic sympathomimetic action. Orally administered beta-adrenergic blocking agents reduce cardiac output in healthy subjects and patients with heart disease. In patients with severe impairment of myocardial function, beta-adrenergic receptor antagonists may inhibit the sympathetic stimulatory effect necessary to maintain adequate cardiac function.
When instilled in the eye, BETOPTIC S® Ophthalmic Suspension 0.25% has the action of reducing elevated intraocular pressure, whether or not accompanied by glaucoma. Ophthalmic betaxolol has minimal effect on pulmonary and cardiovascular parameters.
Elevated IOP presents a major risk factor in glaucomatous field loss. The higher the level of IOP, the greater the likelihood of optic nerve damage and visual field loss. Betaxolol has the action of reducing elevated as well as normal intraocular pressure and the mechanism of ocular hypotensive action appears to be a reduction of aqueous production as demonstrated by tonography and aqueous fluorophotometry. The onset of action with betaxolol can generally be noted within 30 minutes and the maximal effect can usually be detected 2 hours after topical administration. A single dose provides a 12-hour reduction in intraocular pressure.
In controlled, double-masked studies, the magnitude and duration of the ocular hypotensive effect of BETOPTIC S® Ophthalmic Suspension 0.25% and BETOPTIC® Ophthalmic Solution 0.5% were clinically equivalent. BETOPTIC S® Suspension was significantly more comfortable than BETOPTIC® Solution. Ophthalmic betaxolol solution at 1% (one drop in each eye) was compared to placebo in a crossover study challenging nine patients with reactive airway disease. Betaxolol HCl had no significant effect on pulmonary function as measured by FEV_1, Forced Vital Capacity (FVC), FEV_1/FVC and was not significantly different from placebo. The action of isoproterenol, a beta stimulant, administered at the end of the study was not inhibited by ophthalmic betaxolol.
No evidence of cardiovascular beta adrenergic-blockade during exercise was observed with betaxolol in a double-masked, crossover study in 24 normal subjects comparing ophthalmic betaxolol and placebo for effects on blood pressure and heart rate.

Indications and Usage: BETOPTIC S® Ophthalmic Suspension 0.25% has been shown to be effective in lowering intraocular pressure and may be used in patients with chronic open-angle glaucoma and ocular hypertension. It may be used alone or in combination with other intraocular pressure lowering medications.

Contraindications: Hypersensitivity to any component of this product. BETOPTIC S® Ophthalmic Suspension 0.25% is contraindicated in patients with sinus bradycardia, greater than a first degree atrioventricular block, cardiogenic shock, or patients with overt cardiac failure.

Warning: FOR TOPICAL OPHTHALMIC USE ONLY. Topically applied beta-adrenergic blocking agents may be absorbed systemically.

The same adverse reactions found with systemic administration of beta-adrenergic blocking agents may occur with topical administration. For example, severe respiratory reactions and cardiac reactions, including death due to bronchospasm in patients with asthma, and rarely death in association with cardiac failure, have been reported with topical application of beta-adrenergic blocking agents.
BETOPTIC S® Ophthalmic Suspension 0.25% has been shown to have a minor effect on heart rate and blood pressure in clinical studies. Caution should be used in treating patients with a history of cardiac failure or heart block. Treatment with BETOPTIC S® Ophthalmic Suspension 0.25% should be discontinued at the first signs of cardiac failure.

Precautions:

General: Diabetes Mellitus. Beta-adrenergic blocking agents should be administered with caution in patients subject to spontaneous hypoglycemia or to diabetic patients (especially those with labile diabetes) who are receiving insulin or oral hypoglycemic agents. Beta-adrenergic receptor blocking agents may mask the signs and symptoms of acute hypoglycemia.

Thyrotoxicosis.   Beta-adrenergic blocking agents may mask certain clinical signs (e.g., tachycardia) of hyperthyroidism. Patients suspected of developing thyrotoxicosis should be managed carefully to avoid abrupt withdrawal of beta-adrenergic blocking agents, which might precipitate a thyroid storm.

Muscle Weakness.   Beta-adrenergic blockade has been reported to potentiate muscle weakness consistent with certain myasthenic symptoms (e.g., diplopia, ptosis and generalized weakness).

Major Surgery.   Consideration should be given to the gradual withdrawal of beta-adrenergic blocking agents prior to general anesthesia because of the reduced ability of the heart to respond to beta-adrenergically mediated sympathetic reflex stimuli.

Pulmonary.   Caution should be exercised in the treatment of glaucoma patients with excessive restriction of pulmonary function. There have been reports of asthmatic attacks and pulmonary distress during betaxolol treatment. Although rechallenges of some such patients with ophthalmic betaxolol has not adversely affected pulmonary function test results, the possibility of adverse pulmonary effects in patients sensitive to beta blockers cannot be ruled out.

Information for Patients: Do not touch dropper tip to any surface, as this may contaminate the contents. Do not use with contact lenses in eyes.

Drug Interactions: Patients who are receiving a beta-adrenergic blocking agent orally and BETOPTIC S® Ophthalmic Suspension 0.25% should be observed for a potential additive effect either on the intraocular pressure or on the known systemic effects of beta blockade.
Close observation of the patient is recommended when a beta blocker is administered to patients receiving catecholamine-depleting drugs such as reserpine, because of possible additive effects and the production of hypotension and/or bradycardia.
Betaxolol is an adrenergic blocking agent; therefore, caution should be exercised in patients using concomitant adrenergic psychotropic drugs.

Risk from anaphylactic reaction: While taking beta-blockers, patients with a history of atopy or a history of severe anaphylactic reaction to a variety of allergens may be more reactive to repeated accidental, diagnostic, or therapeutic challenge with such allergens. Such patients may be unresponsive to the usual doses of epinephrine used to treat anaphylactic reactions.

Continued on next page

Betoptic S—Cont.

Ocular: In patients with angle-closure glaucoma, the immediate treatment objective is to reopen the angle by constriction of the pupil with a miotic agent. Betaxolol has little or no effect on the pupil. When BETOPTIC S® Ophthalmic Suspension 0.25% is used to reduce elevated intraocular pressure in angle-closure glaucoma, it should be used with a miotic and not alone.

Carcinogenesis, Mutagenesis, Impairment of Fertility: Lifetime studies with betaxolol HCl have been completed in mice at oral doses of 6, 20 or 60 mg/kg/day and in rats at 3, 12 or 48 mg/kg/day; betaxolol HCl demonstrated no carcinogenic effect. Higher dose levels were not tested.

In a variety of *in vitro* and *in vivo* bacterial and mammalian cell assays, betaxolol HCl was nonmutagenic.

Pregnancy: Pregnancy Category C. Reproduction, teratology, and peri- and postnatal studies have been conducted with orally administered betaxolol HCl in rats and rabbits. There was evidence of drug related postimplantation loss in rabbits and rats at dose levels above 12 mg/kg and 128 mg/kg, respectively. Betaxolol HCl was not shown to be teratogenic, however, and there were no other adverse effects on reproduction at subtoxic dose levels. There are no adequate and well-controlled studies in pregnant women. BETOPTIC S® should be used during pregnancy only if the potential benefit justifies the potential risk to the fetus.

Nursing Mothers: It is not known whether betaxolol HCl is excreted in human milk. Because many drugs are excreted in human milk, caution should be exercised when BETOPTIC S® Ophthalmic Suspension 0.25% is administered to nursing women.

Pediatric Use: Safety and effectiveness in pediatric patients have not been established.

Geriatric Use: No overall differences in safety or effectiveness have been observed between elderly and younger patients.

Adverse Reactions:

Ocular: In clinical trials, the most frequent event associated with the use of BETOPTIC S® Ophthalmic Suspension 0.25% has been transient ocular discomfort. The following other conditions have been reported in small numbers of patients: blurred vision, corneal punctate keratitis, foreign body sensation, photophobia, tearing, itching, dryness of eyes, erythema, inflammation, discharge, ocular pain, decreased visual acuity and crusty lashes.

Additional medical events reported with other formulations of betaxolol include allergic reactions, decreased corneal sensitivity, corneal punctate staining which may appear in dendritic formations, edema and anisocoria.

Systemic: Systemic reactions following administration of BETOPTIC S® Ophthalmic Suspension 0.25% or BETOPTIC® Ophthalmic Solution 0.5% have been rarely reported. These include:

Cardiovascular: Bradycardia, heart block and congestive failure.

Pulmonary: Pulmonary distress characterized by dyspnea, bronchospasm, thickened bronchial secretions, asthma and respiratory failure.

Central Nervous System: Insomnia, dizziness, vertigo, headaches, depression, lethargy, and increase in signs and symptoms of myasthenia gravis.

Other: Hives, toxic epidermal necrolysis, hair loss, and glossitis. Perversions of taste and smell have been reported.

Overdosage: No information is available on overdosage of humans. The oral LD50 of the drug ranged from 350–920 mg/kg in mice and

860–1050 mg/kg in rats. The symptoms which might be expected with an overdose of a systemically administered beta-1-adrenergic receptor blocking agent are bradycardia, hypotension and acute cardiac failure.

A topical overdose of BETOPTIC S® Ophthalmic Suspension 0.25% may be flushed from the eye(s) with warm tap water.

Dosage and Administration: The recommended dose is one to two drops of BETOPTIC S® Ophthalmic Suspension 0.25% in the affected eye(s) twice daily. In some patients, the intraocular pressure lowering responses to BETOPTIC S® may require a few weeks to stabilize. As with any new medication, careful monitoring of patients is advised.

If the intraocular pressure of the patient is not adequately controlled on this regimen, concomitant therapy with pilocarpine and other miotics, and/or epinephrine and/or carbonic anhydrase inhibitors can be instituted.

How Supplied: BETOPTIC S® Ophthalmic Suspension 0.25% is supplied as follows: 2.5, 5, 10 and 15 mL in plastic ophthalmic DROP-TAINER® dispensers.

2.5 mL: **NDC** 0065-0246-20
5 mL: **NDC** 0065-0246-05
10 mL: **NDC** 0065-0246-10
15 mL: **NDC** 0065-0246-15

Storage: Store upright at room temperature. Shake well before using.

℞ Only

U.S. Patent No. 4,911,920

©2003 Alcon Laboratories, Inc.

BSS® ℞

Sterile Irrigating Solution
(balanced salt solution)

Description: BSS® Sterile Irrigating Solution is a sterile balanced salt solution.

How Supplied:

15 mL Sterile DROP-TAINER® Bottle—**NDC** 0065-0795-15

30 mL Sterile DROP-TAINER® Bottle—**NDC** 0065-0795-30

250 mL Bottle—**NDC** 0065-0795-25

500 mL Bottle—**NDC** 0065-0795-50

Storage: Store at 36° - 77°F (2° - 25°C). DO NOT FREEZE.

BSS PLUS® ℞

(balanced salt solution
enriched with bicarbonate, dextrose, and glutathione)
STERILE INTRAOCULAR IRRIGATING SOLUTION

Description: BSS PLUS® is a sterile intraocular irrigating solution for use during all intraocular surgical procedures, including those requiring a relatively long intraocular perfusion time (e.g., pars plana vitrectomy, phacoemulsification, extracapsular cataract extraction/lens aspiration, anterior segment reconstruction, etc.). The solution does not contain a preservative and should be prepared just prior to use in surgery.

How Supplied: BSS PLUS is supplied in two packages for reconstitution prior to use: a 250 mL glass bottle containing 240 mL (Part I) and a 10 mL glass vial (Part II)—NDC 0065-0800-25; a 500 mL glass bottle containing 480 mL (Part I) and a 20 mL glass vial (Part II)—NDC 0065-0800-50. See the **Precautions** section regarding reconstitution of the solution.

Storage: Store Part I and Part II at 36°–77°F (2°–25°C). DO NOT FREEZE. Discard prepared solution after six hours.

CILOXAN® ℞

(ciprofloxacin hydrochloride
ophthalmic ointment) 0.3% as Base
Sterile Ophthalmic Ointment

Description: CILOXAN® (ciprofloxacin hydrochloride ophthalmic ointment) is a synthetic, sterile, multiple dose, antimicrobial for topical use. Ciprofloxacin is a fluoroquinolone antibacterial. It is available as the monohydrochloride monohydrate salt of 1-cyclopropyl-6-fluoro-1,4-dihydro-4-oxo-7-(1-piperazinyl)-3-quinolinecarboxylic acid. Ciprofloxacin is a faint to light yellow crystalline powder with a molecular weight of 385.82. Its empirical formula is $C_{17}H_{18}FN_3O_3 \cdot HCl \cdot H_2O$.

Ciprofloxacin differs from other quinolones in that it has a fluorine atom at the 6-position, a piperazine moiety at the 7-position, and a cyclopropyl ring at the 1-position.

Each gram of CILOXAN (ciprofloxacin hydrochloride ophthalmic ointment) contains:
Active: Ciprofloxacin HCl 3.33 mg equivalent to 3 mg base. **Inactives:** mineral oil, white petrolatum.

Clinical Pharmacology:

Systemic Absorption: Absorption studies in humans with the ciprofloxacin ointment have not been conducted, however, based on studies with ciprofloxacin solution, 0.3%, mean maximal concentrations are expected to be less than 2.5 ng/mL.

Microbiology: Ciprofloxacin has *in vitro* activity against a wide range of gram-negative and gram-positive organisms. The bactericidal action of ciprofloxacin results from interference with the enzyme DNA gyrase which is needed for the synthesis of bacterial DNA.

Ciprofloxacin has been shown to be active against most strains of the following microorganisms both *in vitro* and in clinical infections (**See Indications and Usage** section).

Aerobic gram-positive microorganisms:

Staphylococcus aureus (methicillin-susceptible strains)

Staphylococcus epidermidis (methicillin-susceptible strains)

Streptococcus pneumoniae

Streptococcus Viridans Group

Aerobic gram-negative microorganisms:

Haemophilus influenzae

The following *in vitro* data are available; **but their clinical significance in ophthalmologic infections is unknown**. The safety and effectiveness of ciprofloxacin in treating conjunctivitis due to these microorganisms have not been established in adequate and well controlled trials.

The following organisms are considered susceptible when evaluated using systemic breakpoints. However, a correlation between the *in vitro* systemic breakpoint and ophthalmological efficacy has not been established.

Ciprofloxacin exhibits *in vitro* minimal inhibitory concentrations (MIC's) of 1µg/mL or less (systemic susceptible breakpoint) against most (≥90%) strains of the following ocular pathogens.

Aerobic gram-positive microorganisms:

Bacillus species

Corynebacterium species

Staphylococcus haemolyticus

Staphylococcus hominis

Aerobic gram-negative microorganisms:

Acinetobacter calcoaceticus

Enterobacter aerogenes

Escherichia coli

Haemophilus parainfluenzae

Klebsielle pneumoniae

Moraxella catarrhalis

Neisseria gonorrhoeae

Proteus mirabilis

Pseudomonas aeruginosa

Serratia marcesens

Most strains of *Burkholderia cepacia* and some strains of *Stenotrophomonas maltophilia* are resistant to ciprofloxacin as are most anaerobic bacteria, including *Bacteroides fragilis* and *Clostridium difficile*.

The minimal bactericidal concentration (MBC) generally does not exceed the minimal inhibitory concentration (MIC) by more than a factor of 2. Resistance to ciprofloxacin *in vitro* usually develops slowly (multiple-step mutation).

Ciprofloxacin does not cross-react with other antimicrobial agents such as beta-lactams or aminoglycosides; therefore, organisms resistant to these drugs may be susceptible to ciprofloxacin. Organisms resistant to ciprofloxacin may be susceptible to beta-lactams or aminoglycosides.

Clinical Studies: In multicenter clinical trials, approximately 75% of the patients with signs and symptoms of bacterial conjunctivitis and positive conjunctival cultures were clinically cured and approximately 80% had presumed pathogens eradicated by the end of treatment (day 7).

Indications and Usage: CILOXAN® (ciprofloxacin hydrochloride ophthalmic ointment) is indicated for the treatment of bacterial conjunctivitis caused by susceptible strains of the microorganisms listed below:

Gram-Positive:
Staphylococcus aureus
Staphylococcus epidermidis
Streptococcus pneumoniae
Streptococcus Viridans Group
Gram-Negative:
Haemophilus influenzae

Contraindications: A history of hypersensitivity to ciprofloxacin or any other component of the medication is a contraindication to its use. A history of hypersensitivity to other quinolones may also contraindicate the use of ciprofloxacin.

Warnings:
FOR TOPICAL OPHTHALMIC USE ONLY.
NOT FOR INJECTION INTO THE EYE.
Serious and occasionally fatal hypersensitivity (anaphylactic) reactions, some following the first dose, have been reported in patients receiving systemic quinolone therapy. Some reactions were accompanied by cardiovascular collapse, loss of consciousness, tingling, pharyngeal or facial edema, dyspnea, urticaria, and itching. Only a few patients had a history of hypersensitivity reactions. Serious anaphylactic reactions require immediate emergency treatment with epinephrine and other resuscitation measures, including oxygen, intravenous fluids, intravenous antihistamines, corticosteroids, pressor amines and airway management, as clinically indicated.

Precautions:
General: As with other antibacterial preparations, prolonged use of ciprofloxacin may result in overgrowth of nonsusceptible organisms, including fungi. If superinfection occurs, appropriate therapy should be initiated. Whenever clinical judgment dictates, the patient should be examined with the aid of magnification, such as slit lamp biomicroscopy and, where appropriate, fluorescein staining.

Ciprofloxacin should be discontinued at the first appearance of a skin rash or any other sign of hypersensitivity reaction.

Ophthalmic ointments may retard corneal healing and cause visual blurring.

Patients should be advised not to wear contact lenses if they have signs and symptoms of bacterial conjunctivitis.

Information For Patients: Do not touch tip to any surface as this may contaminate the ointment.

Do not use the product if the imprinted carton seals have been damaged, or removed.

Drug Interactions: Specific drug interaction studies have not been conducted with ophthalmic ciprofloxacin. However, the systemic administration of some quinolones has been shown to elevate plasma concentrations of theophylline, interfere with the metabolism of caf-

feine, enhance the effects of the oral anticoagulant, warfarin, and its derivatives, and has been associated with transient elevations in serum creatinine in patients receiving cyclosporine concomitantly.

Carcinogenesis, Mutagenesis, Impairment of Fertility: Eight *in vitro* mutagenicity tests have been conducted with ciprofloxacin and the test results are listed below:
Salmonella/Microsome Test (Negative)
E. coli DNA Repair Assay (Negative)
Mouse Lymphoma Cell Forward Mutation Assay (Positive)
Chinese Hamster V79 Cell HGPRT Test (Negative)
Syrian Hamster Embryo Cell Transformation Assay (Negative)
Saccharomyces cerevisiae Point Mutation Assay (Negative)
Saccharomyces cerevisiae Mitotic Crossover and Gene Conversion Assay (Negative)
Rat Hepatocyte DNA Repair Assay (Positive)
Thus, two of the eight tests were positive, but the results of the following three *in vivo* test systems gave negative results:
Rat Hepatocyte DNA Repair Assay
Micronucleus Test (Mice)
Dominant Lethal Test (Mice)
Long-term carcinogenicity studies in mice and rats have been completed. After daily oral dosing for up to two years, there is no evidence that ciprofloxacin had any carcinogenic or tumorigenic effects in these species.

Pregnancy: Pregnancy Category C. Reproduction studies have been performed in rats and mice at doses up to six times the usual daily human oral dose and have revealed no evidence of impaired fertility or harm to the fetus due to ciprofloxacin. In rabbits, as with most antimicrobial agents, ciprofloxacin (30 and 100 mg/kg orally) produced gastrointestinal disturbances resulting in maternal weight loss and an increased incidence of abortion. No teratogenicity was observed at either dose. After intravenous administration, at doses up to 20 mg/kg, no maternal toxicity was produced and no embryotoxicity or teratogenicity was observed. There are no adequate and well controlled studies in pregnant women. CILOXAN® (ciprofloxacin hydrochloride ophthalmic ointment) should be used during pregnancy only if the potential benefit justifies the potential risk to the fetus.

Nursing Mothers: It is not known whether topically applied ciprofloxacin is excreted in human milk. However, it is known that orally administered ciprofloxacin is excreted in the milk of lactating rats and oral ciprofloxacin has been reported in human breast milk after a single 500 mg dose. Caution should be exercised when CILOXAN® (ciprofloxacin hydrochloride ophthalmic ointment) is administered to a nursing mother.

Pediatric Use: Safety and effectiveness of CILOXAN (ciprofloxacin hydrochloride ophthalmic ointment) 0.3% in pediatric patients below the age of two years have not been established. Although ciprofloxacin and other quinolones may cause arthropathy in immature Beagle dogs after oral administration, topical ocular administration of ciprofloxacin to immature animals did not cause any arthropathy and there is no evidence that the ophthalmic dosage form has any effect on the weight bearing joints.

Geriatric Use: No overall clinical differences in safety or effectiveness have been observed between the elderly and other adult patients.

Adverse Reactions: The following adverse reactions (incidences) were reported in 2% of the patients in clinical studies for CILOXAN (ciprofloxacin hydrochloride ophthalmic ointment): discomfort, keratopathy. Other reactions associated with ciprofloxacin therapy occurring in less than 1% of patients included allergic reactions, blurred vision, corneal staining, de-

creased visual acuity, dry eye, edema, epitheliopathy, eye pain, foreign body sensation, hyperemia, irritation, keratoconjunctivitis, lid erythema, lid margin hyperemia, photophobia, pruritus, and tearing.

Systemic adverse reactions related to ciprofloxacin therapy occurred at an incidence below 1% and included dermatitis, nausea and taste perversion.

Dosage and Administration: Apply a 1/2'' ribbon into the conjunctival sac three times a day on the first two days, then apply a 1/2'' ribbon two times a day for the next five days.

How Supplied: 3.5 g STERILE ointment supplied in an aluminum tube with a white polyethylene tip and white polyethylene cap. 3.5 g - NDC 0065-0654-35

Storage: Store at 2° - 25°C (36° - 77°F).

Animal Pharmacology: Ciprofloxacin and related drugs have been shown to cause arthropathy in immature animals of most species tested following oral administration. However, a one month topical ocular study using immature Beagle dogs did not demonstrate any articular lesions.

℞ Only

©2002 - 2005 Alcon, Inc.

CILOXAN®   ℞
(ciprofloxacin HCl ophthalmic solution)
0.3% as base
Sterile

Description: CILOXAN® (ciprofloxacin HCl ophthalmic solution) is a synthetic, sterile, multiple dose, antimicrobial for topical ophthalmic use. Ciprofloxacin is a fluoroquinolone antibacterial active against a broad spectrum of gram-positive and gram-negative ocular pathogens. It is available as the monohydrochloride monohydrate salt of 1-cyclopropyl-6-fluoro-1,4-dihydro-4-oxo - 7 - (1 - piperazinyl) - 3 -quinolinecarboxylic acid. It is a faint to light yellow crystalline powder with a molecular weight of 385.8. Its empirical formula is $C_{17}H_{18}FN_3O_3 \bullet HCl \bullet H_2O$

Ciprofloxacin differs from other quinolones in that it has a fluorine atom at the 6-position, a piperazine moiety at the 7-position, and a cyclopropyl ring at the 1-position.

Each mL of CILOXAN Ophthalmic Solution contains: **Active:** Ciprofloxacin HCl 3.5 mg equivalent to 3 mg base. **Preservative:** Benzalkonium Chloride 0.006%. **Inactives:** Sodium Acetate, Acetic Acid, Mannitol 4.6%, Edetate Disodium 0.05%, Hydrochloric Acid and/or Sodium Hydroxide (to adjust pH) and Purified Water. The pH is approximately 4.5 and the osmolality is approximately 300 mOsm.

Clinical Pharmacology:

Systemic Absorption: A systemic absorption study was performed in which CILOXAN Ophthalmic Solution was administered in each eye every two hours while awake for two days followed by every four hours while awake for an additional 5 days. The maximum reported plasma concentration of ciprofloxacin was less than 5 ng/mL. The mean concentration was usually less than 2.5 ng/mL.

Microbiology: Ciprofloxacin has *in vitro* activity against a wide range of gram-negative and gram-positive organisms. The bactericidal action of ciprofloxacin results from interference with the enzyme DNA gyrase which is needed for the synthesis of bacterial DNA.

Ciprofloxacin has been shown to be active against most strains of the following organisms both *in vitro* and in clinical infections. (See Indications and Usage section).

Continued on next page

Ciloxan Solution—Cont.

Gram-Positive:
Staphylococcus aureus
Staphylococcus epidermidis
Streptococcus pneumoniae
Streptococcus (Viridans Group)
Gram-Negative:
Haemophilus influenzae
Pseudomonas aeruginosa
Serratia marcescens
Ciprofloxacin has been shown to be active *in vitro* against most strains of the following organisms, however, *the clinical significance of these data is unknown:*
Gram-Positive:
Enterococcus faecalis (Many strains are only moderately susceptible)
Staphylococcus haemolyticus
Staphylococcus hominis
Staphylococcus saprophyticus
Streptococcus pyogenes
Gram-Negative:
Acinetobacter calcoaceticus subsp. anitratus
Aeromonas caviae
Aeromonas hydrophila
Brucella melitensis
Campylobacter coli
Campylobacter jejuni
Citrobacter diversus
Citrobacter freundii
Edwardsiella tarda
Enterobacter aerogenes
Enterobacter cloacae
Escherichia coli
Haemophilus ducreyi
Haemophilus parainfluenzae
Klebsiella pneumoniae
Klebsiella oxytoca
Legionella pneumophila
Moraxella (Branhamella) catarrhalis
Morganella morganii
Neisseria gonorrhoeae
Neisseria meningitidis
Pasteurella multocida
Proteus mirabilis
Proteus vulgaris
Providencia rettgeri
Providencia stuartii
Salmonella enteritidis
Salmonella typhi
Shigella sonnei
Shigella flexneri
Vibrio cholerae
Vibrio parahaemolyticus
Vibrio vulnificus
Yersinia enterocolitica
Other Organisms: *Chlamydia trachomatis* (only moderately susceptible) and *Mycobacterium tuberculosis* (only moderately susceptible).
Most strains of *Pseudomonas cepacia* and some strains of *Pseudomonas maltophilia* are resistant to ciprofloxacin as are most anaerobic bacteria, including *Bacteroides fragilis* and *Clostridium difficile*.
The minimal bactericidal concentration (MBC) generally does not exceed the minimal inhibitory concentration (MIC) by more than a factor of 2. Resistance to ciprofloxacin *in vitro* usually develops slowly (multiple-step mutation).
Ciprofloxacin does not cross-react with other antimicrobial agents such as beta-lactams or aminoglycosides; therefore, organisms resistant to these drugs may be susceptible to ciprofloxacin.
Clinical Studies: Following therapy with CILOXAN® Ophthalmic Solution, 76% of the patients with corneal ulcers and positive bacterial cultures were clinically cured and complete re-epithelialization occurred in about 92% of the ulcers.
In 3 and 7 day multicenter clinical trials, 52% of the patients with conjunctivitis and positive conjunctival cultures were clinically cured and 70–80% had all causative pathogens eradicated by the end of treatment.
Indications and Usage: CILOXAN Ophthalmic Solution is indicated for the treatment of infections caused by susceptible strains of the designated microorganisms in the conditions listed below:
Corneal Ulcers: *Pseudomonas aeruginosa*
*Serratia marcescens**
Staphylococcus aureus
Staphylococcus epidermidis
Streptococcus pneumoniae
Streptococcus (Viridans Group)**
Conjunctivitis: *Haemophilus influenzae*
Staphylococcus aureus
Staphylococcus epidermidis
Streptococcus pneumoniae

---

*Efficacy for this organism was studied in fewer than 10 infections.
Contraindications: A history of hypersensitivity to ciprofloxacin or any other component of the medication is a contraindication to its use. A history of hypersensitivity to other quinolones may also contraindicate the use of ciprofloxacin.
Warnings: NOT FOR INJECTION INTO THE EYE.
Serious and occasionally fatal hypersensitivity (anaphylactic) reactions, some following the first dose, have been reported in patients receiving systemic quinolone therapy. Some reactions were accompanied by cardiovascular collapse, loss of consciousness, tingling, pharyngeal or facial edema, dyspnea, urticaria, and itching. Only a few patients had a history of hypersensitivity reactions. Serious anaphylactic reactions require immediate emergency treatment with epinephrine and other resuscitation measures, including oxygen, intravenous fluids, intravenous antihistamines, corticosteroids, pressor amines and airway management, as clinically indicated.
Remove contact lenses before using.
Precautions: General: As with other antibacterial preparations, prolonged use of ciprofloxacin may result in overgrowth of non-susceptible organisms, including fungi. If superinfection occurs, appropriate therapy should be initiated. Whenever clinical judgment dictates, the patient should be examined with the aid of magnification, such as slit lamp biomicroscopy and, where appropriate, fluorescein staining.
Ciprofloxacin should be discontinued at the first appearance of a skin rash or any other sign of hypersensitivity reaction.
In clinical studies of patients with bacterial corneal ulcer, a white crystalline precipitate located in the superficial portion of the corneal defect was observed in 35 (16.6%) of 210 patients. The onset of the precipitate was within 24 hours to 7 days after starting therapy. In one patient, the precipitate was immediately irrigated out upon its appearance. In 17 patients, resolution of the precipitate was seen in 1 to 8 days (seven within the first 24–72 hours), in five patients, resolution was noted in 10–13 days. In nine patients, exact resolution days were unavailable; however, at follow-up examinations, 18–44 days after onset of the event, complete resolution of the precipitate was noted. In three patients, outcome information was unavailable. The precipitate did not preclude continued use of ciprofloxacin, nor did it adversely affect the clinical course of the ulcer or visual outcome. (See Adverse Reactions.)
Information for patients: Do not touch dropper tip to any surface, as this may contaminate the solution.
Drug Interactions: Specific drug interaction studies have not been conducted with ophthalmic ciprofloxacin. However, the systemic administration of some quinolones has been shown to elevate plasma concentrations of theophylline, interfere with the metabolism of caffeine, enhance the effects of the oral anticoagulant, warfarin, and its derivatives and has been associated with transient elevations in serum creatinine in patients receiving cyclosporine concomitantly.
Carcinogenesis, Mutagenesis, Impairment of Fertility: Eight *in vitro* mutagenicity tests have been conducted with ciprofloxacin and the test results are listed below:
Salmonella/Microsome Test (Negative)
E. coli DNA Repair Assay (Negative)
Mouse Lymphoma Cell Forward Mutation Assay (Positive)
Chinese Hamster V_{79} Cell HGPRT Test (Negative)
Syrian Hamster Embryo Cell Transformation Assay (Negative)
Saccharomyces cerevisiae Point Mutation Assay (Negative)
Saccharomyces cerevisiae Mitotic Crossover and Gene Conversion Assay (Negative)
Rat Hepatocyte DNA Repair Assay (Positive)
Thus, two of the eight tests were positive, but the results of the following three *in vivo* test systems gave negative results:
Rat Hepatocyte DNA Repair Assay
Micronucleus Test (Mice)
Dominant Lethal Test (Mice)
Long term carcinogenicity studies in mice and rats have been completed. After daily oral dosing for up to two years, there is no evidence that ciprofloxacin had any carcinogenic or tumorigenic effects in these species.
Pregnancy—Pregnancy Category C: Reproduction studies have been performed in rats and mice at doses up to six times the usual daily human oral dose and have revealed no evidence of impaired fertility or harm to the fetus due to ciprofloxacin. In rabbits, as with most antimicrobial agents, ciprofloxacin (30 and 100 mg/kg orally) produced gastrointestinal disturbances resulting in maternal weight loss and an increased incidence of abortion. No teratogenicity was observed at either dose. After intravenous administration, at doses up to 20 mg/kg, no maternal toxicity was produced and no embryotoxicity or teratogenicity was observed. There are no adequate and well controlled studies in pregnant women. CILOXAN® Ophthalmic Solution should be used during pregnancy only if the potential benefit justifies the potential risk to the fetus.
Nursing Mothers: It is not known whether topically applied ciprofloxacin is excreted in human milk; however, it is known that orally administered ciprofloxacin is excreted in the milk of lactating rats and oral ciprofloxacin has been reported in human breast milk after a single 500 mg dose. Caution should be exercised when CILOXAN Ophthalmic Solution is administered to a nursing mother.
Pediatric Use: Safety and effectiveness in pediatric patients below the age of 1 year have not been established. Although ciprofloxacin and other quinolones cause arthropathy in immature animals after oral administration, topical ocular administration of ciprofloxacin to immature animals did not cause any arthropathy and there is no evidence that the ophthalmic dosage form has any effect on the weight bearing joints.
Geriatric Use: No overall differences in safety or effectiveness have been observed between elderly and younger patients.
Adverse Reactions: The most frequently reported drug related adverse reaction was local burning or discomfort. In corneal ulcer studies with frequent administration of the drug, white crystalline precipitates were seen in approximately 17% of patients (See Precautions). Other reactions occurring in less than 10% of patients included lid margin crusting, crystals/scales, foreign body sensation, itching, conjunctival hyperemia and a bad taste following instillation. Additional events occurring in less

than 1% of patients included corneal staining, keratopathy/keratitis, allergic reactions, lid edema, tearing, photophobia, corneal infiltrates, nausea and decreased vision.

Overdosage: A topical overdose of CILOXAN® Ophthalmic Solution may be flushed from the eye(s) with warm tap water.

Dosage and Administration:

Corneal Ulcers: The recommended dosage regimen for the treatment of **corneal ulcers** is two drops into the affected eye every 15 minutes for the first six hours and then two drops into the affected eye every 30 minutes for the remainder of the first day. On the second day, instill two drops in the affected eye hourly. On the third through the fourteenth day, place two drops in the affected eye every four hours. Treatment may be continued after 14 days if corneal re-epithelialization has not occurred.

Bacterial Conjunctivitis: The recommended dosage regimen for the treatment of **bacterial conjunctivitis** is one or two drops instilled into the conjunctival sac(s) every two hours while awake for two days and one or two drops every four hours while awake for the next five days.

How Supplied: As a sterile ophthalmic solution in Alcon's DROP-TAINER® dispensing system consisting of a natural low density polyethylene bottle and dispensing plug and tan polypropylene closure. Tamper evidence is provided with a shrink band around the closure and neck area of the package.

2.5 mL in 8 mL bottle – **NDC** 0065-0656-25
5 mL in 8 mL bottle – **NDC** 0065-0656-05
10 mL in 10 mL bottle – **NDC** 0065-0656-10

Storage: Store at 2° - 25°C (36° - 77°F). Protect from light.

Animal Pharmacology: Ciprofloxacin and related drugs have been shown to cause arthropathy in immature animals of most species tested following oral administration. However, a one-month topical ocular study using immature Beagle dogs did not demonstrate any articular lesions.

Rx Only

FLUORESCITE® ℞
(fluorescein injection, USP) 10%
Sterile

Description:

FLUORESCITE® (fluorescein injection, USP) 10% contains fluorescein sodium (equivalent to fluorescein 10% w/v). It is a sterile solution for use intravenously as a diagnostic aid. Its chemical name is spiro[isobenzofuran-1(3H), 9'-[9H]xanthene]-3-one, 3'6'-dihydroxy, disodium salt. The active ingredient is represented by the chemical structure:

376.27 MW
FLUORESCITE® (fluorescein injection, USP) 10% is supplied as a sterile, unpreserved, single-use aqueous solution, that has a pH of 8.0 – 9.8 and an osmolality of 572-858 mOsm/kg.

Active ingredient: fluorescein sodium

Inactive Ingredients
Sodium hydroxide and/or hydrochloric acid (to adjust pH), and water for injection.

Clinical Pharmacology:

Mechanism of Action
Fluorescein sodium responds to electromagnetic radiation and light between the wave-lengths of 465-490 nm and fluoresces, i.e., emits light at wavelengths of 520-530 nm. Thus, the hydrocarbon is excited by blue light and emits light that appears yellowish-green. Following intravenous injection of fluorescein sodium in an aqueous solution, the unbound fraction of the fluorescein can be excited with a blue light flash from a fundus camera as it circulates through the ocular vasculature, and the yellowish green fluorescence of the dye is captured by the camera. In the fundus, the fluorescence of the dye demarcates the retinal and/or choroidal vasculature under observation, distinguishing it from adjacent areas/structures.

Pharmacokinetics

Distribution:
Within 7 to 14 seconds after IV administration into antecubital vein, fluorescein usually appears in the central artery of the eye. Within a few minutes of IV administration of fluorescein sodium, a yellowish discoloration of the skin occurs, which begins to fade after 6 to 12 hours of dosing. Various estimates of volume of distribution indicate that fluorescein distributes well into interstitial space (0.5 L/kg).

Metabolism:
Fluorescein undergoes rapid metabolism to fluorescein monoglucuronide. After IV administration of fluorescein sodium (14 mg/kg) to 7 healthy subjects, approximately 80% of fluorescein in plasma was converted to glucuronide conjugate after a period of 1 hour post dose, indicating relatively rapid conjugation.

Excretion:
Fluorescein and its metabolites are mainly eliminated via renal excretion. After IV administration, the urine remains slightly fluorescent for 24 to 36 hours. A renal clearance of 1.75 mL/min/kg and a hepatic clearance (due to conjugation) of 1.50 mL/min/kg have been estimated. The systemic clearance of fluorescein was essentially complete by 48 to 72 hours after administration of 500 mg fluorescein.

Indications and Usage:
FLUORESCITE® (fluorescein injection, USP) 10% is indicated in diagnostic fluorescein angiography or angioscopy of the retina and iris vasculature.

Contraindications:
FLUORESCITE® (fluorescein injection, USP) 10% is contraindicated in patients with known hypersensitivity to fluorescein sodium or any other ingredients in this product.

Warnings:
FOR INTRAVENOUS USE
Care must be taken to avoid extravasation during injection as the high pH of fluorescein solution can result in severe local tissue damage. The following complications resulting from extravasation of fluorescein have been noted to occur: Sloughing of the skin, superficial phlebitis, subcutaneous granuloma, and toxic neuritis along the median curve in the antecubital area. Complications resulting from extravasation can cause severe pain in the arm for up to several hours. When significant extravasation occurs, the injection should be discontinued and conservative measures to treat damaged tissue and to relieve pain should be implemented. Rare cases of death due to anaphylaxis have been reported (See PRECAUTIONS).

Precautions:

General
Caution is to be exercised in patients with a history of allergy or bronchial asthma. An emergency tray should be available in the event of possible reaction to **FLUORESCITE®** (fluorescein injection, USP) 10%. Use only if the container is undamaged.

Information for Patients
Skin will attain a temporary yellowish discoloration. Urine attains a bright yellow color. Discoloration of the skin usually fades in 6 to 12 hours and usually fades in urine in 24 to 36 hours.

Laboratory Information
If a potential allergy is suspected, an intradermal skin test may be performed prior to intravenous administration, i.e., 0.05 mL injected intradermally to be evaluated 30 to 60 minutes following injection. Given the sensitivity and specificity of skin testing, a negative skin test is not proof that a patient is not allergic to fluorescein.

Carcinogenesis, Mutagenesis, Impairment of Fertility
There have been no long-term studies done using fluorescein in animals to evaluate carcinogenic potential.

Pregnancy

Teratogenic Effects: Pregnancy Category C
Adequate animal reproduction studies have not been conducted with fluorescein sodium. It is also not known whether fluorescein sodium can cause fetal harm when administered to a pregnant woman. Fluorescein sodium should be given to a pregnant woman only if clearly needed.

Nursing Mothers
Fluorescein sodium has been demonstrated to be excreted in human milk. Caution should be exercised when fluorescein sodium is administered to a nursing woman.

Pediatric Use
Safety and effectiveness in pediatric patients have been established.

Geriatric Use
No overall differences in safety or effectiveness have been observed between elderly and other adult patients.

ADVERSE REACTIONS (see **WARNINGS** and **PRECAUTIONS**)
Nausea, vomiting, gastrointestinal distress, headache, syncope, hypotension, and symptoms and signs of hypersensitivity have occurred. Cardiac arrest, basilar artery ischemia, severe shock, convulsions, thrombophlebitis at the injection site, and rare cases of death have been reported. Extravasation of the solution at the injection site causes intense pain at the site and a dull aching pain in the injected arm (see **WARNINGS**). Generalized hives and itching, bronchospasm and anaphylaxis have been reported. A strong taste may develop after injection.

Dosage and Administration:
The normal adult dose of **FLUORESCITE®** (fluorescein injection, USP) 10% is 500 mg (100 mg/mL) via intravenous administration. For children, the dose should be calculated on the basis of 35 mg for each ten pounds of body weight (7.7 mg/kg body weight).

Parenteral drug products should be inspected visually for particulate matter and discoloration prior to administration. Do not mix or dilute with other solutions or drugs. Flush intravenous cannulas before and after drugs are injected to avoid physical incompatibility reactions.

Inject the dose rapidly (1 mL per second is normally recommended) into the antecubital vein, after taking precautions to avoid extravasation. A syringe, filled with **FLUORESCITE®** (fluorescein injection, USP) 10%, may be attached to transparent tubing and a 23 gauge butterfly needle for injection. Insert the needle and draw the patient's blood to the hub of the syringe so that a small air bubble separates the patient's blood in the tubing from the fluorescein. With the room lights on, slowly inject the blood back into the vein while watching the skin over the needle tip. If the needle has extravasated, the patient's blood will be seen to bulge the skin and the injection should be stopped before any fluorescein is injected. When assured that extravasation has not

Continued on next page

Fluorescite—Cont.

occurred, the room light may be turned off and the fluorescein injection completed. Luminescence usually appears in the retina and choroidal vessels in 7 to 14 seconds and can be observed by standard viewing equipment.

Reduction in dose from 5 ml to 2 ml of **FLUORESCITE®** (fluorescein injection, USP) 10% may be appropriate in cases when a highly sensitive imaging system e.g., scanning laser ophthalmoscope is used.

How Supplied:
FLUORESCITE® (fluorescein injection, USP) 10% is supplied in a single-use 5 mL glass vial with a gray FluroTec coated chlorobutyl (latex free) stopper and purple flip-off aluminum seal. It contains a sterile, red-orange solution of fluorescein sodium.
NDC 0065-0092-05
Storage
Store at 2°- 25°C (36°- 77°F).
Do Not Freeze
Rx Only
Mfd. for:
ALCON LABORATORIES, INC.
Fort Worth, Texas 76134 USA
Mfd. by:
International Medication Systems, Limited
South El Monte, CA 91733 USA
Printed in USA
© 2006 Alcon, Inc.

NATACYN®   ℞
(natamycin ophthalmic suspension)
5% Sterile

Description: NATACYN® (natamycin ophthalmic suspension) 5% is a sterile, antifungal drug for topical ophthalmic administration.
Established name: Natamycin
  Chemical name:
    Stereoisomer of 22-[(3-amino-3,6-dideoxy-β-D-mannopyranosyl) oxy]-1, 3, 26-trihydroxy-12-methyl-10-oxo-6,   11,   28-trioxatricyclo [22. 3. 1. 0$^{5, 7}$] octacosa-8, 14, 16, 18, 20-pentaene-25-carboxylic acid.
    Other: Pimaricin
Each mL of the suspension contains: **Active:** Natamycin 5% (50mg). **Preservative:** Benzalkonium Chloride 0.02%. **Inactive:** Sodium Hydroxide and/or Hydrochloric Acid (neutralized to adjust the pH), Purified Water.
Clinical Pharmacology: Natamycin is a tetraene polyene antibiotic derived from *Streptomyces natalensis*. It possesses *in vitro* activity against a variety of yeast and filamentous fungi, including *Candida, Aspergillus, Cephalosporium, Fusarium* and *Penicillium*. The mechanism of action appears to be through binding of the molecule to the sterol moiety of the fungal cell membrane. The polyenesterol complex alters the permeability of the membrane to produce depletion of essential cellular constituents. Although the activity against fungi is dose-related, natamycin is predominantly fungicidal.* Natamycin is not effective *in vitro* against gram-positive or gram-negative bacteria. Topical administration appears to produce effective concentrations of natamycin within the corneal stroma but not in intraocular fluid. Systemic absorption should not be expected following topical administration of NATACYN (natamycin ophthalmic suspension) 5%. As with other polyene antibiotics, absorption from the gastrointestinal tract is very poor. Studies in rabbits receiving topical natamycin revealed no measurable compound in the aqueous humor or sera, but the sensitivity of the measurement was no greater than 2 mg/mL.
Indications and Usage: NATACYN (natamycin ophthalmic suspension) 5% is indicated for the treatment of fungal blepharitis, conjunctivitis, and keratitis caused by suscepti-

ble organisms including *Fusarium solani* keratitis. As in other forms of suppurative keratitis, initial and sustained therapy of fungal keratitis should be determined by the clinical diagnosis, laboratory diagnosis by smear and culture of corneal scrapings and drug response. Whenever possible, the *in vitro* activity of natamycin against the responsible fungus should be determined. The effectiveness of natamycin as a single agent in fungal endophthalmitis has not been established.

Contraindications: NATACYN® (natamycin ophthalmic suspension) 5% is contraindicated in individuals with a history of hypersensitivity to any of its components.
Precautions: General. For topical eye use only—NOT FOR INJECTION. Failure of improvement of keratitis following 7–10 days of administration of the drug suggests that the infection may be caused by a microorganism not susceptible to natamycin.
Continuation of therapy should be based on clinical re-evaluation and additional laboratory studies.
Adherence of the suspension to areas of epithelial ulceration or retention of the suspension in the fornices occurs regularly. There have only been a limited number of cases in which natamycin has been used; therefore, it is possible that adverse reactions of which we have no knowledge at present may occur. For this reason, patients on this drug should be monitored at least twice weekly. Should suspicion of drug toxicity occur, the drug should be discontinued.
Information for Patients: Do not touch dropper tip to any surface, as this may contaminate the suspension.
Carcinogenesis, Mutagenesis, Impairment of Fertility: There have been no long term studies done using natamycin in animals to evaluate carcinogenesis, mutagenesis, or impairment of fertility.
Pregnancy: Pregnancy Category C. Animal reproduction studies have not been conducted with natamycin. It is also not known whether natamycin can cause fetal harm when administered to a pregnant woman or can affect reproduction capacity. NATACYN® (natamycin ophthalmic suspension) 5% should be given to a pregnant woman only if clearly needed.
Nursing Mothers: It is not known whether these drugs are excreted in human milk. Because many drugs are excreted in human milk, caution should be exercised when natamycin is administered to a nursing woman.
Pediatric Use: Safety and effectiveness in pediatric patients have not been established.
Adverse Reactions: One case of conjunctival chemosis and hyperemia, thought to be allergic in nature, has been reported.
Dosage and Administration: SHAKE WELL BEFORE USING. The preferred initial dosage in fungal keratitis is one drop of NATACYN (natamycin ophthalmic suspension) 5% instilled in the conjunctival sac at hourly or two-hourly intervals. The frequency of application can usually be reduced to one drop 6 to 8 times daily after the first 3 to 4 days. Therapy should generally be continued for 14 to 21 days or until there is resolution of active fungal keratitis. In many cases, it may be helpful to reduce the dosage gradually at 4 to 7 day intervals to assure that the replicating organism has been eliminated. Less frequent initial dosage (4 to 6 daily applications) may be sufficient in fungal blepharitis and conjunctivitis.
How Supplied: 15 mL in glass bottles with sterile dropper assembly.
NDC 0065-0645-15.
Storage: May be stored in refrigerator [(36°–46°F) (2°–8°C)] or at room temperature [(46°–75°F) (8°–24°C)]. *Do not freeze*. Avoid exposure to light and excessive heat.
℞ **Only**

*Laupen, J.O.; McLellan, W.L.; El Nakeeb, M.A.: "Antibiotics and Fungal Physiology," Antimicrobial Agents and Chemotherapy, 1965: 1006, 1965.
References:
1. Barckhausen, B.: Die Behandlung der Probleminfektionen das vorderen Augenabschnittes in der Praxis. Landarzt 46: 842, 1970.
2. Cuendet, J.F.; Nouri, A.: Traitement local en ophthalmologie par un nouvel antibiotique fungicide, la "pimaricine". Ophthalmologica 145: 297, 1963.
3. Forster, R.K.; Rebell, G.: "The Diagnosis and Management of Keratomycoses", Arch. Ophth. 93: 1134, 1975.
4. Francois, J.; de Vos, El: Traitement des mycoses oculaires par la pimaricine. Bull. Soc. Belge Ophthal. 131: 382, 1962.
5. Jones, D.B.; Sexton, R.; Rebell, G.: "Mycotic keratitis in South Florida: A Review of Thirty-nine Cases." Transactions ophthal. Soc. U.K. 89: 781, 1969.
6. Jones, D.B.; Forster, R.K.; Rebell, G.: "*Fusarium solani* keratitis treated with Natamycin (pimaricin), 18 consecutive cases." Arch. Ophth. 88: 147, 1972.
7. L'Editeur: Traitement des mycoses oculaires. Presse med. 77: 147, 1969.
8. Vozza, R.; Bagolini, B.: Su di un caso di grave ulcerazione bilaterale delle palpebra de Candida albicans. Bol. Oculist. 43: 433, 1964.

NEVANAC®   ℞
(nepanfenac opthlamic suspension 0.1%)

Description:
NEVANAC® (nepafenac ophthalmic suspension) 0.1% is a sterile, topical, nonsteroidal anti-inflammatory (NSAID) prodrug for ophthalmic use. Each mL of NEVANAC® suspension contains 1 mg of nepafenac. Nepafenac is designated chemically as 2-amino-3-benzoylbenzeneacetamide with an empirical formula of $C_{15}H_{14}N_2O_2$. The structural formula of nepafenac is:

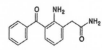

Nepafenac is a yellow crystalline powder. The molecular weight of nepafenac is 254.28. NEVANAC® ophthalmic suspension is supplied as a sterile, aqueous 0.1% suspension with a pH approximately of 7.4. The osmolality of NEVANAC® ophthalmic suspension is approximately 305 mOsmol/kg. Each mL of NEVANAC® contains: **Active:** nepafenac 0.1% **Inactives:** mannitol, carbomer 974P, sodium chloride, tyloxapol, edetate disodium benzalkonium chloride 0.005% (preservative), sodium hydroxide and/or hydrochloric acid to adjust pH and purified water, USP.
Clinical Pharmacology:
Pharmacodynamics: NEVANAC® suspension contains nepafenac (0.1%), a nonsteroidal anti-inflammatory and analgesic prodrug. After topical ocular dosing, nepafenac penetrates the cornea and is converted by ocular tissue hydrolases to amfenac, a nonsteroidal anti-inflammatory drug. Amfenac is thought to inhibit the action of prostaglandin H synthase (cyclooxygenase), an enzyme required for prostaglandin production.
Pharmacokinetics:
Drug-Drug Interaction: Nepafenac at concentrations up to 300 ng/mL did not inhibit the *in vitro* metabolism of 6 specific marker substrates of cytochrome P450 (CYP) isozymes (CYP1A2, CYP2C9, CYP2C19, CYP2D6,

CYP2E1, and CYP3A4). Therefore, drug-drug interactions involving CYP-mediated metabolism of concomitantly administered drugs are unlikely. Drug-drug interactions mediated by protein binding are also unlikely.

Gender: Data in healthy subjects indicate no clinically relevant or significant gender difference in the steady-state pharmacokinetics of amfenac following three-times-daily dosing of NEVANAC®.

Low but quantifiable plasma concentrations of nepafenac and amfenac were observed in the majority of subjects 2 and 3 hours postdose, respectively, following bilateral topical ocular TID dosing of nepafenac ophthalmic suspension, 0.1%. The mean steady-state C_{max} for nepafenac and for amfenac were 0.310 ± 0.104 ng/ml and 0.422 ± 0.121 ng/ml, respectively, following ocular administration.

Clinical Studies: In two double-masked, randomized clinical trials in which patients were dosed three-times-daily beginning one day prior to cataract surgery, continued on the day of surgery and for the first two weeks of the postoperative period, NEVANAC® ophthalmic suspension demonstrated clinical efficacy, compared to its vehicle in treating postoperative inflammation.

Patients treated with NEVANAC® ophthalmic suspension were less likely to have ocular pain and measurable signs of inflammation (cells and flare) in the early postoperative period through the end of treatment than those treated with its vehicle.

For ocular pain in both studies a significantly higher percentage of patients (approximately 80%) in the nepafenac group reported no ocular pain on the day following cataract surgery (Day 1) compared to those in the vehicle group (approximately 50%).

Results from clinical studies indicated that NEVANAC® has no significant effect upon intraocular pressure; however, changes in intraocular pressure may occur following cataract surgery.

Indications and Usage:
NEVANAC® ophthalmic suspension is indicated for the treatment of pain and inflammation associated with cataract surgery.

Contraindications:
NEVANAC® ophthalmic suspension is contraindicated in patients with previously demonstrated hypersensitivity to any of the ingredients in the formulation or to other NSAIDs.

Warnings:
There is the potential for cross-sensitivity to acetylsalicylic acid, phenylacetic acid derivatives, and other nonsteroidal anti-inflammatory agents. Therefore, caution should be used when treating individuals who have previously exhibited sensitivities to these drugs.

With some nonsteroidal anti-inflammatory drugs including NEVANAC®, there exists the potential for increased bleeding time due to interference with thrombocyte aggregation. There have been reports that ocularly applied nonsteroidal anti-inflammatory drugs may cause increased bleeding of ocular tissues (including hyphemas) in conjunction with ocular surgery.

Precautions:
General: Topical nonsteroidal anti-inflammatory drugs (NSAIDs) including NEVANAC®, may slow or delay healing. Topical corticosteroids are also known to slow or delay healing. Concomitant use of topical NSAIDs and topical steroids may increase the potential for healing problems.

Use of topical NSAIDs may result in keratitis. In some susceptible patients, continued use of topical NSAIDs may result in epithelial breakdown, corneal thinning, corneal erosion, corneal ulceration or corneal perforation. These events may be sight threatening. Patients with evidence of corneal epithelial breakdown

should immediately discontinue use of topical NSAIDs including NEVANAC® and should be closely monitored for corneal health.

Postmarketing experience with topical NSAIDs suggests that patients with complicated ocular surgeries, corneal denervation, corneal epithelial defects, diabetes mellitus, ocular surface diseases (e.g., dry eye syndrome), rheumatoid arthritis, or repeat ocular surgeries within a short period of time may be at increased risk for corneal adverse events which may become sight threatening. Topical NSAIDs should be used with caution in these patients.

Postmarketing experience with topical NSAIDs also suggests that use more than 1 day prior to surgery or use beyond 14 days post surgery may increase patient risk for occurrence and severity of corneal adverse events.

It is recommended that NEVANAC® ophthalmic suspension be used with caution in patients with known bleeding tendencies or who are receiving other medications which may prolong bleeding time.

Information for Patients: NEVANAC® ophthalmic suspension should not be administered while wearing contact lenses.

Carcinogenesis, Mutagenesis, Impairment of Fertility: Nepafenac has not been evaluated in long-term carcinogenicity studies. Increased chromosomal aberrations were observed in Chinese hamster ovary cells exposed *in vitro* to nepafenac suspension. Nepafenac was not mutagenic in the Ames assay or in the mouse lymphoma forward mutation assay. Oral doses up to 5,000 mg/kg did not result in an increase in the formation of micronucleated polychromatic erythrocytes *in vivo* in the mouse micronucleus assay in the bone marrow of mice.

Nepafenac did not impair fertility when administered orally to male and female rats at 3 mg/kg (approximately 90 and 380 times the plasma exposure to the parent drug, nepafenac, and the active metabolite, amfenac, respectively, at the recommended human topical ophthalmic dose).

Pregnancy: Teratogenic Effects.

Pregnancy Category C: Reproduction studies performed with nepafenac in rabbits and rats at oral doses up to 10 mg/kg/day have revealed no evidence of teratogenicity due to nepafenac, despite the induction of maternal toxicity. At this dose, the animal plasma exposure to nepafenac and amfenac was approximately 260 and 2400 times human plasma exposure at the recommended human topical ophthalmic dose for rats and 80 and 680 times human plasma exposure for rabbits, respectively. In rats, maternally toxic doses ≥ 10 mg/kg were associated with dystocia, increased post-implantation loss, reduced fetal weights and growth, and reduced fetal survival.

Nepafenac has been shown to cross the placental barrier in rats. There are no adequate and well-controlled studies in pregnant women. Because animal reproduction studies are not always predictive of human response, NEVANAC® should be used during pregnancy only if the potential benefit justifies the potential risk to the fetus.

Non-teratogenic Effects: Because of the known effects of prostaglandin biosynthesis inhibiting drugs on the fetal cardiovascular system (closure of the ductus arteriosus), the use of NEVANAC® ophthalmic suspension during late pregnancy should be avoided.

Nursing Mothers: NEVANAC® ophthalmic suspension is excreted in the milk of pregnant rats. It is not known whether this drug is excreted in human milk. Because many drugs are excreted in human milk, caution should be exercised when NEVANAC® ophthalmic suspension is administered to a nursing woman.

Pediatric Use: The safety and effectiveness of NEVANAC® in pediatric patients below the age of 10 years have not been established.

Geriatric Use: No overall differences in safety and effectiveness have been observed between elderly and younger patients.

Adverse Reactions:
In controlled clinical studies, the most frequently reported ocular adverse events following cataract surgery were capsular opacity, decreased visual acuity, foreign body sensation, increased intraocular pressure, and sticky sensation. These events occurred in approximately 5 to 10% of patients.

Other ocular adverse events occurring at an incidence of approximately 1 to 5% included conjunctival edema, corneal edema, dry eye, lid margin crusting, ocular discomfort, ocular hyperemia, ocular pain, ocular pruritus, photophobia, tearing and vitreous detachment. Some of these events may be the consequence of the cataract surgical procedure.

Nonocular adverse events reported at an incidence of 1 to 4% included headache, hypertension, nausea/vomiting, and sinusitis.

Dosage and Administration:
Shake well before use. One drop of NEVANAC® ophthalmic suspension should be applied to the affected eye(s) three-times-daily beginning 1 day prior to cataract surgery, continued on the day of surgery and through the first 2 weeks of the postoperative period.

NEVANAC® ophthalmic suspension may be administered in conjunction with other topical ophthalmic medications such as beta-blockers, carbonic anhydrase inhibitors, alpha-agonists, cycloplegics, and mydriatics.

How Supplied:
NEVANAC® (nepafenac ophthalmic suspension) is supplied in a natural, oval, low density polyethylene DROP-TAINER® dispenser with a natural low density polyethylene dispensing plug and gray polypropylene cap. Tamper evidence is provided with a shrink band around the closure and neck area of the package.

3 mL in 4 mL bottle **NDC** 0065–0002–03

Storage: Store at 2 – 25°C (36 – 77°F).

Rx Only

Manufactured by:
Alcon Laboratories, Inc.
Fort Worth, TX 76134 USA
U.S. Patent No: 5,475,034
©2005 Alcon, Inc.

PATADAY™ ℞
(olopatadine hydrochloride ophthalmic solution) 0.2%

DESCRIPTION
PATADAY™ (olopatadine hydrochloride ophthalmic solution) 0.2% is a sterile ophthalmic solution containing olopatadine for topical administration to the eyes. Olopatadine hydrochloride is a white, crystalline, water-soluble powder with a molecular weight of 373.88 and a molecular formula of $C_{21}H_{23}NO_3$ • HCl. The chemical structure is presented below:

Chemical Name: 11-[(Z)-3-(Dimethylamino) propylidene]-6-11-dihydrodibenz[b,e] oxepin-2-acetic acid, hydrochloride.

Continued on next page

Pataday—Cont.

Each mL of PATADAY™ solution contains: **Active:** 2.22 mg olopatadine hydrochloride equivalent to 2 mg olopatadine.
Inactives: povidone; dibasic sodium phosphate; sodium chloride; edetate disodium; benzalkonium chloride 0.01% **(preservative)** hydrochloric acid / sodium hydroxide (adjust pH); and purified water.
It has a pH of approximately 7 and an osmolality of approximately 300 mOsm/kg.

CLINICAL PHARMACOLOGY
Olopatadine is a relatively selective histamine H_1 antagonist and an inhibitor of the release of histamine from the mast cells. Decreased chemotaxis and inhibition of eosinophil activation has also been demonstrated. Olopatadine is devoid of effects on alpha-adrenergic, dopaminergic, and muscarinic type 1 and 2 receptors. Systemic bioavailability data upon topical ocular administration of PATADAY™ solution are not available. Following topical ocular administration of olopatadine 0.15% ophthalmic solution in man, olopatadine was shown to have a low systemic exposure. Two studies in normal volunteers (totaling 24 subjects) dosed bilaterally with olopatadine 0.15% ophthalmic solution once every 12 hours for 2 weeks demonstrated plasma concentrations to be generally below the quantitation limit of the assay (< 0.5 ng/mL). Samples in which olopatadine was quantifiable were typically found within 2 hours of dosing and ranged from 0.5 to 1.3 ng/mL. The elimination half-life in plasma following oral dosing was 8 to 12 hours, and elimination was predominantly through renal excretion. Approximately 60–70% of the dose was recovered in the urine as parent drug. Two metabolites, the mono-desmethyl and the N-oxide, were detected at low concentrations in the urine.

CLINICAL STUDIES
Results from clinical studies of up to 12 weeks duration demonstrate that PATADAY™ solution when dosed once a day is effective in the treatment of ocular itching associated with allergic conjunctivitis.

INDICATIONS AND USAGE
PATADAY™ solution is indicated for the treatment of ocular itching associated with allergic conjunctivitis.

CONTRAINDICATIONS
Hypersensitivity to any components of this product.

WARNINGS
For topical ocular use only. Not for injection or oral use.

PRECAUTIONS
Information for Patients
As with any eye drop, to prevent contaminating the dropper tip and solution, care should be taken not to touch the eyelids or surrounding areas with the dropper tip of the bottle. Keep bottle tightly closed when not in use. Patients should be advised not to wear a contact lens if their eye is red.
PATADAY™ (olopatadine hydrochloride ophthalmic solution) 0.2% should not be used to treat contact lens related irritation. The preservative in PATADAY™ solution, benzalkonium chloride, may be absorbed by soft contact lenses. Patients who wear soft contact lenses and **whose eyes are not red**, should be instructed to wait at least ten minutes after instilling PATADAY™ (olopatadine hydrochloride ophthalmic solution) 0.2% before they insert their contact lenses.

Carcinogenesis, Mutagenesis, Impairment of Fertility
Olopatadine administered orally was not carcinogenic in mice and rats in doses up to 500 mg/kg/day and 200 mg/kg/day, respectively. Based on a 40 μL drop size and a 50 kg person, these doses were approximately 150,000 and 50,000 times higher than the maximum recommended ocular human dose (MROHD). No mutagenic potential was observed when olopatadine was tested in an *in vitro* bacterial reverse mutation (Ames) test, an *in vitro* mammalian chromosome aberration assay or an *in vivo* mouse micronucleus test.
Olopatadine administered to male and female rats at oral doses of approximately 100,000 times MROHD level resulted in a slight decrease in the fertility index and reduced implantation rate; no effects on reproductive function were observed at doses of approximately 15,000 times the MROHD level.

Pregnancy:

Teratogenic effects: Pregnancy Category C
Olopatadine was found not to be teratogenic in rats and rabbits. However, rats treated at 600 mg/kg/day, or 150,000 times the MROHD and rabbits treated at 400 mg/kg/day, or approximately 100,000 times the MROHD, during organogenesis showed a decrease in live fetuses. In addition, rats treated with 600 mg/kg/day of olopatadine during organogenesis showed a decrease in fetal weight. Further, rats treated with 600 mg/kg/day of olopatadine during late gestation through the lactation period showed a decrease in neonatal survival and body weight.
There are, however, no adequate and well-controlled studies in pregnant women. Because animal studies are not always predictive of human responses, this drug should be used in pregnant women only if the potential benefit to the mother justifies the potential risk to the embryo or fetus.

Nursing Mothers:
Olopatadine has been identified in the milk of nursing rats following oral administration. It is not known whether topical ocular administration could result in sufficient systemic absorption to produce detectable quantities in the human breast milk. Nevertheless, caution should be exercised when PATADAY™ (olopatadine hydrochloride ophthalmic solution) 0.2% is administered to a nursing mother.

Pediatric Use:
Safety and effectiveness in pediatric patients below the age of 3 years have not been established.

Geriatric Use:
No overall differences in safety and effectiveness have been observed between elderly and younger patients.

ADVERSE REACTIONS
Symptoms similar to cold syndrome and pharyngitis were reported at an incidence of approximately 10%.
The following adverse experiences have been reported in 5% or less of patients:
Ocular: blurred vision, burning or stinging, conjunctivitis, dry eye, foreign body sensation, hyperemia, hypersensitivity, keratitis, lid edema, pain and ocular pruritus.
Non-ocular: asthenia, back pain, flu syndrome, headache, increased cough, infection, nausea, rhinitis, sinusitis and taste perversion. Some of these events were similar to the underlying disease being studied.

DOSAGE AND ADMINISTRATION
The recommended dose is one drop in each affected eye once a day.

HOW SUPPLIED
PATADAY™ (olopatadine hydrochloride ophthalmic solution) 0.2% is supplied in a white, oval, low density polyethylene DROP-TAINER® dispenser with a natural low density polyethylene dispensing plug and a white polypropylene cap. Tamper evidence is provided with a shrink band around the closure and neck area of the package.
NDC 0065-0272-25   2.5 mL fill in 4 mL oval bottle
Storage:
Store at 2°C to 25°C (36°F to 77°F)

U.S. Patents Nos. 4,871,865; 4,923,892; 5,116,863; 5,641,805; 6,995,186
Rx Only

ALCON LABORATORIES, INC.
Fort Worth, Texas 76134 USA
© 2005-2006 Alcon, Inc.

PATANOL®   ℞
[pă'tə-nŏl]
(olopatadine hydrochloride ophthalmic solution) 0.1%

Description: PATANOL® (olopatadine hydrochloride ophthalmic solution) 0.1% is a sterile ophthalmic solution containing olopatadine, a relatively selective H_1-receptor antagonist and inhibitor of histamine release from the mast cell for topical administration to the eyes. Olopatadine hydrochloride is a white, crystalline, water-soluble powder with a molecular weight of 373.88.
Chemical Name: 11-[(Z)-3-(Dimethylamino) propylidene]-6-11-dihydrodibenz[b,e] oxepin-2-acetic acid hydrochloride.
Each mL of PATANOL contains: **Active:** 1.11 mg olopatadine hydrochloride equivalent to 1 mg olopatadine. **Preservative:** benzalkonium chloride 0.01%. **Inactives:** dibasic sodium phosphate; sodium chloride; hydrochloric acid/sodium hydroxide (adjust pH); and purified water. It has a pH of approximately 7 and an osmolality of approximately 300 mOsm/kg.
Clinical Pharmacology: Olopatadine is an inhibitor of the release of histamine from the mast cell and a relatively selective histamine H_1-antagonist that inhibits the *in vivo* and *in vitro* type 1 immediate hypersensitivity reaction including inhibition of histamine induced effects on human conjunctival epithelial cells. Olopatadine is devoid of effects on alpha-adrenergic, dopamine and muscarinic type 1 and 2 receptors. Following topical ocular administration in man, olopatadine was shown to have low systemic exposure. Two studies in normal volunteers (totaling 24 subjects) dosed bilaterally with olopatadine 0.15% ophthalmic solution once every 12 hours for 2 weeks demonstrated plasma concentrations to be generally below the quantitation limit of the assay (<0.5 ng/mL). Samples in which olopatadine was quantifiable were typically found within 2 hours of dosing and ranged from 0.5 to 1.3 ng/mL. The half-life in plasma was approximately 3 hours, and elimination was predominantly through renal excretion. Approximately 60–70% of the dose was recovered in the urine as parent drug. Two metabolites, the mono-desmethyl and the N-oxide, were detected at low concentrations in the urine.
Results from an environmental study demonstrated that PATANOL was effective in the treatment of the signs and symptoms of allergic conjunctivitis when dosed twice daily for up to 6 weeks. Results from conjunctival antigen challenge studies demonstrated that PATANOL®, when subjects were challenged with antigen both initially and up to 8 hours after dosing, was significantly more effective than its vehicle in preventing ocular itching associated with allergic conjunctivitis.
Indications and Usage: PATANOL (olopatadine hydrochloride ophthalmic solution) 0.1% is indicated for the treatment of the signs and symptoms of allergic conjunctivitis.
Contraindications: PATANOL (olopatadine hydrochloride ophthalmic solution) 0.1% is contraindicated in persons with a known hypersensitivity to olopatadine hydrochloride or any components of PATANOL.
Warnings: PATANOL (olopatadine hydrochloride ophthalmic solution) 0.1% is for topical use only and not for injection or oral use.
Precautions:
Information for Patients: To prevent contaminating the dropper tip and solution, care

should be taken not to touch the eyelids or surrounding areas with the dropper tip of the bottle. Keep bottle tightly closed when not in use. Patients should be advised not to wear a contact lens if their eye is red. PATANOL® (olopatadine hydrochloride ophthalmic solution) 0.1% should not be used to treat contact lens related irritation. The preservative in PATANOL, benzalkonium chloride, may be absorbed by soft contact lenses. Patients who wear soft contact lenses and **whose eyes are not red** should be instructed to wait at least ten minutes after instilling PATANOL (olopatadine hydrochloride ophthalmic solution) 0.1% before they insert their contact lenses.

Carcinogenesis, Mutagenesis, Impairment of Fertility: Olopatadine administered orally was not carcinogenic in mice and rats in doses up to 500 mg/kg/day and 200 mg/kg/day, respectively. Based on a 40 μL drop size, these doses were 78,125 and 31,250 times higher than the maximum recommended ocular human dose (MROHD). No mutagenic potential was observed when olopatadine was tested in an *in vitro* bacterial reverse mutation (Ames) test, an *in vitro* mammalian chromosome aberration assay or an *in vivo* mouse micronucleus test. Olopatadine administered to male and female rats at oral doses of 62,500 times MROHD level resulted in a slight decrease in the fertility index and reduced implantation rate; no effects on reproductive function were observed at doses of 7,800 times the maximum recommended ocular human use level.

Pregnancy: Pregnancy Category C. Olopatadine was found not to be teratogenic in rats and rabbits. However, rats treated at 600 mg/kg/day, or 93,750 times the MROHD and rabbits treated at 400 mg/kg/day, or 62,500 times the MROHD, during organogenesis showed a decrease in live fetuses. There are, however, no adequate and well-controlled studies in pregnant women. Because animal studies are not always predictive of human responses, this drug should be used in pregnant women only if the potential benefit to the mother justifies the potential risk to the embryo or fetus.

Nursing Mothers: Olopatadine has been identified in the milk of nursing rats following oral administration. It is not known whether topical ocular administration could result in sufficient systemic absorption to produce detectable quantities in the human breast milk. Nevertheless, caution should be exercised when PATANOL® (olopatadine hydrochloride ophthalmic solution) 0.1% is administered to a nursing mother.

Pediatric Use: Safety and effectiveness in pediatric patients below the age of 3 years have not been established.

Geriatric Use: No overall differences in safety or effectiveness have been observed between elderly and younger patients.

Adverse Reactions: Headaches have been reported at an incidence of 7%. The following adverse experiences have been reported in less than 5% of patients: asthenia, blurred vision, burning or stinging, cold syndrome, dry eye, foreign body sensation, hyperemia, hypersensitivity, keratitis, lid edema, nausea, pharyngitis, pruritus, rhinitis, sinusitis, and taste perversion. Some of these events were similar to the underlying disease being studied.

Dosage and Administration: The recommended dose is one drop in each affected eye two times per day at an interval of 6 to 8 hours.

How Supplied: PATANOL (olopatadine hydrochloride ophthalmic solution) 0.1% is supplied as follows: 5 mL in plastic DROP-TAINER® dispenser.

　　5 mL: **NDC** 0065-0271-05

Storage: Store at 39°F–77°F (4°C–25°C)

Rx Only
U.S. Patent Nos. 5,116,863; 5,641,805.
©2000, 2003, 2007 Alcon, Inc.

SYSTANE®　　　　　　　　　　**OTC**
[sĭstān]
Lubricant Eye Drops

Description: SYSTANE® is scientifically formulated to shield eyes from dry eye discomfort so that eyes feel moist and refreshed longer. For the temporary relief of burning and irritation due to dryness of the eye.

Active Ingredients: Polyethylene Glycol 400 0.4% and Propylene Glycol 0.3% as lubricants.

Inactive Ingredients: boric acid, calcium chloride, hydroxypropyl guar, magnesium chloride, polyquaternium-1 as a preservative, potassium chloride, purified water, sodium chloride, zinc chloride. May contain hydrochloric acid and/or sodium hydroxide to adjust pH.

Warnings: For external use only
Do not use
• if this product changes color or becomes cloudy
• if you are sensitive to any ingredient in this product

When using this product
• do not touch tip of container to any surface to avoid contamination
• replace cap after each use

Stop use and ask a doctor if
• you feel eye pain
• changes in vision occur
• redness or irritation of the eye(s) gets worse or lasts more than 72 hours

Keep out of reach of children
If swallowed, get medical help or contact a Poison Control Center right away.

Directions:
• Instill 1 or 2 drops in the affected eye(s) as needed.

Other Information:
• Store at room temperature.

How Supplied: SYSTANE® Lubricant Eye Drops are supplied in 15 mL and 30 mL bottles. Systane® is also available in convenient preservative-free vials (0.4 mL each).

TOBRADEX®　　　　　　　　　　Rx
(tobramycin and dexamethasone ophthalmic suspension)
Sterile

Description: TOBRADEX® (tobramycin and dexamethasone ophthalmic suspension) is a sterile, multiple dose antibiotic and steroid combination for topical ophthalmic use.

Each mL of TOBRADEX® (tobramycin and dexamethasone ophthalmic suspension) contains: Actives: tobramycin 0.3% (3 mg) and dexamethasone 0.1% (1 mg). **Preservative:** benzalkonium chloride 0.01%. **Inactives:** tyloxapol, edetate disodium, sodium chloride, hydroxyethyl cellulose, sodium sulfate, sulfuric acid and/or sodium hydroxide (to adjust pH) and purified water.

Clinical Pharmacology: Corticoids suppress the inflammatory response to a variety of agents and they probably delay or slow healing. Since corticoids may inhibit the body's defense mechanism against infection, a concomitant antimicrobial drug may be used when this inhibition is considered to be clinically significant. Dexamethasone is a potent corticoid.

The antibiotic component in the combination (tobramycin) is included to provide action against susceptible organisms. *In vitro* studies have demonstrated that tobramycin is active against susceptible strains of the following microorganisms:

Staphylococci, including *S. aureus* and *S. epidermidis* (coagulase-positive and coagulase-negative), including penicillin-resistant strains.

Streptococci, including some of the Group A beta-hemolytic species, some nonhemolytic species, and some *Streptococcus pneumoniae*. *Pseudomonas aeruginosa, Escherichia coli, Klebsiella pneumoniae, Enterobacter aerogenes, Proteus mirabilis, Morganella morganii,* most *Proteus vulgaris* strains, *Haemophilus influenzae* and *H. aegyptius, Moraxella lacunata, Acinetobacter calcoaceticus* and some *Neisseria* species.

Bacterial susceptibility studies demonstrate that in some cases microorganisms resistant to gentamicin remain susceptible to tobramycin. No data are available on the extent of systemic absorption from TOBRADEX® (tobramycin and dexamethasone ophthalmic suspension); however, it is known that some systemic absorption can occur with ocularly applied drugs. If the maximum dose of TOBRADEX® (tobramycin and dexamethasone ophthalmic suspension) is given for the first 48 hours (two drops in each eye every 2 hours) and complete systemic absorption occurs, which is highly unlikely, the daily dose of dexamethasone would be 2.4 mg. The usual physiologic replacement dose is 0.75 mg daily. If TOBRADEX® (tobramycin and dexamethasone ophthalmic suspension) is given after the first 48 hours as two drops in each eye every 4 hours, the administered dose of dexamethasone would be 1.2 mg daily.

Indications and Usage: TOBRADEX® (tobramycin and dexamethasone ophthalmic suspension) is indicated for steroid-responsive inflammatory ocular conditions for which a corticosteroid is indicated and where superficial bacterial ocular infection or a risk of bacterial ocular infection exists.

Ocular steroids are indicated in inflammatory conditions of the palpebral and bulbar conjunctiva, cornea and anterior segment of the globe where the inherent risk of steroid use in certain infective conjunctivitides is accepted to obtain a diminution in edema and inflammation. They are also indicated in chronic anterior uveitis and corneal injury from chemical, radiation or thermal burns, or penetration of foreign bodies.

The use of a combination drug with an anti-infective component is indicated where the risk of superficial ocular infection is high or where there is an expectation that potentially dangerous numbers of bacteria will be present in the eye.

The particular anti-infective drug in this product is active against the following common bacterial eye pathogens:

Staphylococci, including *S. aureus* and *S. epidermidis*(coagulase-positive and coagulase-negative), including penicillin-resistant strains.

Streptococci, including some of the Group A beta-hemolytic species, some nonhemolytic species, and some *Streptococcus pneumoniae*. *Pseudomonas aeruginosa, Escherichia coli, Klebsiella pneumoniae, Enterobacter aerogenes, Proteus mirabilis, Morganella morganii,* most *Proteus vulgaris* strains, *Haemophilus influenzae* and *H. aegyptius, Moraxella lacunata, Acinetobacter calcoaceticus* and some *Neisseria* species.

Contraindications: Epithelial herpes simplex keratitis (dendritic keratitis), vaccinia, varicella, and many other viral diseases of the cornea and conjunctiva. Mycobacterial infection of the eye. Fungal diseases of ocular structures. Hypersensitivity to a component of the medication.

Continued on next page

TobraDex Suspension—Cont.

Warnings: FOR TOPICAL OPHTHALMIC USE ONLY. NOT FOR INJECTION INTO THE EYE. Sensitivity to topically applied aminoglycosides may occur in some patients. If a sensitivity reaction does occur, discontinue use.

Prolonged use of steroids may result in glaucoma, with damage to the optic nerve, defects in visual acuity and fields of vision, and posterior subcapsular cataract formation. Intraocular pressure should be routinely monitored even though it may be difficult in pediatric patients and uncooperative patients. Prolonged use may suppress the host response and thus increase the hazard of secondary ocular infections. In those diseases causing thinning of the cornea or sclera, perforations have been known to occur with the use of topical steroids. In acute purulent conditions of the eye, steroids may mask infection or enhance existing infection.

Precautions:

General. The possibility of fungal infections of the cornea should be considered after long-term steroid dosing. As with other antibiotic preparations, prolonged use may result in overgrowth of nonsusceptible organisms, including fungi. If superinfection occurs, appropriate therapy should be initiated. When multiple prescriptions are required, or whenever clinical judgement dictates, the patient should be examined with the aid of magnification, such as slit lamp biomicroscopy and, where appropriate, fluorescein staining.

Cross-sensitivity to other aminoglycoside antibiotics may occur; if hypersensitivity develops with this product, discontinue use and institute appropriate therapy.

Information for Patients: Do not touch dropper tip to any surface, as this may contaminate the contents. Contact lenses should not be worn during the use of this product.

Carcinogenesis, Mutagenesis, Impairment of Fertility: No studies have been conducted to evaluate the carcinogenic or mutagenic potential. No impairment of fertility was noted in studies of subcutaneous tobramycin in rats at doses of 50 and 100 mg/kg/day.

Pregnancy Category C. Corticosteroids have been found to be teratogenic in animal studies. Ocular administration of 0.1% dexamethasone resulted in 15.6% and 32.3% incidence of fetal anomalies in two groups of pregnant rabbits. Fetal growth retardation and increased mortality rates have been observed in rats with chronic dexamethasone therapy. Reproduction studies have been performed in rats and rabbits with tobramycin at doses up to 100 mg/kg/day parenterally and have revealed no evidence of impaired fertility or harm to the fetus. There are no adequate and well controlled studies in pregnant women. TOBRADEX® (tobramycin and dexamethasone ophthalmic suspension) should be used during pregnancy only if the potential benefit justifies the potential risk to the fetus.

Nursing Mothers. Systemically administered corticosteroids appear in human milk and could suppress growth, interfere with endogenous corticosteroid production, or cause other untoward effects. It is not known whether topical administration of corticosteroids could result in sufficient systemic absorption to produce detectable quantities in human milk. Because many drugs are excreted in human milk, caution should be exercised when TOBRADEX® (tobramycin and dexamethasone ophthalmic suspension) is administered to a nursing woman.

Pediatric Use. Safety and effectiveness in pediatric patients below the age of 2 years have not been established.

Geriatric Use: No overall differences in safety or effectiveness have been observed between elderly and younger patients.

Adverse Reactions: Adverse reactions have occurred with steroid/anti-infective combination drugs which can be attributed to the steroid component, the anti-infective component, or the combination. Exact incidence figures are not available. The most frequent adverse reactions to topical ocular tobramycin [(TOBREX®) (tobramycin ophthalmic solution)] are hypersensitivity and localized ocular toxicity, including lid itching and swelling, and conjunctival erythema. These reactions occur in less than 4% of patients. Similar reactions may occur with the topical use of other aminoglycoside antibiotics. Other adverse reactions have not been reported; however, if topical ocular tobramycin is administered concomitantly with systemic aminoglycoside antibiotics, care should be taken to monitor the total serum concentration. The reactions due to the steroid component are: elevation of intraocular pressure (IOP) with possible development of glaucoma, and infrequent optic nerve damage; posterior subcapsular cataract formation; and delayed wound healing.

Secondary Infection. The development of secondary infection has occurred after use of combinations containing steroids and antimicrobials. Fungal infections of the cornea are particularly prone to develop coincidentally with long-term applications of steroids. The possibility of fungal invasion must be considered in any persistent corneal ulceration where steroid treatment has been used. Secondary bacterial ocular infection following suppression of host responses also occurs.

Overdosage: Clinically apparent signs and symptoms of an overdosage of TOBRADEX® (tobramycin and dexamethasone ophthalmic suspension) punctate keratitis, erythema, increased lacrimation, edema and lid itching) may be similar to adverse reaction effects seen in some patients.

Dosage and Administration: One or two drops instilled into the conjunctival sac(s) every four to six hours. During the initial 24 to 48 hours, the dosage may be increased to one or two drops every two (2) hours. Frequency should be decreased gradually as warranted by improvement in clinical signs. Care should be taken not to discontinue therapy prematurely. Not more than 20 mL should be prescribed initially and the prescription should not be refilled without further evaluation as outlined in PRECAUTIONS above.

How Supplied: Sterile ophthalmic suspension in 2.5 mL (**NDC** 0065-0647-25), 5 mL (**NDC** 0065-0647-05) and 10 mL (**NDC** 0065-0647-10) DROP-TAINER® dispensers.

Storage: Store at 8°-27°C (46°-80°F). Store suspension upright and shake well before using.

℞ Only

U.S. Patent No. 5,149,694

TOBRADEX®
(tobramycin and dexamethasone ophthalmic ointment)
Sterile   ℞

Description: TOBRADEX® (tobramycin and dexamethasone ophthalmic ointment) is a sterile, multiple dose antibiotic and steroid combination for topical ophthalmic use.

Each gram of TOBRADEX® (tobramycin and dexamethasone ophthalmic ointment) contains: **Actives:** tobramycin 0.3% (3mg) and dexamethasone 0.1% (1mg). **Preservative:** chlorobutanol 0.5%. **Inactives:** mineral oil and white petrolatum.

Clinical Pharmacology: Corticoids suppress the inflammatory response to a variety of agents and they probably delay or slow healing.

Since corticoids may inhibit the body's defense mechanism against infection, a concomitant antimicrobial drug may be used when this inhibition is considered to be clinically significant. Dexamethasone is a potent corticoid.

The antibiotic component in the combination (tobramycin) is included to provide action against susceptible organisms. *In vitro* studies have demonstrated that tobramycin is active against susceptible strains of the following microorganisms:

Staphylococci, including *S. aureus* and *S. epidermidis* (coagulase-positive and coagulase-negative), including penicillin-resistant strains.

Streptococci, including some of the Group A-beta-hemolytic species, some nonhemolytic species, and some *Streptococcus pneumoniae.* *Pseudomonas aeruginosa, Escherichia coli, Klebsiella pneumoniae, Enterobacter aerogenes, Proteus mirabilis, Morganella morganii,* most *Proteus vulgaris* strains, *Haemophilus influenzae* and *H. aegyptius, Moraxella lacunata, Acinetobacter calcoaceticus* and some *Neisseria* species.

Bacterial susceptibility studies demonstrate that in some cases microorganisms resistant to gentamicin remain susceptible to tobramycin. No data are available on the extent of systemic absorption from TOBRADEX® (tobramycin and dexamethasone ophthalmic ointment); however, it is known that some systemic absorption can occur with ocularly applied drugs. The usual physiologic replacement dose is 0.75 mg daily. The administered dose for TOBRADEX® (tobramycin and dexamethasone ophthalmic ointment) in both eyes four times daily would be 0.4 mg of dexamethasone daily.

Indications and Usage: TOBRADEX® (tobramycin and dexamethasone ophthalmic ointment) is indicated for steroid-responsive inflammatory ocular conditions for which a corticosteroid is indicated and where superficial bacterial ocular infection or a risk of bacterial ocular infection exists.

Ocular steroids are indicated in inflammatory conditions of the palpebral and bulbar conjunctiva, cornea and anterior segment of the globe where the inherent risk of steroid use in certain infective conjunctivitides is accepted to obtain a diminution in edema and inflammation. They are also indicated in chronic anterior uveitis and corneal injury from chemical, radiation or thermal burns, or penetration of foreign bodies.

The use of a combination drug with an anti-infective component is indicated where the risk of superficial ocular infection is high or where there is an expectation that potentially dangerous numbers of bacteria will be present in the eye.

The particular anti-infective drug in this product is active against the following common bacterial eye pathogens:

Staphylococci, including *S. aureus* and *S. epidermidis* (coagulase-positive and coagulase-negative), including penicillin-resistant strains.

Streptococci, including some of the Group A-beta-hemolytic species, some nonhemolytic species, and some *Streptococcus pneumoniae.* *Pseudomonas aeruginosa, Escherichia coli, Klebsiella pneumoniae, Enterobacter aerogenes, Proteus mirabilis, Morganella morganii,* most *Proteus vulgaris* strains, *Haemophilus influenzae* and *H. aegyptius, Moraxella lacunata, Acinetobacter calcoaceticus* and some *Neisseria* species.

Contraindications: Epithelial herpes simplex keratitis (dendritic keratitis), vaccinia, varicella, and many other viral diseases of the cornea and conjunctiva. Mycobacterial infection of the eye. Fungal diseases of ocular structures. Hypersensitivity to a component of the medication.

Warnings: NOT FOR INJECTION INTO THE EYE. Sensitivity to topically applied aminoglycosides may occur in some patients. If a sensitivity reaction does occur, discontinue use. Prolonged use of steroids may result in glaucoma, with damage to the optic nerve, defects in visual acuity and fields of vision, and posterior subcapsular cataract formation. Intraocular pressure should be routinely monitored even though it may be difficult in pediatric patients and uncooperative patients. Prolonged use may suppress the host response and thus increase the hazard of secondary ocular infections. In those diseases causing thinning of the cornea or sclera, perforations have been known to occur with the use of topical steroids. In acute purulent conditions of the eye, steroids may mask infection or enhance existing infection.

Precautions:

General. The possibility of fungal infections of the cornea should be considered after long-term steroid dosing. As with other antibiotic preparations, prolonged use may result in overgrowth of nonsusceptible organisms, including fungi. If superinfection occurs, appropriate therapy should be initiated. When multiple prescriptions are required, or whenever clinical judgement dictates, the patient should be examined with the aid of magnification, such as slit lamp biomicroscopy and, where appropriate, fluorescein staining.

Cross-sensitivity to other aminoglycoside antibiotics may occur; if hypersensitivity develops with this product, discontinue use and institute appropriate therapy.

Ophthalmic ointment may retard corneal wound healing.

Patients should be advised not to wear contact lenses if they have signs and symptoms of bacterial ocular infection.

Information for Patients: Do not touch tube tip to any surface, as this may contaminate the contents. Contact lenses should not be worn during the use of this product.

Do not use the product if the imprinted carton seals have been damaged, or removed.

Carcinogenesis, Mutagenesis, Impairment of Fertility. No studies have been conducted to evaluate the carcinogenic or mutagenic potential. No impairment of fertility was noted in studies of subcutaneous tobramycin in rats at doses of 50 and 100 mg/kg/day.

Pregnancy Category C. Corticosteroids have been found to be teratogenic in animal studies. Ocular administration of 0.1% dexamethasone resulted in 15.6% and 32.3% incidence of fetal anomalies in two groups of pregnant rabbits. Fetal growth retardation and increased mortality rates have been observed in rats with chronic dexamethasone therapy. Reproduction studies have been performed in rats and rabbits with tobramycin at doses up to 100 mg/kg/day parenterally and have revealed no evidence of impaired fertility or harm to the fetus. There are no adequate and well controlled studies in pregnant women. TOBRADEX® (tobramycin and dexamethasone ophthalmic ointment) should be used during pregnancy only if the potential benefit justifies the potential risk to the fetus.

Nursing Mothers. Systemically administered corticosteroids appear in human milk and could suppress growth, interfere with endogenous corticosteroid production, or cause other untoward effects. It is not known whether topical administration of corticosteroids could result in sufficient systemic absorption to produce detectable quantities in human milk. Because many drugs are excreted in human milk, caution should be exercised when TOBRADEX® (tobramycin and dexamethasone ophthalmic ointment) is administered to a nursing woman.

Pediatric Use: Safety and effectiveness in pediatric patients below the age of 2 years have not been established.

Geriatric Use: No overall clinical differences in safety or effectiveness have been observed between the elderly and other adult patients.

Adverse Reactions: Adverse reactions have occurred with steroid/anti-infective combination drugs which can be attributed to the steroid component, the anti-infective component, or the combination. Exact incidence figures are not available. The most frequent adverse reactions to topical ocular tobramycin (TOBREX® tobramycin ophthalmic ointment) are hypersensitivity and localized ocular toxicity, including lid itching and swelling, and conjunctival erythema. These reactions occur in less than 4% of patients. Similar reactions may occur with the topical use of other aminoglycoside antibiotics. Other adverse reactions have not been reported; however, if topical ocular tobramycin is administered concomitantly with systemic aminoglycoside antibiotics, care should be taken to monitor the total serum concentration. The reactions due to the steroid component are: elevation of intraocular pressure (IOP) with possible development of glaucoma, and infrequent optic nerve damage; posterior subcapsular cataract formation; and delayed wound healing.

Secondary Infection. The development of secondary infection has occurred after use of combinations containing steroids and antimicrobials. Fungal infections of the cornea are particularly prone to develop coincidentally with long-term applications of steroids. The possibility of fungal invasion must be considered in any persistent corneal ulceration where steroid treatment has been used. Secondary bacterial ocular infection following suppression of host responses also occurs.

Overdosage: Clinically apparent signs and symptoms of an overdose of TOBRADEX® (tobramycin and dexamethasone ophthalmic ointment) (punctate keratitis, erythema, increased lacrimation, edema and lid itching) may be similar to adverse reaction effects seen in some patients.

Dosage and Administration: Apply a small amount (approximately ½ inch ribbon) into the conjunctival sac(s) up to three or four times daily.

How to apply TOBRADEX® (tobramycin and dexamethasone ophthalmic ointment):

1. Tilt your head back.
2. Place a finger on your cheek just under your eye and gently pull down until a "V" pocket is formed between your eyeball and your lower lid.
3. Place a small amount (about ½ inch) of TOBRADEX® (tobramycin and dexamethasone ophthalmic ointment) in the "V" pocket. Do not let the tip of the tube touch your eye.
4. Look downward before closing your eye.

Not more than 8 g should be prescribed initially and the prescription should not be refilled without further evaluation as outlined in PRECAUTIONS above.

How Supplied: 3.5 g STERILE ointment supplied in an aluminum tube with a white polyethylene tip and white polyethylene cap. (NDC 0065-0648-35).

Storage: Store at 8°–27°C (46°–80°F).

℞ Only

U.S. Patent No. 5,149,694

©2002, 2003 Alcon, Inc.

Alcon®

Manufactured for:

Alcon Laboratories, Inc.

Fort Worth, Texas 76134 USA

Manufactured by:

S.A. Alcon-Couvieur N.V.

Puurs, Belgium

TRAVATAN® ℞

[*tra-va-tan*]

(travoprost ophthalmic solution) 0.004%

Sterile

Description: Travoprost is a synthetic prostaglandin $F_{2\alpha}$ analogue. Its chemical name is isopropyl (Z)-7-[(1R,2R,3R,5 S)-3, 5-dihydroxy-2-[(1E, 3R)-3-hydroxy-4-[(α,α,α-trifluoro-m-tolyl)oxy]-1-butenyl]cyclopentyl]-5-heptenoate. It has a molecular formula of $C_{26}H_{35}F_3O_6$ and a molecular weight of 500.56.

Travoprost is a clear, colorless to slightly yellow oil that is very soluble in acetonitrile, methanol, octanol, and chloroform. It is practically insoluble in water.

TRAVATAN® 0.004% is supplied as sterile, buffered aqueous solution of travoprost with a pH of approximately 6.0 and an osmolality of approximately 290 mOsmol/kg.

Each mL of TRAVATAN® Ophthalmic Solution 0.004% contains 40 μg travoprost. Benzalkonium chloride 0.015% is added as a preservative. Inactive ingredients are: polyoxyl 40 hydrogenated castor oil, tromethamine, boric acid, mannitol, edetate disodium, sodium hydroxide and/or hydrochloric acid (to adjust pH) and purified water.

Clinical Pharmacology:

Mechanism of Action

Travoprost free acid is a selective FP prostanoid receptor agonist which is believed to reduce intraocular pressure by increasing uveoscleral outflow. The exact mechanism of action is unknown at this time.

Pharmacokinetics/Pharmacodynamics

Absorption: Travoprost is absorbed through the cornea and is hydrolyzed to the active free acid. Data from four multiple dose pharmacokinetic studies (totaling 107 subjects) have shown that plasma concentrations of the free acid are below 0.01 ng/mL (the quantitation limit of the assay) in two-thirds of the subjects. In those individuals with quantifiable plasma concentrations (N=38), the mean plasma C_{max} was 0.018 ± 007 ng/mL (ranged 0.01 to 0.052 ng/mL) and was reached within 30 minutes. From these studies, travoprost is estimated to have a plasma half-life of 45 minutes. There was no difference in plasma concentrations between Days 1 and 7, indicating steady-state was reached early and that there was no significant accumulation.

Metabolism: Travoprost, an isopropyl ester prodrug, is hydrolyzed by esterases in the cornea to its biologically active free acid. Systemically, travoprost free acid is metabolized to inactive metabolites via beta-oxidation of the α(carboxylic acid) chain to give the 1,2-dinor and 1,2,3,4-tetranor analogs, via oxidation of the 15-hydroxyl moiety, as well as via reduction of the 13,14 double bond.

Elimination: The elimination of travoprost free acid from plasma was rapid and levels were generally below the limit of quantification within one hour after dosing. The terminal elimination half-life of travoprost free acid was estimated from fourteen subjects and ranged from 17 minutes to 86 minutes with the mean half-life of 45 minutes. Less than 2% of the topical ocular dose of travoprost was excreted in the urine within 4 hours as the travoprost free acid.

Clinical Studies

In clinical studies, patients with open-angle glaucoma or ocular hypertension and baseline pressure of 25–27 mm Hg who were treated with TRAVATAN® 0.004% dosed once-daily in the evening demonstrated 7–8 mm Hg reductions in intraocular pressure. In subgroup analyses of these studies, mean IOP reduction in black patients was up to 1.8 mm Hg greater

Continued on next page

Travatan—Cont.

than in non-black patients. It is not known at this time whether this difference is attributed to race or to heavily pigmented irides.

In a multi-center, randomized, controlled trial, patients with mean baseline intraocular pressure of 24–26 mm Hg on TIMOPTIC*0.5% BID who were treated with TRAVATAN® Ophthalmic Solution 0.004% dosed QD adjunctively to TIMOPTIC* 0.5% BID demonstrated 6–7 mm Hg reductions in intraocular pressure.

TRAVATAN® has been studied in patients with hepatic impairment and also in patients with renal impairment. No clinically relevant changes in hematology, blood chemistry, or urinalysis laboratory data were observed in these patients.

Indications and Usage: TRAVATAN® Ophthalmic Solution is indicated for the reduction of elevated intraocular pressure in patients with open-angle glaucoma or ocular hypertension who are intolerant of other intraocular pressure lowering medications or insufficiently responsive (failed to achieve target IOP determined after multiple measurements over time) to another intraocular pressure lowering medication.

Contraindications: TRAVATAN® is contraindicated in patients with hypersensitivity to travoprost, benzalkonium chloride or any other ingredients in this product.

Warnings: TRAVATAN® has been reported to cause changes to pigmented tissues. The most frequently reported changes have been increased pigmentation of the iris and periorbital tissue (eyelid) and increased pigmentation and growth of eyelashes. These changes may be permanent.

TRAVATAN® may gradually change eye color, increasing the amount of brown pigmentation in the iris by increasing the number of melanosomes (pigment granules) in melanocytes. The long term effects on the melanocytes and the consequences of potential injury to the melanocytes and/or deposition of pigment granules to other areas of the eye are currently unknown. The change in iris color occurs slowly and may not be noticeable for months to years. Patients should be informed of the possibility of iris color change.

Eyelid skin darkening has been reported in association with the use of TRAVATAN®.

TRAVATAN® Ophthalmic Solution may gradually change eyelashes in the treated eye; these changes include increased length, thickness, pigmentation, and/or number of lashes. Patients who are expected to receive treatment in only one eye should be informed about the potential for increased brown pigmentation of the iris, periorbital and/or eyelid tissue, and eyelashes in the treated eye and thus heterochromia between the eyes. They should also be advised of the potential for a disparity between the eyes in length, thickness, and/or number of eyelashes.

Precautions:
General

There have been reports of bacterial keratitis associated with the use of multiple-dose containers of topical ophthalmic products. These containers had been inadvertently contaminated by patients who, in most cases, had a concurrent corneal disease or a disruption of the epithelial surface (see Information for Patients).

Patients may slowly develop increased brown pigmentation of the iris. This change may not be noticeable for months to years (see Warnings). Iris pigmentation changes may be more noticeable in patients with mixed colored irides, i.e., blue-brown, grey-brown, yellow-brown, and green-brown; however, it has also been observed in patients with brown eyes. The color change is believed to be due to increased melanin content in the stromal mel-

anocytes of the iris. The exact mechanism of action is unknown at this time. Typically the brown pigmentation around the pupil spreads concentrically towards the periphery in affected eyes, but the entire iris or parts of it may become more brownish. Until more information about increased brown pigmentation is available, patients should be examined regularly and, depending on the situation, treatment may be stopped if increased pigmentation ensues.

TRAVATAN® should be used with caution in patients with a history of intraocular inflammation (iritis/uveitis) and should generally not be used in patients with active intraocular inflammation.

Macular edema, including cystoid macular edema, has been reported during treatment with prostaglandin $F_{2\alpha}$ analogues. These reports have mainly occurred in aphakic patients, pseudophakic patients with a torn posterior lens capsule, or in patients with known risk factors for macular edema. TRAVATAN® Ophthalmic Solution should be used with caution in these patients.

TRAVATAN® has not been evaluated for the treatment of angle closure, inflammatory or neovascular glaucoma.

TRAVATAN® Ophthalmic Solution should not be administered while wearing contact lenses. Patients should be advised that TRAVATAN® contains benzalkonium chloride which may be absorbed by contact lenses. Contact lenses should be removed prior to the administration of the solution. Lenses may be reinserted 15 minutes following administration of TRAVATAN®.

Information for Patients
Patients should be advised concerning all the information contained in the Warnings and Precautions sections.

Patients should also be instructed to avoid allowing the tip of the dispensing container to contact the eye or surrounding structures because this could cause the tip to become contaminated by common bacteria known to cause ocular infections. Serious damage to the eye and subsequent loss of vision may result from using contaminated solutions.

Patients also should be advised that if they develop an intercurrent ocular condition (e.g., trauma, or infection) or have ocular surgery, they should immediately seek their physician's advice concerning the continued use of the multi-dose container.

Patients should be advised that if they develop any ocular reactions, particularly conjunctivitis and lid reactions, they should immediately seek their physician's advice.

If more than one topical ophthalmic drug is being used, the drugs should be administered at least five (5) minutes apart.

Carcinogenesis, Mutagenesis, Impairment of Fertility
Two-year carcinogenicity studies in mice and rats at subcutaneous doses of 10, 30, or 100 µg/kg/day did not show any evidence of carcinogenic potential. However, at 100 µg/kg/day, male rats were only treated for 82 weeks, and the maximum tolerated dose (MTD) was not reached in the mouse study. The high dose (100 µg/kg) corresponds to exposure levels over 400 times the human exposure at the maximum recommended human ocular dose (MRHOD) of 0.04 µg/kg, based on plasma active drug levels.

Travoprost was not mutagenic in the Ames test, mouse micronucleus test or rat chromosome aberration assay. A slight increase in the mutant frequency was observed in one of two mouse lymphoma assays in the presence of rat S-9 activation enzymes.

Travoprost did not affect mating or fertility indices in male or female rats at subcutaneous doses up to 10 µg/kg/day [250 times the maximum recommended human ocular dose of

0.04 µg/kg/day on a µg/kg basis (MRHOD)]. At 10 µg/kg/day, the mean number of corpora lutea was reduced, and the post-implantation losses were increased. These effects were not observed at 3 µg/kg/day (75 times the MRHOD).

Pregnancy: Teratogenic Effects
Pregnancy Category: C
Travoprost was teratogenic in rats, at an intravenous (IV) dose up to 10 µg/kg/day (250 times the MRHOD), evidenced by an increase in the incidence of skeletal malformations as well as external and visceral malformations, such as fused sternebrae, domed head and hydrocephaly. Travoprost was not teratogenic in rats at IV doses up to 3 µg/kg/day (75 times the MRHOD), and in mice at subcutaneous doses up to 1.0 µg/kg/day (25 times the MRHOD). Travoprost produced an increase in post-implantation losses and a decrease in fetal viability in rats at IV doses >3 µg/kg/day (75 times the MRHOD) and in mice at subcutaneous doses >0.3 µg/kg/day (7.5 times the MRHOD). In the offspring of female rats that received travoprost subcutaneously from Day 7 of pregnancy to lactation Day 21 at the doses of ≥ 0.12 µg/kg/day (3 times the MRHOD), the incidence of postnatal mortality was increased, and neonatal body weight gain was decreased. Neonatal development was also affected, evidenced by delayed eye opening, pinna detachment and preputial separation, and by decreased motor activity.

There are no adequate and well-controlled studies in pregnant women. TRAVATAN® should be used during pregnancy only if the potential benefit justifies the potential risk to the fetus.

Nursing Mothers
A study in lactating rats demonstrated that radiolabeled travoprost and/or its metabolites were excreted in milk. It is not known whether this drug or its metabolites are excreted in human milk. Because many drugs are excreted in human milk, caution should be exercised when TRAVATAN® is administered to a nursing woman.

Pediatric Use
Safety and effectiveness in pediatric patients have not been established.

Geriatric Use
No overall differences in safety or effectiveness have been observed between elderly and other adult patients.

Adverse Reactions: The most common ocular adverse event observed in controlled clinical studies with TRAVATAN® 0.004% was ocular hyperemia which was reported in 35 to 50% of patients. Approximately 3% of patients discontinued therapy due to conjunctival hyperemia.

Ocular adverse events reported at an incidence of 5 to 10% included decreased visual acuity, eye discomfort, foreign body sensation, pain, and pruritus.

Ocular adverse events reported at an incidence of 1 to 4% included abnormal vision, blepharitis, blurred vision, cataract, cells, conjunctivitis, dry eye, eye disorder, flare, iris discoloration, keratitis, lid margin crusting, photophobia, subconjunctival hemorrhage, and tearing.

Nonocular adverse events reported at a rate of 1 to 5% were accidental injury, angina pectoris, anxiety, arthritis, back pain, bradycardia, bronchitis, chest pain, cold syndrome, depression, dyspepsia, gastrointestinal disorder, headache, hypercholesterolemia, hypertension, hypotension, infection, pain, prostate disorder, sinusitis, urinary incontinence, and urinary tract infection.

Dosage and Administration: The recommended dosage is one drop in the affected eye(s) once-daily in the evening. The dosage of TRAVATAN® should not exceed once-daily since it has been shown that more frequent administration may decrease the intraocular pressure lowering effect.

Reduction of intraocular pressure starts approximately 2 hours after administration and the maximum effect is reached after 12 hours. TRAVATAN® may be used concomitantly with other topical ophthalmic drug products to lower intraocular pressure. If more than one topical ophthalmic drug is being used, the drugs should be administered at least five (5) minutes apart.

How Supplied: TRAVATAN® (travoprost ophthalmic solution) 0.004% is a sterile, isotonic, buffered, preserved, aqueous solution of travoprost (0.04 mg/mL) supplied in Alcon's oval DROP-TAINER® package system.

TRAVATAN® is supplied as a 2.5 mL solution in a 4 mL and a 5 mL solution in a 7.5 mL natural polypropylene dispenser bottle with a natural polypropylene dropper tip and a turquoise polypropylene overcap. Tamper evidence is provided with a shrink band around the closure and neck area of the package.

NDC 0065-0266-25, 2.5 mL fill
NDC 0065-0266-17, 2 units, 2.5 mL fill each
NDC 0065-0266-34, 5 mL fill

Storage
Store at 2°-25°C (36°-77°F).

Rx Only
U.S. Patent Nos. 5,631,287; 5,849,792; 5,889,052; 6,011,062 and 6,235,781.

*TIMOPTIC is a registered trademark of Merck & Co., Inc.
© 2004 Alcon, Inc.

TRAVATAN® Z   Rx

[tra-va-tan]
(travoprost ophthalmic solution) 0.004%
Sterile

Description: Travoprost is a synthetic prostaglandin $F_{2\alpha}$ analogue. Its chemical name is $[1R-[1\alpha(Z),2\beta(1E,3R^*),3\alpha,5\alpha]]$-7-[3,5-Dihydroxy-2-[3-hydroxy-4-[3-(trifluoromethyl)phenoxy]-1-butenyl]cyclopentyl]-5-heptenoic acid, 1-methylethylester. It has a molecular formula of $C_{26}H_{35}F_3O_6$ and a molecular weight of 500.55. Travoprost is a clear, colorless to slightly yellow oil that is very soluble in acetonitrile, methanol, octanol, and chloroform. It is practically insoluble in water.

TRAVATAN® Z ophthalmic solution is supplied as sterile, buffered aqueous solution of travoprost with a pH of approximately 5.7 and an osmolality of approximately 290 mOsmol/kg. Each mL of TRAVATAN® Z contains: Active: travoprost 0.004%. Inactives: polyoxyl 40 hydrogenated castor oil, *sof*Zia™ (boric acid, propylene glycol, sorbitol, zinc chloride), sodium hydroxide and/or hydrochloric acid to adjust pH, and purified water, USP. Preserved in the bottle with an ionic buffered system, *sof*Zia™.

Clinical Pharmacology:
Mechanism of Action
Travoprost free acid is a selective FP prostanoid receptor agonist which is believed to reduce intraocular pressure by increasing trabecular meshwork and uveoscleral outflow. The exact mechanism of action is unknown at this time.

Pharmacokinetics/Pharmacodynamics
Absorption:
Travoprost is absorbed through the cornea and is hydrolyzed to the active free acid. Data from four multiple dose pharmacokinetic studies (totaling 107 subjects) have shown that plasma concentrations of the free acid are below 0.01 ng/mL (the quantitation limit of the assay) in two-thirds of the subjects. In those individuals with quantifiable plasma concentrations (N = 38), the mean plasma C_{max} was

0.018 ± 007 ng/mL (ranged 0.01 to 0.052 ng/mL) and was reached within 30 minutes. From these studies, travoprost is estimated to have a plasma half-life of 45 minutes. There was no difference in plasma concentrations between Days 1 and 7, indicating that there was no significant accumulation.

Metabolism:
Travoprost, an isopropyl ester prodrug, is hydrolyzed by esterases in the cornea to its biologically active free acid. Systemically, travoprost free acid is metabolized to inactive metabolites via beta-oxidation of the α(carboxylic acid) chain to give the 1,2-dinor and 1,2,3,4-tetranor analogs, via oxidation of the 15-hydroxyl moiety, as well as via reduction of the 13,14 double bond.

Elimination:
The elimination of travoprost free acid from plasma was rapid and levels were generally below the limit of quantification within one hour after dosing. The terminal elimination half-life of travoprost free acid was estimated from fourteen subjects and ranged from 17 minutes to 86 minutes with the mean half-life of 45 minutes. Less than 2% of the topical ocular dose of travoprost was excreted in the urine within 4 hours as the travoprost free acid.

Clinical Studies
In clinical studies, patients with open-angle glaucoma or ocular hypertension and baseline pressure of 25–27 mm Hg, who were treated with TRAVATAN® (travoprost ophthalmic solution) or TRAVATAN®Z (travoprost ophthalmic solution) dosed once-daily in the evening demonstrated 7–8 mm Hg reduction in intraocular pressure. In subgroup analysis of this study, mean IOP reduction in black patients was up to 1.8 mm Hg greater than in nonblack patients. It is not known at this time whether this difference is attributed to race or to heavily pigmented irides.

In a multi-center, randomized, controlled trial, patients with mean baseline intraocular pressure of 24–26 mm Hg on TIMOPTIC* 0.5% BID who were treated with travoprost 0.004% dosed QD adjunctively to TIMOPTIC* 0.5% BID demonstrated 6–7 mm Hg reductions in intraocular pressure.

Travoprost ophthalmic solution, 0.004% has been studied in patients with hepatic impairment and also in patients with renal impairment. No clinically relevant changes in hematology, blood chemistry, or urinalysis laboratory data were observed in these patients.

Indications and Usage: TRAVATAN® Z ophthalmic solution is indicated for the reduction of elevated intraocular pressure in patients with open-angle glaucoma or ocular hypertension who are intolerant of other intraocular pressure lowering medications or insufficiently responsive (failed to achieve target IOP determined after multiple measurements over time) to another intraocular pressure lowering medication.

Contraindications: TRAVATAN® Z is contraindicated in patients with hypersensitivity to travoprost or any other ingredients in this product.

Warnings: Prostaglandin analogues, including travoprost ophthalmic solution, 0.004% have been reported to cause changes to pigmented tissues. The most frequently reported changes have been increased pigmentation of the iris and periorbital tissue (eyelid) and increased pigmentation and growth of eyelashes. These changes may be permanent.

Prostaglandin analogues, including travoprost ophthalmic solution, 0.004% may gradually change eye color, increasing the amount of brown pigmentation in the iris by increasing the number of melanosomes (pigment granules) in melanocytes. The long term effects on the melanocytes and the consequences of potential injury to the melanocytes and/or deposition of pigment granules to other areas of the eye are currently unknown. The change in iris color occurs slowly and may not be noticeable for months to years. Patients should be informed of the possibility of iris color change. Eyelid skin darkening has been reported in association with the use of prostaglandin analogues, including travoprost ophthalmic solution, 0.004%.

Prostaglandin analogues, including travoprost ophthalmic solution, 0.004% may gradually change eyelashes in the treated eye; these changes include increased length, thickness, pigmentation, and/or number of lashes.

Patients who are expected to receive treatment in only one eye should be informed about the potential for increased brown pigmentation of the iris, periorbital and/or eyelid tissue, and eyelashes in the treated eye and thus heterochromia between the eyes. They should also be advised of the potential for a disparity between the eyes in length, thickness, and/or number of eyelashes.

Precautions:
General
There have been reports of bacterial keratitis associated with the use of multiple-dose containers of topical ophthalmic products. These containers had been inadvertently contaminated by patients who, in most cases, had a concurrent corneal disease or a disruption of the epithelial surface (see **Information for Patients**).

Patients may slowly develop increased brown pigmentation of the iris. This change may not be noticeable for months to years (see **WARNINGS**). Iris pigmentation changes may be more noticeable in patients with mixed colored irides, i.e., blue-brown, grey-brown, yellow-brown, and green-brown; however, it has also been observed in patients with brown eyes. The color change is believed to be due to increased melanin content in the stromal melanocytes of the iris. The exact mechanism of action is unknown at this time. Typically the brown pigmentation around the pupil spreads concentrically towards the periphery in affected eyes, but the entire iris or parts of it may become more brownish. Until more information about increased brown pigmentation is available, patients should be examined regularly and, depending on the situation, treatment may be stopped if increased pigmentation ensues.

TRAVATAN® Z ophthalmic solution should be used with caution in patients with a history of intraocular inflammation (iritis/uveitis) and should generally not be used in patients with active intraocular inflammation.

Macular edema, including cystoid macular edema, has been reported during treatment with prostaglandin $F_{2\alpha}$ analogues. These reports have mainly occurred in aphakic patients, pseudophakic patients with a torn posterior lens capsule, or in patients with known risk factors for macular edema. TRAVATAN® Z should be used with caution in these patients. TRAVATAN® Z has not been evaluated for the treatment of angle closure, inflammatory or neovascular glaucoma.

Information for Patients
Patients should be advised concerning all the information contained in the Warnings and Precautions sections. Patients should also be instructed to avoid allowing the tip of the dispensing container to contact the eye or surrounding structures because this could cause the tip to become contaminated by common bacteria known to cause ocular infections. Serious damage to the eye and subsequent loss of vision may result from using contaminated solutions.

Patients also should be advised that if they develop an intercurrent ocular condition (e.g.,

Continued on next page

Travatan Z—Cont.

trauma, or infection) or have ocular surgery, they should immediately seek their physician's advice concerning the continued use of the multi-dose container.

Patients should be advised that if they develop any ocular reactions, particularly conjunctivitis and lid reactions, they should immediately seek their physician's advice.

If more than one topical ophthalmic drug is being used, the drugs should be administered at least five (5) minutes apart.

Carcinogenesis, Mutagenesis, Impairment of Fertility

Two-year carcinogenicity studies in mice and rats at subcutaneous doses of 10, 30, or 100 µg/kg/day did not show any evidence of carcinogenic potential. However, at 100 µg/kg/day, male rats were only treated for 82 weeks, and the maximum tolerated dose (MTD) was not reached in the mouse study. The high dose (100 µg/kg) corresponds to exposure levels over 400 times the human exposure at the maximum recommended human ocular dose (MRHOD) of 0.04 µg/kg, based on plasma active drug levels.

Travoprost was not mutagenic in the Ames test, mouse micronucleus test and rat chromosome aberration assay. A slight increase in the mutant frequency was observed in one of two mouse lymphoma assays in the presence of rat S-9 activation enzymes.

Travoprost did not affect mating or fertility indices in male or female rats at subcutaneous doses up to 10 µg/kg/day [250 times the maximum recommended human ocular dose of 0.04 µg/kg/day on a µg/kg basis (MRHOD)]. At 10 µg/kg/day, the mean number of corpora lutea was reduced, and the post-implantation losses were increased. These effects were not observed at 3 µg/kg/day (75 times the MRHOD).

Pregnancy: Teratogenic Effects
Pregnancy Category: C
Travoprost was teratogenic in rats, at an intravenous (IV) dose up to 10 µg/kg/day (250 times the MRHOD), evidenced by an increase in the incidence of skeletal malformations as well as external and visceral malformations, such as fused sternebrae, domed head and hydrocephaly.

Travoprost was not teratogenic in rats at IV doses up to 3 µg/kg/day (75 times the MRHOD), or in mice at subcutaneous doses up to 1.0 µg/kg/day (25 times the MRHOD). Travoprost produced an increase in post-implantation losses and a decrease in fetal viability in rats at IV doses > 3 µg/kg/day (75 times the MRHOD) and in mice at subcutaneous doses > 0.3 µg/kg/day (7.5 times the MRHOD). In the offspring of female rats that received travoprost subcutaneously from Day 7 of pregnancy to lactation Day 21 at the doses of ≥ 0.12 µg/kg/day (3 times the MRHOD), the incidence of postnatal mortality was increased, and neonatal body weight gain was decreased. Neonatal development was also affected, evidenced by delayed eye opening, pinna detachment and preputial separation, and by decreased motor activity.

There are no adequate and well-controlled studies in pregnant women. TRAVATAN® Z should be used during pregnancy only if the potential benefit justifies the potential risk to the fetus.

Nursing Mothers
A study in lactating rats demonstrated that radiolabeled travoprost and/or its metabolites were excreted in milk. It is not known whether this drug or its metabolites are excreted in human milk. Because many drugs are excreted in

human milk, caution should be exercised when TRAVATAN® Z ophthalmic solution is administered to a nursing woman.

Pediatric Use
Safety and effectiveness in pediatric patients have not been established.

Geriatric Use
No overall differences in safety or effectiveness have been observed between elderly and other adult patients.

Adverse Reactions: The most common adverse event observed in controlled clinical studies with TRAVATAN® (travoprost ophthalmic solution) 0.004% and TRAVATAN® Z (travoprost ophthalmic solution) 0.004% was ocular hyperemia which was reported in 30 to 50% of patients. Up to 3% of patients discontinued therapy due to subconjunctival hyperemia.

Ocular adverse events reported at an incidence of 5 to 10% in these clinical studies included decreased visual acuity, eye discomfort, foreign body sensation, pain and pruritus.

Ocular adverse events reported at an incidence of 1 to 4% in clinical studies with TRAVATAN® or TRAVATAN® Z included abnormal vision, blepharitis, blurred vision, cataract, cells, conjunctivitis, corneal staining, dry eye, eye disorder, flare, iris discoloration, keratitis, lid margin crusting, photophobia, subconjunctival hemorrhage, and tearing.

Nonocular adverse events reported at an incidence of 1 to 5% in these clinical studies were accidental injury, allergy, angina pectoris, anxiety, arthritis, back pain, bradycardia, bronchitis, chest pain, cold/flu syndrome, depression, dyspepsia, gastrointestinal disorder, headache, hypercholesterolemia, hypertension, hypotension, infection, pain, prostate disorder, sinusitis, urinary incontinence, and urinary tract infection.

Dosage and Administration: The recommended dosage is one drop in the affected eye(s) once-daily in the evening. The dosage of TRAVATAN®Z ophthalmic solution should not exceed once-daily since it has been shown that more frequent administration of travoprost may decrease the intraocular pressure lowering effect.

Reduction of intraocular pressure starts approximately 2 hours after administration of travoprost. The maximum effect is observed 12 hours after administration and is maintained throughout the day.

TRAVATAN® Z may be used concomitantly with other topical ophthalmic drug products to lower intraocular pressure. If more than one topical ophthalmic drug is being used, the drugs should be administered at least five (5) minutes apart.

How Supplied: TRAVATAN® Z (travoprost ophthalmic solution) 0.004% is a sterile, isotonic, buffered, preserved, aqueous solution of travoprost (0.04 mg/mL) supplied in Alcon's oval DROP-TAINER® package system.

TRAVATAN® Z is supplied as a 2.5 mL solution in a 4 mL and a 5 mL solution in a 7.5 mL natural polypropylene dispenser bottle with a natural polypropylene dropper tip and a turquoise polypropylene overcap. Tamper evidence is provided with a shrink band around the closure and neck area of the package.

2.5 mL fill in 4 mL bottle **NDC** 0065-0260-25
5 mL fill in 7.5 mL bottle **NDC** 0065-0260-05
Storage: Store at 2° - 25°C (36° - 77°F).
Rx Only
U.S. Patent Nos. 5,889,052 and 6,235,781

---

* TIMOPTIC is a registered trademark of Merck & Co., Inc.
Alcon®
ALCON LABORATORIES, INC.
Fort Worth, Texas 76134 USA
© 2005-2006 Alcon, Inc.

VIGAMOX®   ℞
[*vi-ga-mox*]
**(moxifloxacin hydrochloride ophthalmic solution) ·
0.5% as base**

Description: VIGAMOX® (moxifloxacin HCl ophthalmic solution) 0.5% is a sterile ophthalmic solution. It is an 8-methoxy fluoroquinolone anti-infective for topical ophthalmic use.

Chemical Name: 1-Cyclopropyl-6-fluoro-1,4-dihydro-8-methoxy-7-[(4aS, 7aS)-octahydro-6H-pyrrolol [3, 4-b] pyridin-6-yl]-4-oxo-3-quinolinecarboxylic acid, monohydrochloride. Moxifloxacin hydrochloride is a slightly yellow to yellow crystalline powder. Each mL of VIGAMOX® contains 5.45 mg moxifloxacin hydrochloride equivalent to 5 mg moxifloxacin base.

Contains:
Active: Moxifloxacin 0.5% (5 mg/mL); **Inactives:** Boric acid, sodium chloride, and purified water. May also contain hydrochloric acid/sodium hydroxide to adjust pH to approximately 6.8.

VIGAMOX® solution is an isotonic solution with an osmolality of approximately 290 mOsm/kg.

Clinical Pharmacology:

Pharmacokinetics: Plasma concentrations of moxifloxacin were measured in healthy adult male and female subjects who received bilateral topical ocular doses of VIGAMOX® solution 3 times a day. The mean steady-state C_{max} (2.7 ng/mL) and estimated daily exposure AUC (45 ng·hr/ mL) values were 1,600 and 1,000 times lower than the mean C_{max} and AUC reported after therapeutic 400 mg oral doses of moxifloxacin. The plasma half-life of moxifloxacin was estimated to be 13 hours.

Microbiology:

Moxifloxacin is an 8-methoxy fluoroquinolone with a diazabicyclononyl ring at the C7 position. The antibacterial action of moxifloxacin results from inhibition of the topoisomerase II (DNA gyrase) and topoisomerase IV. DNA gyrase is an essential enzyme that is involved in the replication, transcription and repair of bacterial DNA. Topoisomerase IV is an enzyme known to play a key role in the partitioning of the chromosomal DNA during bacterial cell division.

The mechanism of action for quinolones, including moxifloxacin, is different from that of macrolides, aminoglycosides, or tetracyclines. Therefore, moxifloxacin may be active against pathogens that are resistant to these antibiotics and these antibiotics may be active against pathogens that are resistant to moxifloxacin. There is no cross-resistance between moxifloxacin and the aforementioned classes of antibiotics. Cross resistance has been observed between systemic moxifloxacin and some other quinolones.

In vitro resistance to moxifloxacin develops via multiple-step mutations. Resistance to moxifloxacin occurs *in vitro* at a general frequency of between 1.8×10^{-9} to $<1 \times 10^{-11}$ for Gram-positive bacteria.

Moxifloxacin has been shown to be active against most strains of the following microorganisms, both *in vitro* and in clinical infections as described in the INDICATIONS AND USAGE section:

Aerobic Gram-positive microorganisms:
Corynebacterium species*
*Micrococcus luteus**
Staphylococcus aureus
Staphylococcus epidermidis
Staphylococcus haemolyticus
Staphylococcus hominis
*Staphylococcus warneri**
Streptococcus pneumoniae
Streptococcus viridans *group*

Aerobic Gram-negative microorganisms:
*Acinetobacter lwoffii**
Haemophilus influenzae
*Haemophilus parainfluenzae**
Other microorganisms:
Chlamydia trachomatis

---

*Efficacy for this organism was studied in fewer than 10 infections.

The following *in vitro* data are also available, **but their clinical significance in ophthalmic infections is unknown**. The safety and effectiveness of VIGAMOX® solution in treating ophthalmological infections due to these microorganisms have not been established in adequate and well-controlled trials.

The following organisms are considered susceptible when evaluated using systemic breakpoints. However, a correlation between the *in vitro* systemic breakpoint and ophthalmological efficacy has not been established. The list of organisms is provided as guidance only in assessing the potential treatment of conjunctival infections. Moxifloxacin exhibits *in vitro* minimal inhibitory concentrations (MICs) of 2 µg/ml or less (systemic susceptible breakpoint) against most (≥90%) of strains of the following ocular pathogens.

Aerobic Gram-positive microorganisms:
Listeria monocytogenes
Staphylococcus saprophyticus
Streptococcus agalactiae
Streptococcus mitis
Streptococcus pyogenes
Streptococcus Group C, G and F
Aerobic Gram-negative microorganisms:
Acinetobacter baumannii
Acinetobacter calcoaceticus
Citrobacter freundii
Citrobacter koseri
Enterobacter aerogenes
Enterobacter cloacae
Escherichia coli
Klebsiella oxytoca
Klebsiella pneumoniae
Moraxella catarrhalis
Morganella morganii
Neisseria gonorrhoeae
Proteus mirabilis
Proteus vulgaris
Pseudomonas stutzeri
Anaerobic microorganisms:
Clostridium perfringens
Fusobacterium species
Prevotella species
Propionibacterium acnes
Other microorganisms:
Chlamydia pneumoniae
Legionella pneumophila
Mycobacterium avium
Mycobacterium marinum
Mycoplasma pneumoniae
Clinical Studies:
In two randomized, double-masked, multicenter, controlled clinical trials in which patients were dosed 3 times a day for 4 days, VIGAMOX® solution produced clinical cures on day 5–6 in 66% to 69% of patients treated for bacterial conjunctivitis. Microbiological success rates for the eradication of the baseline pathogens ranged from 84% to 94%. Please note that microbiologic eradication does not always correlate with clinical outcome in anti-infective trials.

Indications and Usage: VIGAMOX® solution is indicated for the treatment of bacterial conjunctivitis caused by susceptible strains of the following organisms:
Aerobic Gram-positive microorganisms:
Corynebacterium species*
*Micrococcus luteus**
Staphylococcus aureus
Staphylococcus epidermidis
Staphylococcus haemolyticus
Staphylococcus hominis
*Staphylococcus warneri**

Streptococcus pneumoniae
Streptococcus viridans *group*
Aerobic Gram-negative microorganisms:
*Acinetobacter lwoffii**
Haemophilus influenzae
*Haemophilus parainfluenzae**
Other microorganisms:
Chlamydia trachomatis

---

*Efficacy for this organism was studied in fewer than 10 infections.

Contraindications: VIGAMOX® solution is contraindicated in patients with a history of hypersensitivity to moxifloxacin, to other quinolones, or to any of the components in this medication.

Warnings: NOT FOR INJECTION.
VIGAMOX® solution should not be injected subconjunctivally, nor should it be introduced directly into the anterior chamber of the eye. In patients receiving systemically administered quinolones, including moxifloxacin, serious and occasionally fatal hypersensitivity (anaphylactic) reactions have been reported, some following the first dose. Some reactions were accompanied by cardiovascular collapse, loss of consciousness, angioedema (including laryngeal, pharyngeal or facial edema), airway obstruction, dyspnea, urticaria, and itching. If an allergic reaction to moxifloxacin occurs, discontinue use of the drug. Serious acute hypersensitivity reactions may require immediate emergency treatment. Oxygen and airway management should be administered as clinically indicated.

Precautions:
General: As with other anti-infectives, prolonged use may result in overgrowth of non-susceptible organisms, including fungi. If superinfection occurs, discontinue use and institute alternative therapy. Whenever clinical judgment dictates, the patient should be examined with the aid of magnification, such as slit-lamp biomicroscopy, and, where appropriate, fluorescein staining. Patients should be advised not to wear contact lenses if they have signs and symptoms of bacterial conjunctivitis.

Information for Patients: Avoid contaminating the applicator tip with material from the eye, fingers or other source. Systemically administered quinolones including moxifloxacin have been associated with hypersensitivity reactions, even following a single dose. Discontinue use immediately and contact your physician at the first sign of a rash or allergic reaction.

Drug Interactions: Drug-drug interaction studies have not been conducted with VIGAMOX® solution. *In vitro* studies indicate that moxifloxacin does not inhibit CYP3A4, CYP2D6, CYP2C9, CYP2C19, or CYP1A2 indicating that moxifloxacin is unlikely to alter the pharmacokinetics of drugs metabolized by these cytochrome P450 isozymes.

Carcinogenesis, Mutagenesis, Impairment of Fertility: Long term studies in animals to determine the carcinogenic potential of moxifloxacin have not been performed. However, in an accelerated study with initiators and promoters, moxifloxacin was not carcinogenic in rats following up to 38 weeks of oral dosing at 500 mg/kg/day (approximately 21,700 times the highest recommended total daily human ophthalmic dose for a 50 kg person, on a mg/kg basis).

Moxifloxacin was not mutagenic in four bacterial strains used in the Ames *Salmonella* reversion assay. As with other quinolones, the positive response observed with moxifloxacin in strain TA 102 using the same assay may be due to the inhibition of DNA gyrase. Moxifloxacin was not mutagenic in the CHO/HGPRT mammalian cell gene mutation assay. An equivocal result was obtained in the same assay when v79 cells were used. Moxifloxacin

was clastogenic in the v79 chromosome aberration assay, but it did not induce unscheduled DNA synthesis in cultured rat hepatocytes. There was no evidence of genotoxicity *in vivo* in a micronucleus test or a dominant lethal test in mice.

Moxifloxacin had no effect on fertility in male and female rats at oral doses as high as 500 mg/kg/day, approximately 21,700 times the highest recommended total daily human ophthalmic dose. At 500 mg/kg orally there were slight effects on sperm morphology (head-tail separation) in male rats and on the estrous cycle in female rats.

Pregnancy: Teratogenic Effects.
Pregnancy Category C: Moxifloxacin was not teratogenic when administered to pregnant rats during organogenesis at oral doses as high as 500 mg/kg/day (approximately 21,700 times the highest recommended total daily human ophthalmic dose); however, decreased fetal body weights and slightly delayed fetal skeletal development were observed. There was no evidence of teratogenicity when pregnant Cynomolgus monkeys were given oral doses as high as 100 mg/kg/day (approximately 4,300 times the highest recommended total daily human ophthalmic dose). An increased incidence of smaller fetuses was observed at 100 mg/kg/day.

Since there are no adequate and well-controlled studies in pregnant women, VIGAMOX® solution should be used during pregnancy only if the potential benefit justifies the potential risk to the fetus.

Nursing Mothers: Moxifloxacin has not been measured in human milk, although it can be presumed to be excreted in human milk. Caution should be exercised when VIGAMOX® solution is administered to a nursing mother.

Pediatric Use: The safety and effectiveness of VIGAMOX® solution in infants below 1 year of age have not been established. There is no evidence that the ophthalmic administration of VIGAMOX® has any effect on weight bearing joints, even though oral administration of some quinolones has been shown to cause arthropathy in immature animals.

Geriatric Use: No overall differences in safety and effectiveness have been observed between elderly and younger patients.

Adverse Reactions: The most frequently reported ocular adverse events were conjunctivitis, decreased visual acuity, dry eye, keratitis, ocular discomfort, ocular hyperemia, ocular pain, ocular pruritus, subconjunctival hemorrhage, and tearing. These events occurred in approximately 1-6% of patients.

Nonocular adverse events reported at a rate of 1-4% were fever, increased cough, infection, otitis media, pharyngitis, rash, and rhinitis.

Dosage and Administration: Instill one drop in the affected eye 3 times a day for 7 days.
How Supplied: VIGAMOX® solution is supplied as a sterile ophthalmic solution in Alcon's DROP-TAINER® dispensing system consisting of a natural low density polyethylene bottle and dispensing plug and tan polypropylene closure. Tamper evidence is provided with a shrink band around the closure and neck area of the package.

3 mL in 6 mL bottle - NDC 0065-4013-03
Storage: Store at 2°C-25°C (36°F-77°F).
Rx Only
Manufactured by
Alcon Laboratories, Inc.
Fort Worth, Texas 76134 USA
Licensed to Alcon, Inc. by Bayer Healthcare AG.
U.S. PAT. NO. 4,990,517; 5,607,942; 6,716,830
© 2003-2006 Alcon, Inc.

Allergan, Inc.
**2525 DUPONT DRIVE
P.O. BOX 19534
IRVINE, CA 92623-9534**

Direct Inquiries to:
(714) 246-4500

ACULAR® ℞
(ketorolac tromethamine
ophthalmic solution) 0.5%
Sterile

Description: ACULAR® (ketorolac tromethamine ophthalmic solution) is a member of the pyrrolo-pyrrole group of nonsteroidal anti- inflammatory drugs (NSAIDs) for ophthalmic use. Its chemical name is (±)-5-benzoyl-2,3-dihydro -1H-pyrrolizine-1-carboxylic acid, compound with 2-amino-2-(hydroxymethyl)-1,3-propanediol (1:1)
ACULAR® ophthalmic solution is supplied as a sterile isotonic aqueous 0.5% solution, with a pH of 7.4. ACULAR® ophthalmic solution is a racemic mixture of R-(+)- and S-(−)-ketorolac tromethamine. Ketorolac tromethamine may exist in three crystal forms. All forms are equally soluble in water. The pKa of ketorolac is 3.5. This white to off-white crystalline substance discolors on prolonged exposure to light. The molecular weight of ketorolac tromethamine is 376.41. The osmolality of ACULAR® ophthalmic solution is 290 mOsml/kg. Each mL of ACULAR® ophthalmic solution contains: **Active:** ketorolac tromethamine 0.5%. **Preservative:** benzalkonium chloride 0.01%. **Inactives:** edetate disodium 0.1%; octoxynol 40; purified water; sodium chloride; hydrochloric acid and/or sodium hydroxide to adjust the pH.
Clinical Pharmacology: Ketorolac tromethamine is a nonsteroidal anti-inflammatory drug which, when administered systemically, has demonstrated analgesic, anti-inflammatory, and anti-pyretic activity. The mechanism of its action is thought to be due to its ability to inhibit prostaglandin biosynthesis. Ketorolac tromethamine given systemically does not cause pupil constriction.
Prostaglandins have been shown in many animal models to be mediators of certain kinds of intraocular inflammation. In studies performed in animal eyes, prostaglandins have been shown to produce disruption of the blood-aqueous humor barrier, vasodilation, increased vascular permeability, leukocytosis, and increased intraocular pressure. Prostaglandins also appear to play a role in the miotic response produced during ocular surgery by constricting the iris sphincter independently of cholinergic mechanisms.
Two drops (0.1 mL) of 0.5% ACULAR® ophthalmic solution instilled into the eyes of patients 12 hours and 1 hour prior to cataract extraction achieved measurable levels in 8 of 9 patients' eyes (mean ketorolac concentration 95 ng/mL aqueous humor, range 40 to 170 ng/mL). Ocular administration of ketorolac tromethamine reduces prostaglandin E_2 (PGE$_2$) levels in aqueous humor. The mean concentration of PGE$_2$ was 80 pg/mL in the aqueous humor of eyes receiving vehicle and 28 pg/mL in the eyes receiving ACULAR® 0.5% ophthalmic solution.
One drop (0.05 mL) of 0.5% ACULAR® ophthalmic solution was instilled into one eye and one drop of vehicle into the other eye TID in 26 normal subjects. Only 5 of 26 subjects had a detectable amount of ketorolac in their plasma (range 10.7 to 22.5 ng/mL) at Day 10 during topical ocular treatment. When

ketorolac tromethamine 10 mg is administered systemically every 6 hours, peak plasma levels at steady state are around 960 ng/mL.
Two controlled clinical studies showed that ACULAR® ophthalmic solution was significantly more effective than its vehicle in relieving ocular itching caused by seasonal allergic conjunctivitis.
Two controlled clinical studies showed that patients treated for two weeks with ACULAR® ophthalmic solution were less likely to have measurable signs of inflammation (cell and flare) than patients treated with its vehicle.
Results from clinical studies indicated that ketorolac tromethamine has no significant effect upon intraocular pressure; however, changes in intraocular pressure may occur following cataract surgery.
Indications and Usage: ACULAR® ophthalmic solution is indicated for the temporary relief of ocular itching due to seasonal allergic conjunctivitis. ACULAR® ophthalmic solution is also indicated for the treatment of postoperative inflammation in patients who have undergone cataract extraction.
Contraindications: ACULAR® ophthalmic solution is contraindicated in patients with previously demonstrated hypersensitivity to any of the ingredients in the formulation.
Warnings: There is the potential for cross-sensitivity to acetylsalicylic acid, phenylacetic acid derivatives, and other nonsteroidal anti- inflammatory agents. Therefore, caution should be used when treating individuals who have previously exhibited sensitivities to these drugs. With some nonsteroidal anti-inflammatory drugs, there exists the potential for increased bleeding time due to interference with thrombocyte aggregation. There have been reports that ocularly applied nonsteroidal anti-inflammatory drugs may cause increased bleeding of ocular tissues (including hyphemas) in conjunction with ocular surgery.
Precautions:
General: All topical nonsteroidal anti-inflammatory drugs (NSAIDs) may slow or delay healing. Topical corticosteroids are also known to slow or delay healing. Concomitant use of topical NSAIDs and topical steroids may increase the potential for healing problems.
Use of topical NSAIDs may result in keratitis. In some susceptible patients, continued use of topical NSAIDs may result in epithelial breakdown, corneal thinning, corneal erosion, corneal ulceration or corneal perforation. These events may be sight threatening. Patients with evidence of corneal epithelial breakdown should immediately discontinue use of topical NSAIDs and should be closely monitored for corneal health.
Postmarketing experience with topical NSAIDs suggests that patients with complicated ocular surgeries, corneal denervation, corneal epithelial defects, diabetes mellitus, ocular surface diseases (e.g., dry eye syndrome), rheumatoid arthritis, or repeat ocular surgeries within a short period of time may be at increased risk for corneal adverse events which may become sight threatening. Topical NSAIDs should be used with caution in these patients.
Postmarketing experience with topical NSAIDs also suggests that use more than 24 hours prior to surgery or use beyond 14 days post-surgery may increase patient risk for the occurrence and severity of corneal adverse events.
It is recommended that ACULAR® ophthalmic solution be used with caution in patients with known bleeding tendencies or who are receiving medications which may prolong bleeding time.
Information for Patients: ACULAR® ophthalmic solution should not be administered while wearing contact lenses.

Carcinogenesis, Mutagenesis, and Impairment of Fertility: Ketorolac tromethamine was not carcinogenic in rats given up to 5 mg/kg/day orally for 24 months (151 times the maximum recommended human topical ophthalmic dose, on a mg/kg basis, assuming 100% absorption in humans and animals) nor in mice given 2 mg/kg/day orally for 18 months (60 times the maximum recommended human topical ophthalmic dose, on a mg/kg basis, assuming 100% absorption in humans and animals).
Ketorolac tromethamine was not mutagenic *in vitro* in the Ames assay or in forward mutation assays. Similarly, it did not result in an *in vitro* increase in unscheduled DNA synthesis or an *in vivo* increase in chromosome breakage in mice. However, ketorolac tromethamine did result in an increased incidence in chromosomal aberrations in Chinese hamster ovary cells.
Ketorolac tromethamine did not impair fertility when administered orally to male and female rats at doses up to 272 and 484 times the maximum recommended human topical ophthalmic dose, respectively, on a mg/kg basis, assuming 100% absorption in humans and animals.
Pregnancy: Teratogenic Effects: Pregnancy Category C. Ketorolac tromethamine, administered during organogenesis, was not teratogenic in rabbits or rats at oral doses up to 109 times and 303 times the maximum recommended human topical ophthalmic dose, respectively, on a mg/kg basis assuming 100% absorption in humans and animals. When administered to rats after Day 17 of gestation at oral doses up to 45 times the maximum recommended human topical ophthalmic dose, respectively, on a mg/kg basis, assuming 100% absorption in humans and animals, ketorolac tromethamine resulted in dystocia and increased pup mortality. There are no adequate and well-controlled studies in pregnant women. ACULAR® ophthalmic solution should be used during pregnancy only if the potential benefit justifies the potential risk to the fetus.
Nonteratogenic Effects: Because of the known effects of prostaglandin-inhibiting drugs on the fetal cardiovascular system (closure of the ductus arteriosus), the use of ACULAR® ophthalmic solution during late pregnancy should be avoided.
Nursing Mothers: Caution should be exercised when ACULAR® ophthalmic solution is administered to a nursing woman.
Pediatric Use: Safety and efficacy in pediatric patients below the age of 3 have not been established.
Geriatric Use: No overall differences in safety or effectiveness have been observed between elderly and younger patients.
Adverse Reactions: The most frequent adverse events reported with the use of ketorolac tromethamine ophthalmic solutions have been transient stinging and burning on instillation. These events were reported by up to 40% of patients participating in clinical trials.
Other adverse events occurring approximately 1 to 10% of the time during treatment with ketorolac tromethamine ophthalmic solutions included allergic reactions, corneal edema, iritis, ocular inflammation, ocular irritation, superficial keratitis and superficial ocular infections.
Other adverse events reported rarely with the use of ketorolac tromethamine ophthalmic solutions included: corneal infiltrates, corneal ulcer, eye dryness, headaches, and visual disturbance (blurry vision).
Clinical Practice: The following events have been identified during postmarketing use of ketorolac tromethamine ophthalmic solution 0.5% in clinical practice. Because they are reported voluntarily from a population of unknown size, estimates of frequency cannot be made. The events, which have been chosen for

inclusion due to either their seriousness, frequency of reporting, possible causal connection to topical ketorolac tromethamine ophthalmic solution 0.5%, or a combination of these factors, include corneal erosion, corneal perforation, corneal thinning and epithelial breakdown (see **Precautions, General**).

Dosage and Administration: The recommended dose of ACULAR® ophthalmic solution is one drop (0.25 mg) four times a day for relief of ocular itching due to seasonal allergic conjunctivitis.

For the treatment of postoperative inflammation in patients who have undergone cataract extraction, one drop of ACULAR® ophthalmic solution should be applied to the affected eye(s) four times daily beginning 24 hours after cataract surgery and continuing through the first 2 weeks of the postoperative period. ACULAR® ophthalmic solution has been safely administered in conjunction with other ophthalmic medications such as antibiotics, beta blockers, carbonic anhydrase inhibitors, cycloplegics, and mydriatics.

How Supplied: ACULAR® (ketorolac tromethamine ophthalmic solution) is supplied sterile in opaque white LDPE plastic bottles with droppers with gray high impact polystyrene (HIPS) caps as follows:

3 mL in 5 mL bottle NDC 0023-2181-03
5 mL in 10 mL bottle NDC 0023-2181-05
10 mL in 10 mL bottle NDC 0023-2181-10
Store at 15°C–25°C (59°F–77°F) with protection from light.

℞ only
Revised January 2004
U.S. Patent 5,110,493.
© 2004 Allergan, Inc., Irvine, CA 92612, U.S.A.
ACULAR®, a registered trademark of Roche Palo Alto LLC, is manufactured and distributed by Allergan, Inc. under license from its developer, Roche Palo Alto LLC, Palo Alto, CA, U.S.A.
71590US11P

ACULAR LS® ℞
[ă-kew-lar]
(ketorolac tromethamine ophthalmic solution) 0.4%
Sterile

Description: ACULAR LS® (ketorolac tromethamine ophthalmic solution) 0.4% is a member of the pyrrolo-pyrrole group of nonsteroidal anti-inflammatory drugs (NSAIDs) for ophthalmic use.

Structural and Molecular Formula:

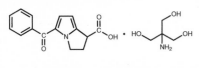

$C_{19}H_{24}N_2O_6$ Mol Wt 376.41

Chemical Name: (±)-5-Benzoyl-2,3-dihydro-1H-pyrrolizine-1-carboxylic acid, compound with 2-amino-2-(hydroxymethyl)-1,3-propanediol (1:1)

Contains: Active: ketorolac tromethamine 0.4%. **Preservative:** benzalkonium chloride 0.006%. **Inactives:** sodium chloride; edetate disodium 0.015%; octoxynol 40; purified water; and hydrochloric acid and/or sodium hydroxide to adjust the pH.

ACULAR LS® ophthalmic solution is supplied as a sterile isotonic aqueous 0.4% solution, with a pH of approximately 7.4. ACULAR LS® ophthalmic solution is a racemic mixture of R-(+) and S-(−)-ketorolac tromethamine. Ketorolac tromethamine may exist in three crystal forms. All forms are equally soluble in water. The pKa of ketorolac is 3.5. This white

to off-white crystalline substance discolors on prolonged exposure to light. The osmolality of ACULAR LS® ophthalmic solution is approximately 290 mOsml/kg.

Clinical Pharmacology:
Mechanism of Action
Ketorolac tromethamine is a nonsteroidal anti-inflammatory drug which, when administered systemically, has demonstrated analgesic, anti-inflammatory, and anti-pyretic activity. The mechanism of its action is thought to be due to its ability to inhibit prostaglandin biosynthesis. Ketorolac tromethamine given systemically does not cause pupil constriction.

Pharmacokinetics
One drop (0.05 mL) of 0.5% ketorolac tromethamine ophthalmic solution was instilled into one eye and one drop of vehicle into the other eye TID in 26 normal subjects. Only 5 of 26 subjects had a detectable amount of ketorolac in their plasma (range 10.7 to 22.5 ng/mL) at day 10 during topical ocular treatment. When ketorolac tromethamine 10 mg is administered systemically every 6 hours, peak plasma levels at steady state are around 960 ng/mL.

Clinical Studies: In two double-masked, multi-centered, parallel-group studies, 313 patients who had undergone photorefractive keratectomy received ACULAR LS® 0.4% or its vehicle QID for up to 4 days. Significant differences favored ACULAR LS® for the reduction of ocular pain and burning/stinging following photorefractive keratectomy surgery.

Results from clinical studies indicate that ketorolac tromethamine has no significant effect upon intraocular pressure.

Indications and Usage: ACULAR LS® ophthalmic solution is indicated for the reduction of ocular pain and burning/stinging following corneal refractive surgery.

Contraindications: ACULAR LS® ophthalmic solution is contraindicated in patients with previously demonstrated hypersensitivity to any of the ingredients in the formulation.

Warnings: There is the potential for cross-sensitivity to acetylsalicylic acid, phenylacetic acid derivatives, and other nonsteroidal anti-inflammatory agents. Therefore, caution should be used when treating individuals who have previously exhibited sensitivities to these drugs. With some nonsteroidal anti-inflammatory drugs there exists the potential for increased bleeding time due to interference with thrombocyte aggregation. There have been reports that ocularly applied nonsteroidal anti-inflammatory drugs may cause increased bleeding of ocular tissues (including hyphemas) in conjunction with ocular surgery.

Precautions:
General: All topical nonsteroidal anti-inflammatory drugs (NSAIDs), including ketorolac tromethamine ophthalmic solution, may slow or delay healing. Topical corticosteroids are also known to slow or delay healing. Concomitant use of topical NSAIDS and topical steroids may increase the potential for healing problems.

Use of topical NSAIDs may result in keratitis. In some susceptible patients, continued use of topical NSAIDs may result in epithelial breakdown, corneal thinning, corneal erosion, corneal ulceration or corneal perforation. These events may be sight threatening. Patients with evidence of corneal epithelial breakdown should immediately discontinue use of topical NSAIDs and should be closely monitored for corneal health.

Postmarketing experience with topical NSAIDs suggests that patients with complicated ocular surgeries, corneal denervation, corneal epithelial defects, diabetes mellitus, ocular surface diseases (e.g., dry eye syndrome), rheumatoid arthritis, or repeat ocular surgeries within a short period of time may be

at increased risk for corneal adverse events which may become sight threatening. Topical NSAIDs should be used with caution in these patients.

Postmarketing experience with topical NSAIDs also suggests that use more than 24 hours prior to surgery or use beyond 14 days post-surgery may increase patient risk for the occurrence and severity of corneal adverse events.

It is recommended that ACULAR LS® ophthalmic solution be used with caution in patients with known bleeding tendencies or who are receiving other medications, which may prolong bleeding time.

Information for Patients: ACULAR LS® ophthalmic solution should not be administered while wearing contact lenses.

Carcinogenesis, Mutagenesis, Impairment of Fertility:
Ketorolac tromethamine was neither carcinogenic in rats given up to 5 mg/kg/day orally for 24 months (156 times the maximum recommended human topical ophthalmic dose, on a mg/kg basis, assuming 100% absorption in humans and animals) nor in mice given 2 mg/kg/day orally for 18 months (62.5 times the maximum recommended human topical ophthalmic dose, on a mg/kg basis, assuming 100% absorption in humans and animals).

Ketorolac tromethamine was not mutagenic *in vitro* in the Ames assay or in forward mutation assays. Similarly, it did not result in an *in vitro* increase in unscheduled DNA synthesis or an *in vivo* increase in chromosome breakage in mice. However, ketorolac tromethamine did result in an increased incidence in chromosomal aberrations in Chinese hamster ovary cells.

Ketorolac tromethamine did not impair fertility when administered orally to male and female rats at doses up to 280 and 499 times the maximum recommended human topical ophthalmic dose, respectively, on a mg/kg basis, assuming 100% absorption in humans and animals.

Pregnancy:
Teratogenic Effects: Pregnancy Category C: Ketorolac tromethamine, administered during organogenesis, was not teratogenic in rabbits or rats at oral doses up to 112 times and 312 times the maximum recommended human topical ophthalmic dose, respectively, on a mg/kg basis assuming 100% absorption in humans and animals. When administered to rats after Day 17 of gestation at oral doses up to 46 times the maximum recommended human topical ophthalmic dose on a mg/kg basis, assuming 100% absorption in humans and animals, ketorolac tromethamine resulted in dystocia and increased pup mortality. There are no adequate and well-controlled studies in pregnant women. ACULAR LS® ophthalmic solution should be used during pregnancy only if the potential benefit justifies the potential risk to the fetus.

Nonteratogenic Effects:
Because of the known effects of prostaglandin-inhibiting drugs on the fetal cardiovascular system (closure of the ductus arteriosus), the use of ACULAR LS® ophthalmic solution during late pregnancy should be avoided.

Nursing Mothers: Caution should be exercised when ACULAR LS® ophthalmic solution is administered to a nursing woman.

Pediatric Use: Safety and effectiveness of ketorolac tromethamine in pediatric patients below the age of 3 have not been established.

Geriatric Use: No overall differences in safety or effectiveness have been observed between elderly and younger patients.

Adverse Reactions: The most frequently reported adverse reactions for ACULAR LS® ophthalmic solution occurring in approximately

Continued on next page

Acular LS—Cont.

1 to 5% of the overall study population were conjunctival hyperemia, corneal infiltrates, headache, ocular edema and ocular pain.

The most frequent adverse events reported with the use of ketorolac tromethamine ophthalmic solutions have been transient stinging and burning on instillation. These events were reported by 20%-40% of patients participating in these other clinical trials.

Other adverse events occurring approximately 1%-10% of the time during treatment with ketorolac tromethamine ophthalmic solutions included allergic reactions, corneal edema, iritis, ocular inflammation, ocular irritation, ocular pain, superficial keratitis, and superficial ocular infections.

Clinical Practice: The following events have been identified during postmarketing use of ketorolac tromethamine ophthalmic solutions in clinical practice. Because they are reported voluntarily from a population of unknown size, estimates of frequency cannot be made. The events, which have been chosen for inclusion due to either their seriousness, frequency of reporting, possible causal connection to topical ketorolac tromethamine ophthalmic solutions, or a combination of these factors, include corneal erosion, corneal perforation, corneal thinning and epithelial breakdown (see **Precautions, General**).

Dosage and Administration: The recommended dose of ACULAR LS® ophthalmic solution is one drop four times a day in the operated eye as needed for pain and burning/stinging for up to 4 days following corneal refractive surgery.

Ketorolac tromethamine ophthalmic solution has been safely administered in conjunction with other ophthalmic medications such as antibiotics, beta blockers, carbonic anhydrase inhibitors, cycloplegics, and mydriatics.

How Supplied: ACULAR LS® (ketorolac tromethamine ophthalmic solution) 0.4% is supplied sterile in an opaque white LDPE plastic bottle with a white dropper with a gray high impact polystyrene (HIPS) cap as follows:

5 mL in 10 mL bottle- NDC 0023-9277-05

Note: Store at 15°C-25°C (59°F-77°F).

℞ only

Revised May 2003

U.S. Pat. 5,110,493

©2003 Allergan, Inc., Irvine, CA 92612, U.S.A.

® marks owned by Allergan, Inc.

ACULAR LS® is a registered trademark of Roche Palto Alto LLC.

This product is manufactured and distributed by Allergan, Inc. under license from its developer, Roche Palo Alto LLC, Palo Alto, CA, U.S.A.

71654US10M

ALBALON® ℞
(naphazoline hydrochloride
ophthalmic solution, USP) 0.1%
Sterile

Description: Naphazoline hydrochloride, an ocular vasoconstrictor, is an imidazoline derivative sympathomimetic amine. It occurs as a white, odorless crystalline powder having a bitter taste and is freely soluble in water and in alcohol.

Chemical Name: 2-(1-Naphthylmethyl)-2-imidazoline monohydrochloride

Contains:

Active: naphazoline HCl 0.1%. **Preservative:** benzalkonium chloride 0.004%.

Inactives: citric acid, monohydrate; edetate disodium; polyvinyl alcohol 1.4%; purified water; sodium chloride; sodium citrate, dihydrate; and sodium hydroxide to adjust the pH. It has a shelf life pH range of 5.5 to 6.5.

Clinical Pharmacology: Naphazoline constricts the vascular system of the conjunctiva. It is presumed that this effect is due to direct stimulation action of the drug upon the alpha-adrenergic receptors in the arterioles of the conjunctiva, resulting in decreased conjunctival congestion. Naphazoline belongs to the imidazoline class of sympathomimetics.

Indications and Usage: ALBALON® (naphazoline hydrochloride ophthalmic solution, USP) 0.1% is indicated for use as a topical ocular vasoconstrictor.

Contraindications: ALBALON® ophthalmic solution is contraindicated in the presence of an anatomically narrow angle or in narrow- angle glaucoma or in persons who have shown hypersensitivity to any component of this preparation.

Warnings: Patients under therapy with MAO inhibitors may experience a severe hypertensive crisis if given a sympathomimetic drug. Use in children, especially infants, may result in CNS depression leading to coma and marked reduction in body temperature.

Precautions:

General: Use with caution in the presence of hypertension, cardiovascular abnormalities, hyperglycemia (diabetes), hyperthyroidism, infection or injury.

Patient Information: Patients should be advised to discontinue the drug and consult a physician if relief is not obtained within 48 hours of therapy, if irritation, blurring or redness persists or increases, or if symptoms of systemic absorption occur, i.e., dizziness, headache, nausea, decrease in body temperature, or drowsiness.

To prevent contaminating the dropper tip and solution, do not touch the eyelids or the surrounding area with the dropper tip of the bottle. If solution changes color or becomes cloudy, do not use.

Drug Interactions: Concurrent use of maprotiline or tricyclic antidepressants and naphazoline may potentiate the pressor effect of naphazoline. Patients under therapy with MAO inhibitors may experience a severe hypertensive crisis if given a sympathomimetic drug. (See **Warnings**).

Pregnancy: Pregnancy Category C: Animal reproduction studies have not been conducted with naphazoline. It is also not known whether naphazoline can cause fetal harm when administered to a pregnant woman or can affect reproduction capacity. Naphazoline should be given to a pregnant woman only if clearly needed.

Nursing Mothers: It is not known whether naphazoline is excreted in human milk. Because many drugs are excreted in human milk, caution should be exercised when naphazoline is administered to a nursing woman.

Pediatric Use: Safety and effectiveness in pediatric patients have not been established. See **"Warnings"** AND **"Contraindications."**

Adverse Reactions:

Ocular: Mydriasis, increased redness, irritation, discomfort, blurring, punctate keratitis, lacrimation, increased intraocular pressure.

Systemic: Dizziness, headache, nausea, sweating, nervousness, drowsiness, weakness, hypertension, cardiac irregularities, and hyperglycemia.

Dosage and Administration: Instill one or two drops in the conjunctival sac(s) every three to four hours as needed.

How Supplied: ALBALON® (naphazoline hydrochloride ophthalmic solution, USP) 0.1% is supplied sterile in opaque white LDPE plastic bottles with dropper tips and white high impact polystyrene (HIPS) caps as follows:

15 mL in 15 mL bottle – **NDC** 11980-154-15

Note: Store between 15° to 25°C (59° to 77°F).

℞ only

Revised January 2003

©2003 Allergan, Inc.

Irvine, CA 92612, U.S.A.

® marks owned by Allergan, Inc.

71583US10M

ALPHAGAN® P ℞
(brimonidine tartrate ophthalmic
solution) 0.1% and 0.15%
Sterile

Description:

ALPHAGAN® P (brimonidine tartrate ophthalmic solution) is a relatively selective alpha-2 adrenergic agonist for ophthalmic use. The chemical name of brimonidine tartrate is 5- bromo-6-(2-imidazolidinylideneamino) quinoxaline L-tartrate. It is an off-white to pale yellow powder. It has a molecular weight of 442.24 as the tartrate salt, and is both soluble in water (0.6 mg/mL) and in the product vehicle (1.4 mg/mL) at pH 7.7. The structural formula is:

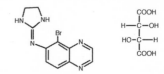

Formula: $C_{11}H_{10}BrN_5 \bullet C_4H_6O_6$ CAS Number: 70359-46-5

In solution, **ALPHAGAN® P** (brimonidine tartrate ophthalmic solution) has a clear, greenish-yellow color. It has an osmolality of 250–350 mOsmol/kg and a pH of 7.4–8.0 (0.1%) or 6.6–7.4 (0.15%).

Each mL of **ALPHAGAN® P** contains:

Active ingredient: brimonidine tartrate 0.1% (1.0 mg/mL) or 0.15% (1.5 mg/mL)

Inactives: sodium carboxymethylcellulose; sodium borate; boric acid; sodium chloride; potassium chloride; calcium chloride; magnesium chloride; Purite® 0.005% (0.05mg/mL) as a preservative; purified water; with hydrochloric acid and/or sodium hydroxide to adjust pH.

Clinical Pharmacology:

Mechanism of action:

ALPHAGAN® P is an alpha adrenergic receptor agonist. It has a peak ocular hypotensive effect occurring at two hours post-dosing. Fluorophotometric studies in animals and humans suggest that brimonidine tartrate has a dual mechanism of action by reducing aqueous humor production and increasing uveoscleral outflow.

Pharmacokinetics:

After ocular administration of either a 0.1% or 0.2% solution, plasma concentrations peaked within 0.5 to 2.5 hours and declined with a systemic half-life of approximately 2 hours.

In humans, systemic metabolism of brimonidine is extensive. It is metabolized primarily by the liver. Urinary excretion is the major route of elimination of the drug and its metabolites. Approximately 87% of an orally-administered radioactive dose was eliminated within 120 hours, with 74% found in the urine.

Clinical Evaluations:

Elevated IOP presents a major risk factor in glaucomatous field loss. The higher the level of IOP, the greater the likelihood of optic nerve damage and visual field loss. Brimonidine tartrate has the action of lowering intraocular pressure with minimal effect on cardiovascular and pulmonary parameters.

Clinical studies were conducted to evaluate the safety, efficacy, and acceptability of **ALPHAGAN® P** (brimonidine tartrate ophthalmic solution) 0.15% compared with **ALPHAGAN®** administered three-times-daily in patients with open-angle glaucoma or ocular hypertension. Those results indicated that **ALPHAGAN® P** (brimonidine tartrate ophthalmic solution) 0.15% is comparable in IOP lowering effect to **ALPHAGAN®** (brimonidine tartrate ophthalmic solution) 0.2%, and effectively lowers IOP in patients with open-angle glaucoma or ocular hypertension by approximately 2–6 mmHg.

A clinical study was conducted to evaluate the safety, efficacy, and acceptability of **ALPHAGAN® P** (brimonidine tartrate ophthalmic solution) 0.1% compared with **ALPHAGAN®** administered three-times-daily in patients with open-angle glaucoma or ocular hypertension. Those results indicated that **ALPHAGAN® P** (brimonidine tartrate ophthalmic solution) 0.1% is equivalent in IOP lowering effect to **ALPHAGAN®** (brimonidine tartrate ophthalmic solution) 0.2%, and effectively lowers IOP in patients with open-angle glaucoma or ocular hypertension by approximately 2–6 mmHg.

Indications and Usage:
ALPHAGAN® P is indicated for the lowering of intraocular pressure in patients with open- angle glaucoma or ocular hypertension.

Contraindications:
ALPHAGAN® P is contraindicated in patients with hypersensitivity to brimonidine tartrate or any component of this medication. It is also contraindicated in patients receiving monoamine oxidase (MAO) inhibitor therapy.

Precautions:
General:
Although brimonidine tartrate ophthalmic solution had minimal effect on the blood pressure of patients in clinical studies, caution should be exercised in treating patients with severe cardiovascular disease.

ALPHAGAN® P has not been studied in patients with hepatic or renal impairment; caution should be used in treating such patients.

ALPHAGAN® P should be used with caution in patients with depression, cerebral or coronary insufficiency, Raynaud's phenomenon, orthostatic hypotension, or thromboangiitis obliterans. Patients prescribed IOP-lowering medication should be routinely monitored for IOP.

Information for Patients:
As with other drugs in this class, **ALPHAGAN® P** may cause fatigue and/or drowsiness in some patients. Patients who engage in hazardous activities should be cautioned of the potential for a decrease in mental alertness.

Drug Interactions:
Although specific drug interaction studies have not been conducted with **ALPHAGAN® P**, the possibility of an additive or potentiating effect with CNS depressants (alcohol, barbiturates, opiates, sedatives, or anesthetics) should be considered. Alpha-agonists, as a class, may reduce pulse and blood pressure. Caution in using concomitant drugs such as anti- hypertensives and/or cardiac glycosides is advised.

Tricyclic antidepressants have been reported to blunt the hypotensive effect of systemic clonidine. It is not known whether the concurrent use of these agents with **ALPHAGAN® P** in humans can lead to resulting interference with the IOP lowering effect. No data on the level of circulating catecholamines after **ALPHAGAN® P** administration are available. Caution, however, is advised in patients taking tricyclic antidepressants which can affect the metabolism and uptake of circulating amines.

Carcinogenesis, Mutagenesis, and Impairment of Fertility:
No compound-related carcinogenic effects were observed in either mice or rats following a 21-month and 24-month study, respectively. In these studies, dietary administration of brimonidine tartrate at doses up to 2.5 mg/kg/day in mice and 1.0 mg/kg/day in rats achieved 150 and 120 times or 90 and 80 times, respectively, the plasma drug concentration (C_{max}) esti-

mated in humans treated with one drop of **ALPHAGAN® P** 0.1% or 0.15% into both eyes 3 times per day.

Brimonidine tartrate was not mutagenic or cytogenic in a series of *in vitro* and *in vivo* studies including the Ames test, chromosomal aberration assay in Chinese Hamster Ovary (CHO) cells, a host-mediated assay and cytogenic studies in mice, and dominant lethal assay.

Pregnancy:
Teratogenic effects: Pregnancy Category B. Reproductive studies performed in rats and rabbits with oral doses of 0.66 mg base/kg revealed no evidence of impaired fertility or harm to the fetus due to **ALPHAGAN® P**. Dosing at this level produced an exposure in rats and rabbits that is 190 and 100 times or 120 and 60 times higher, respectively, than the exposure seen in humans following multiple ophthalmic doses of **ALPHAGAN® P** 0.1% or 0.15%. There are no adequate and well-controlled studies in pregnant women. In animal studies, brimonidine crossed the placenta and entered into the fetal circulation to a limited extent. **ALPHAGAN® P** should be used during pregnancy only if the potential benefit to the mother justifies the potential risk to the fetus.

Nursing Mothers:
It is not known whether this drug is excreted in human milk; although in animal studies brimonidine tartrate was excreted in breast milk. A decision should be made whether to discontinue nursing or to discontinue the drug, taking into account the importance of the drug to the mother.

Pediatric Use:
In a well-controlled clinical study conducted in pediatric glaucoma patients (ages 2 to 7 years) the most commonly observed adverse events with brimonidine tartrate ophthalmic solution 0.2% dosed three times daily were somnolence (50% – 83% in patients ages 2 to 6 years) and decreased alertness. In pediatric patients 7 years of age or older (>20kg), somnolence appears to occur less frequently (25%). Approximately 16% of patients on brimonidine tartrate ophthalmic solution discontinued from the study due to somnolence.

The safety and effectiveness of brimonidine tartrate ophthalmic solution have not been studied in pediatric patients below the age of 2 years. Brimonidine tartrate ophthalmic solution is not recommended for use in pediatric patients under the age of 2 years. (Also refer to Adverse Reactions section.)

Geriatric Use:
No overall differences in safety or effectiveness have been observed between elderly and other adult patients.

Adverse Reactions:
Adverse events occurring in approximately 10– 20% of the subjects receiving brimonidine ophthalmic solution (0.1–0.2%) included: allergic conjunctivitis, conjunctival hyperemia, and eye pruritus. Adverse events occurring in approximately 5–9% included: burning sensation, conjunctival folliculosis, hypertension, ocular allergic reaction, oral dryness, and visual disturbance.

Adverse events occurring in approximately 1–4% of the subjects receiving brimonidine ophthalmic solution (0.1–0.2%) included: allergic reaction, asthenia, blepharitis, blepharoconjunctivitis, blurred vision, bronchitis, cataract, conjunctival edema, conjunctival hemorrhage, conjunctivitis, cough, dizziness, dyspepsia, dyspnea, epiphora, eye discharge, eye dryness, eye irritation, eye pain, eyelid edema, eyelid erythema, fatigue, flu syndrome, follicular conjunctivitis, foreign body sensation, gastrointestinal disorder, headache, hypercholesterolemia, hypotension, infection (primarily colds and respiratory infections), insomnia, keratitis, lid disorder, pharyngitis, photophobia, rash, rhinitis, sinus infection, si-

nusitis, somnolence, stinging, superficial punctate keratopathy, tearing, visual field defect, vitreous detachment, vitreous disorder, vitreous floaters, and worsened visual acuity.

The following events were reported in less than 1% of subjects: corneal erosion, hordeolum, nasal dryness, and taste perversion.

The following events have been identified during post-marketing use of brimonidine tartrate ophthalmic solutions in clinical practice. Because they are reported voluntarily from a population of unknown size, estimates of frequency cannot be made. The events, which have been chosen for inclusion due to either their seriousness, frequency of reporting, possible causal connection to brimonidine tartrate ophthalmic solutions, or a combination of these factors, include: bradycardia; depression; iritis; keratoconjunctivitis sicca; miosis; nausea; skin reactions (including erythema, eyelid pruritus, rash, and vasodilation) and tachycardia. Apnea; bradycardia; hypotension; hypothermia; hypotonia; and somnolence have been reported in infants receiving brimonidine tartrate ophthalmic solutions.

Overdosage:
No information is available on overdosage in humans. Treatment of an oral overdose includes supportive and symptomatic therapy; a patent airway should be maintained.

Dosage and Administration:
The recommended dose is one drop of **ALPHAGAN® P** in the affected eye(s) three times daily, approximately 8 hours apart.

ALPHAGAN® P ophthalmic solution may be used concomitantly with other topical ophthalmic drug products to lower intraocular pressure. If more than one topical ophthalmic product is being used, the products should be administered at least 5 minutes apart.

How Supplied:
ALPHAGAN® P is supplied sterile in opaque teal LDPE plastic bottles and droppers with purple high impact polystyrene (HIPS) caps as follows:

0.1%

5 mL in 10 mL bottle	NDC 0023–9321–05
10 mL in 10 mL bottle	NDC 0023–9321–10
15 mL in 15 mL bottle	NDC 0023–9321–15

0.15%

5 mL in 10 mL bottle	NDC 0023–9177–05
10 mL in 10 mL bottle	NDC 0023–9177–10
15 mL in 15 mL bottle	NDC 0023–9177–15

NOTE: Store at 15°–25° C (59–77°F).

Rx Only
© 2005 Allergan, Inc.
Irvine, CA 92612, U.S.A.
® marks owned by Allergan
US Patents 5,424,078; 5,736,165; 6,194, 415; 6,248,741; 6,465,464; 6,562,873; 6,627,210; 6,641,834; and 6,673,337
71816US10S

Shown in Product Identification Guide, page 103

BETAGAN®   ℞
(levobunolol hydrochloride
ophthalmic solution, USP)
sterile

Description: BETAGAN® (levobunolol hydrochloride ophthalmic solution, USP) sterile is a noncardioselective beta-adrenoceptor blocking agent for ophthalmic use. The solution is colorless to slightly light yellow in appearance with an osmolality range of 250– 360 mOsm/kg. The shelf life pH range is 5.5 to 7.5.

Chemical Name: (-)-5-[3-(tert-Butylamino)-2-hydroxypropoxy]-3, 4-dihydro-1(2H)-naphthalenone hydrochloride.

Contains: Active: levobunolol HCl 0.25% or 0.5%. **Preservative:** benzalkonium chloride

Continued on next page

Betagan—Cont.

0.004% Inactives: edetate disodium; polyvinyl alcohol 1.4%; potassium phosphate, monobasic; purified water; sodium chloride; sodium metabisulfite, sodium phosphate, dibasic; and hydrochloric acid or sodium hydroxide to adjust pH.

Clinical Pharmacology: Levobunolol HCl is a noncardioselective beta-adrenoceptor blocking agent, equipotent at both $beta_1$ and $beta_2$ receptors. Levobunolol HCl is greater than 60 times more potent than its dextro isomer in its beta-blocking activity, yet equipotent in its potential for direct myocardial depression. Accordingly, the levo isomer, levobunolol HCl, is used. Levobunolol HCl does not have significant local anesthetic (membrane- stabilizing) or intrinsic sympathomimetic activity.

Beta-adrenergic receptor blockade reduces cardiac output in both healthy subjects and patients with heart disease. In patients with severe impairment of myocardial function, beta-adrenergic receptor blockade may inhibit the stimulatory effect of the sympathetic nervous system necessary to maintain adequate cardiac function.

Beta-adrenergic receptor blockade in the bronchi and bronchioles results in increased airway resistance from unopposed para-sympathetic activity. Such an effect in patients with asthma or other bronchospastic conditions is potentially dangerous.

BETAGAN® (levobunolol hydrochloride ophthalmic solution, USP) has been shown to be an active agent in lowering elevated as well as normal intraocular pressure (IOP) whether or not accompanied by glaucoma. Elevated IOP presents a major risk factor in glaucomatous field loss. The higher the level of IOP, the greater the likelihood of optic nerve damage and visual field loss.

The onset of action with one drop of BETAGAN® can be detected within one hour after treatment, with maximum effect seen between 2 and 6 hours.

A significant decrease in IOP can be maintained for up to 24 hours following a single dose.

In two separate, controlled studies (one three month and one up to 12 months duration) BETAGAN® ophthalmic solution 0.25% b.i.d. controlled the IOP of approximately 64% and 70% of the subjects.

The overall mean decrease from baseline was 5.4 mm Hg and 5.1 mm Hg respectively. In an open-label study, BETAGAN® ophthalmic solution 0.25% q.d. controlled the IOP of 72% of the subjects while achieving an overall mean decrease of 5.9 mm Hg.

In controlled clinical studies of approximately two years duration, intraocular pressure was well-controlled in approximately 80% of subjects treated with BETAGAN® ophthalmic solution 0.5% b.i.d. The mean IOP decrease from baseline was between 6.87 mm Hg and 7.81 mm Hg. No significant effects on pupil size, tear production or corneal sensitivity were observed. BETAGAN® at the concentrations tested, when applied topically, decreased heart rate and blood pressure in some patients. The IOP-lowering effect of BETAGAN® was well maintained over the course of these studies.

In a three month clinical study, a single daily application of 0.5% BETAGAN® ophthalmic solution controlled the IOP of 72% of subjects achieving an overall mean decrease in IOP of 7.0 mm Hg.

The primary mechanism of the ocular hypotensive action of levobunolol HCl in reducing IOP is most likely a decrease in aqueous humor production. BETAGAN® reduces IOP with little or no effect on pupil size or accommodation in contrast to the miosis which cholinergic agents are known to produce. The blurred vision and night blindness often associated with miotics would not be expected and have not been reported with the use of BETAGAN® ophthalmic solution. This is particularly important in cataract patients with central lens opacities who would experience decreased visual acuity with pupillary constriction.

Indications and Usage: BETAGAN® ophthalmic solution has been shown to be effective in lowering intraocular pressure and may be used in patients with chronic open-angle glaucoma or ocular hypertension.

Contraindications: BETAGAN® ophthalmic solution is contraindicated in those individuals with bronchial asthma or with a history of bronchial asthma, or severe chronic obstructive pulmonary disease (see WARNINGS); sinus bradycardia; second and third degree atrioventricular block; overt cardiac failure (see WARNINGS); cardiogenic shock; or hypersensitivity to any component of these products.

Warnings: As with other topically applied ophthalmic drugs, BETAGAN® may be absorbed systemically. The same adverse reactions found with systemic administration of beta-adrenergic blocking agents may occur with topical administration. For example, severe respiratory reactions and cardiac reactions, including death due to bronchospasm in patients with asthma, and rarely death in association with cardiac failure, have been reported with topical application of beta- adrenergic blocking agents (see CONTRAINDICATIONS).

Cardiac Failure: Sympathetic stimulation may be essential for support of the circulation in individuals with diminished myocardial contractility, and its inhibition by beta-adrenergic receptor blockade may precipitate more severe failure.

In Patients Without a History of Cardiac Failure: Continued depression of the myocardium with beta-blocking agents over a period of time can, in some cases, lead to cardiac failure. At the first sign or symptom of cardiac failure, BETAGAN® ophthalmic solution should be discontinued.

Obstructive Pulmonary Disease:
PATIENTS WITH CHRONIC OBSTRUCTIVE PULMONARY DISEASE (e.g., CHRONIC BRONCHITIS, EMPHYSEMA) OF MILD OR MODERATE SEVERITY, BRONCHOSPASTIC DISEASE OR A HISTORY OF BRONCHOSPASTIC DISEASE (OTHER THAN BRONCHIAL ASTHMA OR A HISTORY OF BRONCHIAL ASTHMA, IN WHICH BETAGAN® IS CONTRAINDICATED, See CONTRAINDICATIONS), SHOULD IN GENERAL NOT RECEIVE BETA BLOCKERS, INCLUDING BETAGAN®. However, if BETAGAN® is deemed necessary in such patients, then it should be administered cautiously since it may block bronchodilation produced by endogenous and exogenous catecholamine stimulation of $beta_2$ receptors.

Major Surgery: The necessity or desirability of withdrawal of beta-adrenergic blocking agents prior to major surgery is controversial. Beta-adrenergic receptor blockade impairs the ability of the heart to respond to beta-adrenergically mediated reflex stimuli. This may augment the risk of general anesthesia in surgical procedures. Some patients receiving beta-adrenergic receptor blocking agents have been subject to protracted severe hypotension during anesthesia. Difficulty in restarting and maintaining the heartbeat has also been reported. For these reasons, in patients undergoing elective surgery, gradual withdrawal of beta-adrenergic receptor blocking agents may be appropriate.

If necessary during surgery, the effects of beta-adrenergic blocking agents may be reversed by sufficient doses of such agonists as isoproterenol, dopamine, dobutamine or levarterenol (See OVERDOSAGE).

Diabetes Mellitus: Beta-adrenergic blocking agents should be administered with caution in patients subject to spontaneous hypoglycemia or to diabetic patients (especially those with labile diabetes) who are receiving insulin or oral hypoglycemic agents. Beta-adrenergic receptor blocking agents may mask the signs and symptoms of acute hypoglycemia.

Thyrotoxicosis: Beta-adrenergic blocking agents may mask certain clinical signs (e.g., tachycardia) of hyperthyroidism. Patients suspected of developing thyrotoxicosis should be managed carefully to avoid abrupt withdrawal of beta-adrenergic blocking agents, which might precipitate a thyroid storm.

These products contain sodium metabisulfite, a sulfite that may cause allergic-type reactions including anaphylactic symptoms and life-threatening or less severe asthmatic episodes in certain susceptible people. The overall prevalence of sulfite sensitivity in the general population is unknown and probably low. Sulfite sensitivity is seen more frequently in asthmatic than in nonasthmatic people.

Precautions
General: BETAGAN® (levobunolol hydrochloride ophthalmic solution, USP) sterile should be used with caution in patients with known hypersensitivity to other beta-adrenoceptor blocking agents.

Use with caution in patients with known diminished pulmonary function.

BETAGAN® should be used with caution in patients who are receiving a beta-adrenergic blocking agent orally, because of the potential for additive effects on systemic beta-blockade or on intraocular pressure. Patients should not typically use two or more topical ophthalmic beta-adrenergic blocking agents simultaneously.

Because of the potential effects of beta- adrenergic blocking agents on blood pressure and pulse rates, these medications must be used cautiously in patients with cerebrovascular insufficiency. Should signs or symptoms develop that suggest reduced cerebral blood flow while using BETAGAN® ophthalmic solution, alternative therapy should be considered.

In patients with angle-closure glaucoma, the immediate objective of treatment is to reopen the angle. This requires, in most cases, constricting the pupil with a miotic. BETAGAN® ophthalmic solution has little or no effect on the pupil. When BETAGAN® is used to reduce elevated intraocular pressure in angle-closure glaucoma, it should be followed with a miotic and not alone.

Muscle Weakness: Beta-adrenergic blockade has been reported to potentiate muscle weakness consistent with certain myasthenic symptoms (e.g., diplopia, ptosis and generalized weakness).

Drug Interactions: Although BETAGAN® ophthalmic solution used alone has little or no effect on pupil size, mydriasis resulting from concomitant therapy with BETAGAN® and epinephrine may occur.

Close observation of the patient is recommended when a beta-blocker is administered to patients receiving catecholamine-depleting drugs such as reserpine, because of possible additive effects and the production of hypotension and/or marked bradycardia, which may produce vertigo, syncope, or postural hypotension.

Patients receiving beta-adrenergic blocking agents along with either oral or intravenous calcium antagonists should be monitored for possible atrioventricular conduction disturbances, left ventricular failure and hypotension. In patients with impaired cardiac function, simultaneous use should be avoided altogether.

The concomitant use of beta-adrenergic blocking agents with digitalis and calcium antagonists may have additive effects on prolonging atrioventricular conduction time.

Phenothiazine-related compounds and beta-adrenergic blocking agents may have additive hypotensive effects due to the inhibition of each other's metabolism.

Risk of anaphylactic reaction: While taking beta-blockers, patients with a history of severe anaphylactic reaction to a variety of allergens may be more reactive to repeated challenge, either accidental, diagnostic, or therapeutic. Such patients may be unresponsive to the usual doses of epinephrine used to treat allergic reaction.

Animal Studies: No adverse ocular effects were observed in rabbits administered BETAGAN® ophthalmic solution topically in studies lasting one year in concentrations up to 10 times the human dose concentration.

Carcinogenesis, mutagenesis, impairment of fertility: In a lifetime oral study in mice, there were statistically significant ($p \leq 0.05$) increases in the incidence of benign leiomyomas in female mice at 200 mg/kg/day (14,000 times the recommended human dose for glaucoma), but not at 12 or 50 mg/kg/day (850 and 3,500 times the human dose). In a two-year oral study of levobunolol HCl in rats, there was a statistically significant ($p \leq 0.05$) increase in the incidence of benign hepatomas in male rats administered 12,800 times the recommended human dose for glaucoma. Similar differences were not observed in rats administered oral doses equivalent to 350 times to 2,000 times the recommended human dose for glaucoma.

Levobunolol did not show evidence of mutagenic activity in a battery of microbiological and mammalian *in vitro* and *in vivo* assays.

Reproduction and fertility studies in rats showed no adverse effect on male or female fertility at doses up to 1,800 times the recommended human dose for glaucoma.

Pregnancy Category C: Fetotoxicity (as evidenced by a greater number of resorption sites) has been observed in rabbits when doses of levobunolol HCl equivalent to 200 and 700 times the recommended dose for the treatment of glaucoma were given. No fetotoxic effects have been observed in similar studies with rats at up to 1,800 times the human dose for glaucoma. Teratogenic studies with levobunolol in rats at doses up to 25 mg/kg/day (1,800 times the recommended human dose for glaucoma) showed no evidence of fetal malformations. There were no adverse effects on postnatal development of offspring. It appears when results from studies using rats and studies with other beta-adrenergic blockers are examined, that the rabbit may be a particularly sensitive species. There are no adequate and well controlled studies in pregnant women. BETAGAN® ophthalmic solution should be used during pregnancy only if the potential benefit justifies the potential risk to the fetus.

Nursing Mothers: It is not known whether this drug is excreted in human milk. Systemic beta-blockers and topical timolol maleate are known to be excreted in human milk. Caution should be exercised when BETAGAN® is administered to a nursing woman.

Pediatric Use: Safety and effectiveness in pediatric patients have not been established.

Geriatric Use: No overall differences in safety or effectiveness have been observed between elderly and younger patients.

Adverse Reactions: In clinical trials, the use of BETAGAN® ophthalmic solution has been associated with transient ocular burning and stinging in up to 1 in 3 patients, and with blepharoconjunctivitis in up to 1 in 20 patients.

Decreases in heart rate and blood pressure have been reported (see CONTRAINDICATIONS and WARNINGS).

The following adverse effects have been reported rarely with the use of BETAGAN®: iridocyclitis, headache, transient ataxia, dizziness, lethargy, urticaria and pruritus.

Decreased corneal sensitivity has been noted in a small number of patients. Although levobunolol has minimal membrane-stabilizing activity, there remains a possibility of decreased corneal sensitivity after prolonged use.

The following additional adverse reactions have been reported either with BETAGAN® ophthalmic solution or ophthalmic use of other beta-adrenergic receptor blocking agents:

BODY AS A WHOLE: Headache, asthenia, chest pain. **CARDIOVASCULAR:** Bradycardia, arrhythmia, hypotension, syncope, heart block, cerebral vascular accident, cerebral ischemia, congestive heart failure, palpitation, cardiac arrest. **DIGESTIVE:** Nausea, diarrhea. **PSYCHIATRIC:** Depression, confusion, increase in signs and symptoms of myasthenia gravis, paresthesia. **SKIN:** Hypersensitivity, including localized and generalized rash, alopecia, Stevens-Johnson Syndrome. **RESPIRATORY:** Bronchospasm (predominantly in patients with pre-existing bronchospastic disease), respiratory failure, dyspnea, nasal congestion. **UROGENITAL:** Impotence. **ENDOCRINE:** Masked symptoms of hypoglycemia in insulin-dependent diabetics (see WARNINGS). **SPECIAL SENSES:** Signs and symptoms of keratitis, blepharoptosis, visual disturbances including refractive changes (due to withdrawal of miotic therapy in some cases), diplopia, ptosis.

Other reactions associated with the oral use of non-selective adrenergic receptor blocking agents should be considered potential effects with ophthalmic use of these agents.

Overdosage: No data are available regarding overdosage in humans. Should accidental ocular overdosage occur, flush eye(s) with water or normal saline. If accidentally ingested, efforts to decrease further absorption may be appropriate (gastric lavage). The most common signs and symptoms to be expected with overdosage with administration of a systemic beta- adrenergic blocking agent are symptomatic bradycardia, hypotension, bronchospasm, and acute cardiac failure. Should these symptoms occur, discontinue BETAGAN® therapy and initiate appropriate supportive therapy. The following supportive measures should be considered:

1. Symptomatic bradycardia: Use atropine sulfate intravenously in a dosage of 0.25 mg to 2 mg to induce vagal blockade. If bradycardia persists, intravenous isoproterenol hydrochloride should be administered cautiously. In refractory cases, the use of a transvenous cardiac pacemaker should be considered.
2. Hypotension: Use sympathomimetic pressor drug therapy, such as dopamine, dobutamine or levarterenol. In refractory cases, the use of glucagon hydrochloride may be useful.
3. Bronchospasm: Use isoproterenol hydrochloride. Additional therapy with aminophylline may be considered.
4. Acute cardiac failure: Conventional therapy with digitalis, diuretics and oxygen should be instituted immediately. In refractory cases, the use of intravenous aminophylline is suggested. This may be followed, if necessary, by glucagon hydrochloride, which may be useful.
5. Heart block (second or third degree): Use isoproterenol hydrochloride or a transvenous cardiac pacemaker.

Dosage and Administration: The recommended starting dose is one to two drops of BETAGAN® ophthalmic solution 0.5% in the af-

fected eye(s) once a day. Typical dosing with BETAGAN® 0.25% ophthalmic solution is one to two drops twice daily. In patients with more severe or uncontrolled glaucoma, BETAGAN® 0.5% can be administered b.i.d. As with any new medication, careful monitoring of patients is advised. Dosages above one drop of BETAGAN® 0.5% b.i.d. are not generally more effective. If the patient's IOP is not at a satisfactory level on this regimen, concomitant therapy with dipivefrin and/or epinephrine, and/or pilocarpine and other miotics, and/or systemically administered carbonic anhydrase inhibitors, such as acetazolamide, can be instituted. Patients should not typically use two or more topical ophthalmic beta-adrenergic blocking agents simultaneously.

How Supplied: BETAGAN® (levobunolol hydrochloride ophthalmic solution, USP) is supplied sterile in white low density polyethylene ophthalmic dispenser bottles and tips.

BETAGAN® 0.25% strength units include a light blue high intensity polystyrene cap.

BETAGAN® 0.5% strength units include a yellow high intensity polystyrene cap.

BETAGAN 0.25%:
10 mL in 15 mL bottle—NDC 0023-4526-10
BETAGAN 0.5%:
5 mL in 10 mL bottle—NDC 0023-4385-05
10 mL in 15 mL bottle—NDC 0023-4385-10
15 mL in 15 mL bottle—NDC 0023-4385-15
NOTE: Protect from light. Store at 15°–25°C (59°–77°F).

℞ only
Revised November 2005
©2006 Allergan, Inc.
Irvine, CA 92612, U.S.A.
71602US12S

BLEPH®–10   ℞
**(sulfacetamide sodium
ophthalmic solution, USP) 10%**

Description: BLEPH®-10 (sulfacetamide sodium ophthalmic solution USP) 10% is a sterile topical antibacterial agent for ophthalmic use.

Chemical Name: N-Sulfanilylacetamide monosodium salt monohydrate.
Contains:

BLEPH®-10 solution: Active: Sulfacetamide sodium 10% (100 mg/mL). **Preservative:** benzalkonium chloride (0.005%). **Inactives:** edetate disodium; polysorbate 80; polyvinyl alcohol 1.4%; purified water; sodium phosphate dibasic; sodium phosphate monobasic; sodium thiosulfate; hydrochloric acid and/or sodium hydroxide to adjust the pH (6.8 to 7.5).

Clinical Pharmacology:
Microbiology: The sulfonamides are bacteriostatic agents and the spectrum of activity is similar for all. Sulfonamides inhibit bacterial synthesis of dihydrofolic acid by preventing the condensation of the pteridine with aminobenzoic acid through competitive inhibition of the enzyme dihydropteroate synthetase. Resistant strains have altered dihydropteroate synthetase with reduced affinity for sulfonamides or produce increased quantities of aminobenzoic acid.

Topically applied sulfonamides are considered active against susceptible strains of the following common bacterial eye pathogens: *Escherichia coli, Staphylococcus aureus, Streptococcus pneumoniae, Streptococcus* (viridans group), *Haemophilus influenzae, Klebsiella* species, and *Enterobacter* species.

Topically applied sulfonamides do not provide adequate coverage against *Neisseria* species, *Serratia marcescens* and *Pseudomonas aerugi-*

Continued on next page

Bleph-10—Cont.

nosa. A significant percentage of staphylococcal isolates are completely resistant to sulfa drugs.

Indications and Usage: BLEPH®-10 solution is indicated for the treatment of conjunctivitis and other superficial ocular infections due to susceptible microorganisms, and as an adjunctive in systemic sulfonamide therapy of trachoma:

Escherichia coli, Staphylococcus aureus, Streptococcus pneumoniae, Streptococcus (viridans group), *Haemophilus influenzae, Klebsiella* species, and *Enterobacter* species.

Topically applied sulfonamides do not provide adequate coverage against *Neisseria* species, *Serratia marcescens* and *Pseudomonas aeruginosa.* A significant percentage of staphylococcal isolates are completely resistant to sulfa drugs.

Contraindications: BLEPH®-10 solution is contraindicated in individuals who have a hypersensitivity to sulfonamides or to any ingredient of the preparations.

Warnings: FOR TOPICAL EYE USE ONLY—NOT FOR INJECTION.

FATALITIES HAVE OCCURRED, ALTHOUGH RARELY, DUE TO SEVERE REACTIONS TO SULFONAMIDES INCLUDING STEVENS-JOHNSON SYNDROME, TOXIC EPIDERMAL NECROLYSIS, FULMINANT HEPATIC NECROSIS, AGRANULOCYTOSIS, APLASTIC ANEMIA AND OTHER BLOOD DYSCRASIAS. Sensitizations may recur when a sulfonamide is readministered, irrespective of the route of administration. Sensitivity reactions have been reported in individuals with no prior history of sulfonamide hypersensitivity. At the first sign of hypersensitivity, skin rash or other serious reaction, discontinue use of these preparations.

Precautions:

General: Prolonged use of topical antibacterial agents may give rise to overgrowth of nonsusceptible organisms including fungi. Bacterial resistance to sulfonamides may also develop.

The effectiveness of sulfonamides may be reduced by the para-aminobenzoic acid present in purulent exudates.

Sensitization may recur when a sulfonamide is readministered irrespective of the route of administration, and cross-sensitivity between different sulfonamides may occur.

At the first sign of hypersensitivity, increase in purulent discharge, or aggravation of inflammation or pain, the patient should discontinue use of the medication and consult a physician (see **Warnings**).

Information for patients: To avoid contamination, do not touch tip of container to the eye, eyelid or any surface.

Drug interactions: Sulfacetamide preparations are incompatible with silver preparations.

Carcinogenesis, Mutagenesis, Impairment of Fertility: No studies have been conducted in animals or in humans to evaluate the possibility of these effects with ocularly administered sulfacetamide. Rats appear to be especially susceptible to the goitrogenic effects of sulfonamides, and long-term oral administration of sulfonamides has resulted in thyroid malignancies in these animals.

Pregnancy: Pregnancy Category C. Animal reproduction studies have not been conducted with sulfonamide ophthalmic preparations. Kernicterus may occur in the newborn as a result of treatment of a pregnant woman at term with orally administered sulfonamides. There are no adequate and well controlled studies of sulfonamide ophthalmic preparations in pregnant women and it is not known whether topically applied sulfonamides can cause fetal harm when administered to a pregnant woman. This product should be used in pregnancy only if the potential benefit justifies the potential risk to the fetus.

Nursing mothers: Systematically administered sulfonamides are capable of producing kernicterus in infants of lactating women. Because of the potential for the development of kernicterus in neonates, a decision should be made whether to discontinue nursing or discontinue the drug taking into account the importance of the drug to the mother.

Pediatric Use: Safety and effectiveness in children below the age of two months have not been established.

Adverse Reactions: Bacterial and fungal corneal ulcers have developed during treatment with sulfonamide ophthalmic preparations.

The most frequently reported reactions are local irritation, stinging and burning. Less commonly reported reactions include non-specific conjunctivitis, conjunctival hyperemia, secondary infections and allergic reactions.

Fatalities have occurred, although rarely, due to severe reactions to sulfonamides including Stevens-Johnson syndrome, toxic epidermal necrolysis, fulminant hepatic necrosis, agranulocytosis, aplastic anemia, and other blood dyscrasias (see **Warnings**).

Dosage and Administration: For conjunctivitis and other superficial ocular infections:

BLEPH-10 solution:

Instill one or two drops into the conjunctival sac(s) of the affected eye(s) every two to three hours initially. Dosages may be tapered by increasing the time interval between doses as the condition responds. The usual duration of treatment is seven to ten days.

For trachoma:

Instill two drops into the conjunctival sac(s) of the affected eye(s) every two hours. Topical administration must be accompanied by systemic administration.

How Supplied: BLEPH®-10 (sulfacetamide sodium ophthalmic solution, USP) 10% is supplied sterile in opaque white LDPE plastic bottles and white dropper tips with white high-impact polystyrene (HIPS) caps as follows:

5 mL in 10 mL bottle—NDC 11980-011-05

Note: Store at 8°–25°C (46°–77°F). Protect from light. Sulfonamide solutions, on long standing, will darken in color and should be discarded.

℞ only

Revised February 2005

©2005 Allergan, Inc.

Irvine, CA 92612, U.S.A.

® marks owned by Allergan, Inc.

71736US11S

BLEPHAMIDE®   ℞
(sulfacetamide sodium—prednisolone acetate ophthalmic suspension USP)
10%/0.2%
sterile

Description: BLEPHAMIDE® ophthalmic suspension is a topical anti-inflammatory/anti-infective combination product for ophthalmic use.

Chemical Names: Sulfacetamide sodium: N-sulfanilylacetamide monosodium salt monohydrate.

Prednisolone acetate: 11β, 17, 21-trihydroxypregna-1, 4-diene-3, 20-dione 21-acetate.**Contains:Actives:** sulfacetamide sodium 10%, prednisolone acetate (microfine suspension) 0.2%. **Preservative:** benzalkonium chloride (0.004%). **Inactives:** edetate disodium; polysorbate 80; polyvinyl alcohol 1.4%; potassium phosphate, monobasic; purified water; sodium phosphate, dibasic; sodium thiosulfate; hydrochloric acid and/or sodium hydroxide to adjust the pH (6.6 to 7.2).

Clinical Pharmacology: Corticosteroids suppress the inflammatory response to a variety of agents and they probably delay or slow healing. Since corticosteroids may inhibit the body's defense mechanism against infection, a concomitant antibacterial drug may be used when this inhibition is considered to be clinically significant in a particular case.

When a decision to administer both a corticosteroid and an antibacterial is made, the administration of such drugs in combination has the advantage of greater patient compliance and convenience, with the added assurance that the appropriate dosage of both drugs is administered. When both types of drugs are in the same formulation, compatibility of ingredients is assured and the correct volume of drug is delivered and retained. The relative potency of corticosteroids depends on the molecular structure, concentration and release from the vehicle.

Microbiology: Sulfacetamide sodium exerts a bacteriostatic effect against susceptible bacteria by restricting the synthesis of folic acid required for growth through competition with p-aminobenzoic acid.

Some strains of these bacteria may be resistant to sulfacetamide or resistant strains may emerge *in vivo*.

The anti-infective component in these products is included to provide action against specific organisms susceptible to it. Sulfacetamide sodium is active *in vitro* against susceptible strains of the following microorganisms: *Escherichia coli, Staphylococcus aureus, Streptococcus pneumoniae, Streptococcus* (viridans group), *Haemophilus influenzae, Klebsiella* species, and *Enterobacter* species. This product does not provide adequate coverage against: *Neisseria* species, *Pseudomonas* species, and *Serratia marcescens* (see **Indications and Usage**).

Indications and Usage: A steroid/anti-infective combination is indicated for steroid-responsive inflammatory ocular conditions for which a corticosteroid is indicated and where superficial bacterial ocular infection or a risk of bacterial ocular infection exists.

Ocular corticosteroids are indicated in inflammatory conditions of the palpebral and bulbar conjunctiva, cornea, and anterior segment of the globe where the inherent risk of corticosteroid use in certain infective conjunctivitides is accepted to obtain diminution in edema and inflammation. They are also indicated in chronic anterior uveitis and corneal injury from chemical, radiation, or thermal burns or penetration of foreign bodies.

The use of a combination drug with an anti-infective component is indicated where the risk of superficial ocular infection is high or where there is an expectation that potentially dangerous numbers of bacteria will be present in the eye.

The particular anti-bacterial drug in this product is active against the following common bacterial eye pathogens: *Escherichia coli, Staphylococcus aureus, Streptococcus pneumoniae, Streptococcus* (viridans group), *Haemophilus influenzae, Klebsiella* species, and *Enterobacter* species. This product does not provide adequate coverage against *Neisseria* species, *Pseudomonas* species, and *Serratia marcescens.*

A significant percentage of staphylococcal isolates are completely resistant to sulfa drugs.

Contraindications: BLEPHAMIDE® ophthalmic suspension is contraindicated in most viral diseases of the cornea and conjunctiva including epithelial herpes simplex keratitis (dendritic keratitis), vaccinia, and varicella, and also in mycobacterial infection of the eye and fungal diseases of ocular structures.

This product is also contraindicated in individuals with known or suspected hypersensitivity to any of the ingredients of this preparation, to other sulfonamides and to other corticosteroids. See **Warnings**. (Hypersensitivity to the antimicrobial component occurs at a higher rate than for other components.)

Warnings:

NOT FOR INJECTION INTO THE EYE.

Prolonged use of corticosteroids may result in ocular hypertension/glaucoma with damage to the optic nerve, defects in visual acuity and fields of vision, and in posterior subcapsular cataract formation.

Acute anterior uveitis may occur in susceptible individuals, primarily Blacks.

Prolonged use of BLEPHAMIDE® ophthalmic suspension may suppress the host response and thus increase the hazard of secondary ocular infections. In those diseases causing thinning of the cornea or sclera, perforation has been known to occur with the use of topical corticosteroids. In acute purulent conditions of the eye, corticosteroids may mask infection or enhance existing infection.

If the product is used for 10 days or longer, intraocular pressure should be routinely monitored even though it may be difficult in children and uncooperative patients. Corticosteroids should be used with caution in the presence of glaucoma. Intraocular pressure should be checked frequently.

A significant percentage of staphylococcal isolates are completely resistant to sulfonamides. The use of steroids after cataract surgery may delay healing and increase the incidence of filtering blebs.

The use of ocular corticosteroids may prolong the course and may exacerbate the severity of many viral infections of the eye (including herpes simplex). Employment of corticosteroid medication in the treatment of herpes simplex requires great caution.

Topical steroids are not effective in mustard gas keratitis and Sjögren's keratoconjunctivitis.

Fatalities have occurred, although rarely, due to severe reactions to sulfonamides including Stevens-Johnson syndrome, toxic epidermal necrolysis, fulminant hepatic necrosis, agranulocytosis, aplastic anemia and other blood dyscrasias. Sensitization may recur when a sulfonamide is readministered, irrespective of the route of administration.

If signs of hypersensitivity or other serious reactions occur, discontinue use of this preparation. Cross-sensitivity among corticosteroids has been demonstrated (see **Adverse Reactions**).

Precautions:

General: The initial prescription and renewal of the medication order beyond 20 milliliters of the suspension should be made by a physician only after examination of the patient with the aid of magnification, such as slit lamp biomicroscopy and, where appropriate, fluorescein staining. If signs and symptoms fail to improve after two days, the patient should be re-evaluated.

The possibility of fungal infections of the cornea should be considered after prolonged corticosteroid dosing. Use with caution in patients with severe dry eye. Fungal cultures should be taken when appropriate.

The p-amino benzoic acid present in purulent exudates competes with sulfonamides and can reduce their effectiveness.

Information for Patients: If inflammation or pain persists longer than 48 hours or becomes aggravated, the patient should be advised to discontinue use of the medication and consult a physician (see **Warnings**).

Contact lenses should not be worn during the use of this product.

This product is sterile when packaged. To prevent contamination, care should be taken to avoid touching the applicator tip to eyelids or to any other surface. The use of this bottle by more than one person may spread infection.

Keep bottle tightly closed when not in use. Protect from light. Sulfonamide solutions darken on prolonged standing and exposure to heat and light. Do not use if solution has darkened. Yellowing does not affect activity. Keep out of the reach of children.

Laboratory Tests: Eyelid cultures and tests to determine the susceptibility of organisms to sulfacetamide may be indicated if signs and symptoms persist or recur in spite of the recommended course of treatment with BLEPHAMIDE® ophthalmic suspension.

Drug Interactions: BLEPHAMIDE® ophthalmic suspension is incompatible with silver preparations. Local anesthetics related to p-amino benzoic acid may antagonize the action of the sulfonamides.

Carcinogenesis, Mutagenesis, Impairment of Fertility: Prednisolone has been reported to be noncarcinogenic. Long-term animal studies for carcinogenic potential have not been performed with sulfacetamide.

One author detected chromosomal nondisjunction in the yeast *Saccharomyces cerevisiae* following application of sulfacetamide sodium. The significance of this finding to topical ophthalmic use of sulfacetamide sodium in the human is unknown.

Mutagenic studies with prednisolone have been negative. Studies on reproduction and fertility have not been performed with sulfacetamide. A long-term chronic toxicity study in dogs showed that high oral doses of prednisolone prevented estrus. A decrease in fertility was seen in male and female rats that were mated following oral dosing with another glucocorticosteroid.

Pregnancy: Teratogenic Effects: Pregnancy Category C. Animal reproduction studies have not been conducted with sulfacetamide sodium. Prednisolone has been shown to be teratogenic in rabbits, hamsters, and mice. In mice, prednisolone has been shown to be teratogenic when given in doses 1 to 10 times the human ocular dose. Dexamethasone, hydrocortisone and prednisolone were ocularly applied to both eyes of pregnant mice five times per day on days 10 through 13 of gestation. A significant increase in the incidence of cleft palate was observed in the fetuses of the treated mice. There are no adequate well-controlled studies in pregnant women dosed with corticosteroids.

Kernicterus may be precipitated in infants by sulfonamides being given systemically during the third trimester of pregnancy. It is not known whether sulfacetamide sodium can cause fetal harm when administered to a pregnant woman or whether it can affect reproductive capacity.

BLEPHAMIDE® ophthalmic suspension should be used during pregnancy only if the potential benefit justifies the potential risk to the fetus.

Nursing Mothers: It is not known whether topical administration of corticosteroids could result in sufficient systemic absorption to produce detectable quantities in human milk. Systemically administered corticosteroids appear in human milk and could suppress growth, interfere with endogenous corticosteroid production, or cause other untoward effects. Systemically administered sulfonamides are capable of producing kernicterus in infants of lactating women. Because of the potential for serious adverse reactions in nursing infants from sulfacetamide sodium and prednisolone acetate ophthalmic suspensions, a decision should be made whether to discontinue nursing or to discontinue the medication.

Pediatric Use: Safety and effectiveness in pediatric patients below the age of six have not been established.

Adverse Reactions: Adverse reactions have occurred with corticosteroid/antibacterial combination drugs which can be attributed to the corticosteroid component, the antibacterial component, or the combination. Exact incidence figures are not available since no denominator of treated patients is available.

Reactions occurring most often from the presence of the antibacterial ingredient are allergic sensitizations. Fatalities have occurred, although rarely, due to severe reactions to sulfonamides including Stevens-Johnson syndrome, toxic epidermal necrolysis, fulminant hepatic necrosis, agranulocytosis, aplastic anemia, and other blood dyscrasias (See **Warnings**).

Sulfacetamide sodium may cause local irritation.

The reactions due to the corticosteroid component in decreasing order of frequency are: elevation of intraocular pressure (IOP) with possible development of glaucoma and infrequent optic nerve damage, posterior subcapsular cataract formation, and delayed wound healing. Although systemic effects are extremely uncommon, there have been rare occurrences of systemic hypercorticoidism after use of topical corticosteroids.

Corticosteroid-containing preparations can also cause acute anterior uveitis or perforation of the globe. Mydriasis, loss of accommodation and ptosis have occasionally been reported following local use of corticosteroids.

Secondary Infection: The development of secondary infection has occurred after use of combinations containing corticosteroids and antibacterials. Fungal and viral infections of the cornea are particularly prone to develop coincidentally with long-term applications of corticosteroid. The possibility of fungal invasion must be considered in any persistent corneal ulceration where corticosteroid treatment has been used.

Secondary bacterial ocular infection following suppression of host responses also occurs.

Dosage and Administration: SHAKE WELL BEFORE USING. Two drops should be instilled into the conjunctival sac every four hours during the day and at bedtime.

Not more than 20 milliliters should be prescribed initially, and the prescription should not be refilled without further evaluation as outlined in **Precautions** above.

BLEPHAMIDE® dosage may be reduced, but care should be taken not to discontinue therapy prematurely. In chronic conditions, withdrawal of treatment should be carried out by gradually decreasing the frequency of application.

If signs and symptoms fail to improve after two days, the patient should be re-evaluated (see **Precautions**).

How Supplied: BLEPHAMIDE® ophthalmic suspension is supplied sterile in opaque white LDPE plastic bottles and white dropper tips with high impact polystyrene (HIPS) caps as follows:

5 mL in 10 mL bottle — NDC 11980-022-05

10 mL in 15 mL bottle — NDC 11980-022-10

Note: Protect from freezing. **Shake well before using.**

Storage: Store BLEPHAMIDE® at 8°–24°C (46°–75°F) in an upright position.

PROTECT FROM LIGHT

Sulfonamide solutions darken on prolonged standing and exposure to heat and light. Do not use if solution has darkened.

Yellowing does not affect activity.

KEEP OUT OF REACH OF CHILDREN

Rx only.

Revised June 2004

©2004 Allergan, Inc.

Irvine, CA 92612, U.S.A.

® marks owned by Allergan, Inc.

71735US10P

Shown in Product Identification Guide, page 103

Continued on next page

BLEPHAMIDE® ℞
(sulfacetamide sodium and prednisolone acetate ophthalmic ointment, USP)
10%/0.2% sterile

Description: BLEPHAMIDE® (sulfacetamide sodium and prednisolone acetate ophthalmic ointment, USP) is a sterile topical ophthalmic ointment combining an antibacterial and a corticosteroid.

Chemical Names: Sulfacetamide sodium: N-sulfanilylacetamide monosodium salt monohydrate.

Prednisolone acetate: 11β, 17, 21-trihydroxypregna-1, 4-diene-3, 20-dione, 21-acetate.

Contains: Actives: sulfacetamide sodium 10% and prednisolone acetate 0.2%. **Preservative:** phenylmercuric acetate (0.0008%). **Inactives:** mineral oil; white petrolatum; and petrolatum (and) lanolin alcohol.

Clinical Pharmacology: Corticosteroids suppress the inflammatory response to a variety of agents and they probably delay or slow healing. Since corticosteroids may inhibit the body's defense mechanism against infection, a concomitant antibacterial drug may be used when this inhibition is considered to be clinically significant in a particular case.

When a decision to administer both a corticosteroid and an antibacterial is made, the administration of such drugs in combination has the advantage of greater patient compliance and convenience, with the added assurance that the appropriate dosage of both drugs is administered, plus assured compatibility of ingredients when both types of drugs are in the same formulation and, particularly, that the correct volume of drug is delivered and retained.

The relative potency of corticosteroids depends on the molecular structure, concentration and release from the vehicle.

Microbiology: Sulfacetamide exerts a bacteriostatic effect against susceptible bacteria by restricting the synthesis of folic acid required for growth through competition with p-amino benzoic acid.

Some strains of these bacteria may be resistant to sulfacetamide or resistant strains may emerge *in vivo*.

The anti-infective component in BLEPHAMIDE® ointment is included to provide action against specific organisms susceptible to it. Sulfacetamide sodium is active *in vitro* against susceptible strains of the following microorganisms: *Escherichia coli, Staphylococcus aureus, Streptococcus pneumoniae, Streptococcus* (*viridans* group), *Haemophilus influenzae, Klebsiella* species, and *Enterobacter* species. This product does not provide adequate coverage against: *Neisseria* species, *Pseudomonas* species, and *Serratia marcescens* (see **Indications and Usage**).

Indications and Usage: BLEPHAMIDE® ophthalmic ointment is indicated for steroid-responsive inflammatory ocular conditions for which a corticosteroid is indicated and where superficial bacterial ocular infection or a risk of bacterial ocular infection exists.

Ocular corticosteroids are indicated in inflammatory conditions of the palpebral and bulbar conjunctiva, cornea, and anterior segment of the globe where the inherent risk of corticosteroid use in certain infective conjunctivitides is accepted to obtain diminution in edema and inflammation. They are also indicated in chronic anterior uveitis and corneal injury from chemical, radiation or thermal burns or penetration of foreign bodies.

The use of a combination drug with an anti-infective component is indicated where the risk of superficial ocular infection is high or where there is an expectation that potentially dangerous numbers of bacteria will be present in the eye.

The particular antibacterial drug in this product is active against the following common bacterial eye pathogens: *Escherichia coli, Staphylococcus aureus, Streptococcus pneumoniae, Streptococcus* (*viridans* group), *Haemophilus influenzae, Klebsiella* species, and *Enterobacter* species.

The product does not provide adequate coverage against: *Neisseria* species, *Pseudomonas* species, and *Serratia marcescens*.

A significant percentage of staphylococcal isolates are completely resistant to sulfa drugs.

Contraindications: BLEPHAMIDE® ophthalmic ointment is contraindicated in most viral diseases of the cornea and conjunctiva including epithelial herpes simplex keratitis (dendritic keratitis), vaccinia, and varicella, and also in mycobacterial infection of the eye and fungal diseases of ocular structures.

This product is also contraindicated in individuals with known or suspected hypersensitivity to any of the ingredients of this preparation, to other sulfonamides and to other corticosteroids. See **Warnings**. (Hypersensitivity to the antimicrobial component occurs at a higher rate than for other components).

Warnings:
NOT FOR INJECTION INTO THE EYE.

Prolonged use of corticosteroids may result in ocular hypertension/glaucoma with damage to the optic nerve, defects in visual acuity and fields of vision, and in posterior subcapsular cataract formation.

Acute anterior uveitis may occur in susceptible individuals, primarily Blacks.

Prolonged use of BLEPHAMIDE® ophthalmic ointment may suppress the host response and thus increase the hazard of secondary ocular infections. In those diseases causing thinning of the cornea or sclera, perforation has been known to occur with the use of topical corticosteroids. In acute purulent conditions of the eye, corticosteroids may mask infection or enhance existing infection.

If the product is used for 10 days or longer, intraocular pressure should be routinely monitored even though it may be difficult in children and uncooperative patients. Corticosteroids should be used with caution in the presence of glaucoma. Intraocular pressure should be checked frequently.

A significant percentage of staphylococcal isolates are completely resistant to sulfonamides. The use of steroids after cataract surgery may delay healing and increase the incidence of filtering blebs.

The use of ocular corticosteroids may prolong the course and may exacerbate the severity of many viral infections of the eye (including herpes simplex). Employment of corticosteroid medication in the treatment of herpes simplex requires great caution.

Topical steroids are not effective in mustard gas keratitis and Sjogren's keratoconjunctivitis.

Fatalities have occurred, although rarely, due to severe reactions to sulfonamides including Stevens-Johnson syndrome, toxic epidermal necrolysis, fulminant hepatic necrosis, agranulocytosis, aplastic anemia and other blood dyscrasias. Sensitization may recur when a sulfonamide is readministered, irrespective of the route of administration.

If signs of hypersensitivity or other serious reactions occur, discontinue use of this preparation. Cross-sensitivity among corticosteroids has been demonstrated (see **Adverse Reactions**).

Precautions:
General: The initial prescription and renewal of the medication order beyond 8 g of ointment should be made by a physician only after examination of the patient with the aid of magnification, such as slit lamp biomicroscopy and, where appropriate, fluorescein staining. If signs and symptoms fail to improve after two

days, the patient should be re-evaluated. The possibility of fungal infections of the cornea should be considered after prolonged corticosteroid dosing. Use with caution in patients with severe dry eye. Fungal cultures should be taken when appropriate.

The p-amino benzoic acid present in purulent exudates competes with sulfonamides and can reduce their effectiveness. Ophthalmic ointments may retard corneal healing.

Information for Patients: If inflammation or pain persists longer than 48 hours or becomes aggravated, the patient should be advised to discontinue use of the medication and consult a physician (see **Warnings**).

This product is sterile when packaged. To prevent contamination, care should be taken to avoid touching the tube tip to eyelids or to any other surface. The use of this tube by more than one person may spread infection. Keep tube tightly closed when not in use. Keep out of the reach of children.

Laboratory Tests: Eyelid cultures and tests to determine the susceptibility of organisms to sulfacetamide may be indicated if signs and symptoms persist or recur in spite of the recommended course of treatment with BLEPHAMIDE® ophthalmic ointment.

Drug Interactions: BLEPHAMIDE® ophthalmic ointment is incompatible with silver preparations. Local anesthetics related to p-amino benzoic acid may antagonize the action of the sulfonamides.

Carcinogenesis, Mutagenesis, Impairment of Fertility: Prednisolone has been reported to be noncarcinogenic. Long-term animal studies for carcinogenic potential have not been performed with sulfacetamide.

One author detected chromosomal nondisjunction in the yeast *Saccharomyces cerevisiae* following application of sulfacetamide sodium. The significance of this finding to topical ophthalmic use of sulfacetamide sodium in the human is unknown.

Mutagenic studies with prednisolone have been negative. Studies on reproduction and fertility have not been performed with sulfacetamide. A long-term chronic toxicity study in dogs showed that high oral doses of prednisolone prevented estrus. A decrease in fertility was seen in male and female rats that were mated following oral dosing with another glucocorticosteroid.

Pregnancy: Teratogenic Effects: Pregnancy Category C. Animal reproduction studies have not been conducted with sulfacetamide sodium. Prednisolone has been shown to be teratogenic in rabbits, hamsters, and mice. In mice, prednisolone has been shown to be teratogenic when given in doses 1 to 10 times the human ocular dose. Dexamethasone, hydrocortisone and prednisolone were ocularly applied to both eyes of pregnant mice five times per day on days 10 through 13 of gestation. A significant increase in the incidence of cleft palate was observed in the fetuses of the treated mice. There are no adequate well-controlled studies in pregnant women dosed with corticosteroids.

Kernicterus may be precipitated in infants by sulfonamides being given systemically during the third trimester of pregnancy. It is not known whether sulfacetamide sodium can cause fetal harm when administered to a pregnant woman or whether it can affect reproductive capacity.

BLEPHAMIDE® ophthalmic ointment should be used during pregnancy only if the potential benefit justifies the potential risk to the fetus.

Nursing Mothers: It is not known whether topical administration of corticosteroids could result in sufficient systemic absorption to produce detectable quantities in human milk. Systemically administered corticosteroids appear in human milk and could suppress growth, interfere with endogenous corticosteroid production, or cause other untoward effects. Systemically administered sulfonamides are capable of producing kernicterus in infants of lactating women. Because of the potential for serious adverse reactions in nursing infants from sulfacetamide sodium and prednisolone acetate ophthalmic ointments, a decision should be made whether to discontinue nursing or to discontinue the medication.

Pediatric Use: Safety and effectiveness in children below the age of six have not been established.

Adverse Reactions: Adverse reactions have occurred with corticosteroid/antibacterial combination drugs which can be attributed to the corticosteroid component, the antibacterial component, or the combination. Exact incidence figures are not available since no denominator of treated patients is available.

Reactions occurring most often from the presence of the antibacterial ingredient are allergic sensitizations. Fatalities have occurred, although rarely, due to severe reactions to sulfonamides including Stevens-Johnson syndrome, toxic epidermal necrolysis, fulminant hepatic necrosis, agranulocytosis, aplastic anemia, and other blood dyscrasias (See **Warnings**).

Sulfacetamide sodium may cause local irritation.

The reactions due to the corticosteroid component in decreasing order of frequency are: elevation of intraocular pressure (IOP) with possible development of glaucoma and infrequent optic nerve damage, posterior subcapsular cataract formation, and delayed wound healing.

Although systemic effects are extremely uncommon, there have been rare occurrences of systemic hypercorticoidism after use of topical steroids.

Corticosteroid-containing preparations can also cause acute anterior uveitis or perforation of the globe. Mydriasis, loss of accommodation and ptosis have occasionally been reported following local use of corticosteroids.

Secondary Infection: The development of secondary infection has occurred after use of combinations containing corticosteroids and antibacterials. Fungal and viral infections of the cornea are particularly prone to develop coincidentally with long-term applications of corticosteroid. The possibility of fungal invasion must be considered in any persistent corneal ulceration where corticosteroid treatment has been used.

Secondary bacterial ocular infection following suppression of host responses also occurs.

Dosage and Administration: A small amount, approximately ½ inch ribbon of ointment, should be applied in the conjunctival sac three or four times daily and once or twice at night.

Not more than 8 g should be prescribed initially.

The dosing of BLEPHAMIDE® ophthalmic ointment may be reduced, but care should be taken not to discontinue therapy prematurely. In chronic conditions, withdrawal of treatment should be carried out by gradually decreasing the frequency of application.

If signs and symptoms fail to improve after two days, the patient should be re-evaluated (see **Precautions**).

How Supplied: BLEPHAMIDE® (sulfacetamide sodium and prednisolone acetate ophthalmic ointment, USP) 10%/0.2% is supplied sterile in ointment tubes of the following size:

3.5 g—NDC 0023-0313-04.

Note: Store between 15–25°C (59–77°F).

℞ only

Revised September 2004
©2004 Allergan, Inc.
Irvine, California 92612, U.S.A.
® marks owned by Allergan, Inc.

71412US11P
Shown in Product Identification Guide, page 103

FML FORTE® ℞
(fluorometholone ophthalmic suspension, USP)
0.25%
sterile

Description: FML FORTE® sterile ophthalmic suspension is a topical anti-inflammatory product for ophthalmic use.

Chemical Name: Fluorometholone: 9-Fluoro-11β, 17-dihydroxy-6α-methylpregna-1,4-diene-3,20-dione.

Contains: Active: fluorometholone 0.25%.
Preservative: benzalkonium chloride 0.005%.
Inactives: edetate disodium; polysorbate 80; polyvinyl alcohol 1.4%; purified water; sodium chloride; sodium phosphate, dibasic; sodium phosphate, monobasic; and sodium hydroxide to adjust the pH. FML Forte® suspension is formulated with a pH from 6.2 to 7.5.

Clinical Pharmacology: Corticosteroids inhibit the inflammatory response to a variety of inciting agents and probably delay or slow healing. They inhibit the edema, fibrin deposition, capillary dilation, leukocyte migration, capillary proliferation, fibroblast proliferation, deposition of collagen, and scar formation associated with inflammation.

There is no generally accepted explanation for the mechanism of action of ocular corticosteroids. However, corticosteroids are thought to act by the induction of phospholipase A$_2$ inhibitory proteins, collectively called lipocortins. It is postulated that these proteins control the biosynthesis of potent mediators of inflammation such as prostaglandins and leukotrienes by inhibiting the release of their common precursor, arachidonic acid. Arachidonic acid is released from membrane phospholipids by phospholipase A$_2$.

Corticosteroids are capable of producing a rise in intraocular pressure. In clinical studies of documented steroid-responders, fluorometholone demonstrated a significantly longer average time to produce a rise in intraocular pressure than dexamethasone phosphate; however, in a small percentage of individuals a significant rise in intraocular pressure occurred within one week. The ultimate magnitude of the rise was equivalent for both drugs.

Indications and Usage: FML FORTE® suspension is indicated for the treatment of corticosteroid-responsive inflammation of the palpebral and bulbar conjunctiva, cornea and anterior segment of the globe.

Contraindications: FML FORTE® suspension is contraindicated in most viral diseases of the cornea and conjunctiva, including epithelial herpes simplex keratitis (dendritic keratitis), vaccinia, and varicella, and also in mycobacterial infection of the eye and fungal diseases of ocular structures. FML FORTE® suspension is also contraindicated in individuals with known or suspected hypersensitivity to any of the ingredients of this preparation and to other corticosteroids.

Warnings: Prolonged use of corticosteroids may result in glaucoma, with damage to the optic nerve, defects in visual acuity and fields of vision, and in posterior subcapsular cataract formation. Prolonged use may also suppress the host immune response and thus increase the hazard of secondary ocular infections.

Various ocular diseases and long-term use of topical corticosteroids have been known to cause corneal and scleral thinning. Use of topical corticosteroids in the presence of thin corneal or scleral tissue may lead to perforation.

Acute purulent infections of the eye may be masked or activity enhanced by the presence of corticosteroid medication.

If this product is used for 10 days or longer, intraocular pressure should be routinely monitored even though it may be difficult in children and uncooperative patients. Steroids should be used with caution in the presence of glaucoma. Intraocular pressure should be checked frequently.

The use of steroids after cataract surgery may delay healing and increase the incidence of bleb formation.

Use of ocular steroids may prolong the course and may exacerbate the severity of many viral infections of the eye (including herpes simplex). Employment of a corticosteroid medication in the treatment of patients with a history of herpes simplex requires great caution; frequent slit lamp microscopy is recommended.

Precautions:
General: The initial prescription and renewal of the medication order beyond 20 milliliters of FML FORTE® suspension should be made by a physician only after examination of the patient with the aid of magnification, such as slit lamp biomicroscopy and, where appropriate, fluorescein staining. If signs and symptoms fail to improve after two days, the patient should be re-evaluated.

As fungal infections of the cornea are particularly prone to develop coincidentally with long-term local corticosteroid applications, fungal invasion should be suspected in any persistent corneal ulceration where a corticosteroid has been used or is in use. Fungal cultures should be taken when appropriate.

If this product is used for 10 days or longer, intraocular pressure should be monitored (see **Warnings**).

Information for Patients: If inflammation or pain persists longer than 48 hours or becomes aggravated, the patient should be advised to discontinue use of the medication and consult a physician.

This product is sterile when packaged. To prevent contamination, care should be taken to avoid touching the bottle tip to eyelids or to any other surface. The use of this bottle by more than one person may spread infection. Keep bottle tightly closed when not in use. Keep out of reach of children.

Carcinogenesis, mutagenesis, impairment of fertility: No studies have been conducted in animals or in humans to evaluate the possibility of these effects with fluorometholone.

Pregnancy: Teratogenic effects. Pregnancy Category C: Fluorometholone has been shown to be embryocidal and teratogenic in rabbits when administered at low multiples of the human ocular dose. Fluorometholone was applied ocularly to rabbits daily on days 6–18 of gestation, and dose-related fetal loss and fetal abnormalities including cleft palate, deformed rib cage, anomalous limbs and neural abnormalities such as encephalocele, craniorachischisis, and spina bifida were observed. There are no adequate and well-controlled studies of fluorometholone in pregnant women, and it is not known whether fluorometholone can cause fetal harm when administered to a pregnant woman. Fluorometholone should be used during pregnancy only if the potential benefit justifies the potential risk to the fetus.

Nursing Mothers: It is not known whether topical ophthalmic adminstration of corticosteroids could result in sufficient systemic absorption to produce detectable quantities in human milk. Systemically administered corticosteroids appear in human milk and could suppress growth, interfere with endogenous corticosteroid production, or cause other untoward effects. Because of the potential for serious adverse reactions in nursing infants from

Continued on next page

FML Forte—Cont.

fluorometholone, a decision should be made whether to discontinue nursing or to discontinue the drug, taking into account the importance of the drug to the mother.

Pediatric Use: Safety and effectiveness in infants below the age of two years have not been established.

Geriatric Use: No overall differences in safety or effectiveness have been observed between elderly and younger patients.

Adverse Reactions: Adverse reactions include, in decreasing order of frequency, elevation of intraocular pressure (IOP) with possible development of glaucoma and infrequent optic nerve damage, posterior subcapsular cataract formation, and delayed wound healing.

Corticosteroid-containing preparations have also been reported to cause acute anterior uveitis and perforation of the globe. Keratitis, conjunctivitis, corneal ulcers, mydriasis, conjunctival hyperemia, loss of accommodation and ptosis have occasionally been reported following local use of corticosteroids.

The development of secondary ocular infection (bacterial, fungal and viral) has occurred. Fungal and viral infections of the cornea are particularly prone to develop coincidentally with long-term applications of steroids. The possibility of fungal invasion should be considered in any persistent corneal ulceration where steroid treatment has been used (see **Warnings**).

Other adverse events reported with the use of FML FORTE® include transient burning and stinging upon instillation, ocular irritation, taste perversion, and visual disturbance (blurry vision).

Dosage and Administration: Instill one drop into the conjunctival sac two to four times daily. Care should be taken not to discontinue therapy prematurely. If signs and symptoms fail to improve after two days, the patient should be re-evaluated (see **Precautions**).

The dosing of FML FORTE® suspension may be reduced, but care should be taken not to discontinue therapy prematurely. In chronic conditions, withdrawal of treatment should be carried out by gradually decreasing the frequency of applications.

How Supplied: FML FORTE® (fluorometholone ophthalmic suspension, USP) 0.25% is supplied sterile in opaque white LDPE plastic bottles with droppers with white high impact polystyrene (HIPS) caps as follows:

5 mL in 10 mL bottle—NDC 11980-228-05
10 mL in 15 mL bottle—NDC 11980-228-10
15 mL in 15 mL bottle—NDC 11980-228-15

Note: Store at or below 25°C (77°F); protect from freezing. **Shake well before using.**

℞ only
Revised June 2004
©2004 Allergan, Inc.
Irvine, CA 92612 U.S.A.
® marks owned by Allergan, Inc.
71744US10P

FML®   ℞
(fluorometholone ophthalmic suspension, USP) 0.1%
Sterile

Description: FML® (fluorometholone ophthalmic suspension, USP) 0.1% is a sterile, topical anti-inflammatory agent for ophthalmic use.

Chemical Name: Fluorometholone:
9-Fluoro-11β, 17-dihydroxy-6α-methylpregna-1, 4-diene-3,20-dione.

Contains:
Active: fluorometholone 0.1%. **Preservative:** benzalkonium chloride 0.004%. **Inactives:** Edetate disodium; polysorbate 80; polyvinyl alcohol 1.4%; purified water; sodium chloride; so-

dium phosphate, dibasic; sodium phosphate, monobasic; and sodium hydroxide to adjust the pH. FML® suspension is formulated with a pH from 6.2 to 7.5. It has an osmolality range of 290–350 mOsm/kg.

Clinical Pharmacology: Corticosteroids inhibit the inflammatory response to a variety of inciting agents and probably delay or slow healing. They inhibit the edema, fibrin deposition, capillary dilation, leukocyte migration, capillary proliferation, fibroblast proliferation, deposition of collagen, and scar formation associated with inflammation.

There is no generally accepted explanation for the mechanism of action of ocular corticosteroids. However, corticosteroids are thought to act by the induction of phospholipase A_2 inhibitory proteins, collectively called lipocortins. It is postulated that these proteins control the biosynthesis of potent mediators of inflammation such as prostaglandins and leukotrienes by inhibiting the release of their common precursor arachidonic acid. Arachidonic acid is released from membrane phospholipids by phospholipase A_2.

Corticosteroids are capable of producing a rise in intraocular pressure. In clinical studies of documented steroid-responders, fluorometholone demonstrated a significantly longer average time to produce a rise in intraocular pressure than dexamethasome phosphate; however, in a small percentage of individuals, a significant rise in intraocular pressure occurred within one week. The ultimate magnitude of the rise was equivalent for both drugs.

Indications and Usage: FML® suspension is indicated for the treatment of corticosteroid-responsive inflammation of the palpebral and bulbar conjunctiva, cornea and anterior segment of the globe.

Contraindications: FML® suspension is contraindicated in most viral diseases of the cornea and conjunctiva, including epithelial herpes simplex keratitis (dendritic keratitis), vaccinia, and varicella, and also in mycobacterial infection of the eye and fungal diseases of ocular structures. FML® suspension is also contraindicated in individuals with known or suspected hypersensitivity to any of the ingredients of this preparation and to other corticosteroids.

Warnings: Prolonged use of corticosteroids may result in glaucoma with damage to the optic nerve, defects in visual acuity and fields of vision, and in posterior subcapsular cataract formation. Prolonged use may also suppress the host immune response and thus increase the hazard of secondary ocular infections.

Various ocular diseases and long-term use of topical corticosteroids have been known to cause corneal and scleral thinning. Use of topical corticosteroids in the presence of thin corneal or scleral tissue may lead to perforation.

Acute purulent infections of the eye may be masked or activity enhanced by the presence of corticosteroid medication.

If this product is used for 10 days or longer, intraocular pressure should be routinely monitored even though it may be difficult in children and uncooperative patients. Steroids should be used with caution in the presence of glaucoma. Intraocular pressure should be checked frequently.

The use of steroids after cataract surgery may delay healing and increase the incidence of bleb formation.

Use of ocular steroids may prolong the course and may exacerbate the severity of many viral infections of the eye (including herpes simplex). Employment of a corticosteroid medication in the treatment of patients with a history of herpes simplex requires great caution; frequent slit lamp microscopy is recommended.

Corticosteroids are not effective in mustard gas keratitis and Sjögren's keratoconjunctivitis.

Precautions:

General: The initial prescription and renewal of the medication order beyond 20 milliliters of FML® suspension should be made by a physician only after examination of the patient with the aid of magnification, such as slit lamp biomicroscopy and, where appropriate, fluorescein staining. If signs and symptoms fail to improve after two days, the patient should be re-evaluated.

As fungal infections of the cornea are particularly prone to develop coincidentally with long-term local corticosteroid applications, fungal invasion should be suspected in any persistent corneal ulceration where a corticosteroid has been used or is in use. Fungal cultures should be taken when appropriate.

If this product is used for 10 days or longer, intraocular pressure should be monitored (see **Warnings**).

Information for Patients: If inflammation or pain persists longer than 48 hours or becomes aggravated, the patient should be advised to discontinue use of the medication and consult a physician.

This product is sterile when packaged. To prevent contamination, care should be taken to avoid touching the bottle tip to eyelids or to any other surface. The use of this bottle by more than one person may spread infection. Keep bottle tightly closed when not in use. Keep out of the reach of children.

The preservative in FML® suspension, benzalkonium chloride, may be absorbed by soft contact lenses. Patients wearing soft contact lenses should be instructed to wait at least 15 minutes after instilling FML® suspension to insert soft contact lenses.

Carcinogenesis, mutagenesis, impairment of fertility:
No studies have been conducted in animals or in humans to evaluate the possibility of these effects with fluorometholone.

Pregnancy: Teratogenic effects. Pregnancy Category C: Fluorometholone has been shown to be embryocidal and teratogenic in rabbits when administered at low multiples of the human ocular dose. Fluorometholone was applied ocularly to rabbits daily on days 6–18 of gestation, and dose-related fetal loss and fetal abnormalities including cleft palate, deformed rib cage, anomalous limbs and neural abnormalities such as encephalocele, craniorachischisis, and spina bifida were observed. There are no adequate and well-controlled studies of fluorometholone in pregnant women, and it is not known whether fluorometholone can cause fetal harm when administered to a pregnant woman. Fluorometholone should be used during pregnancy only if the potential benefit justifies the potential risk to the fetus.

Nursing Mothers: It is not known whether topical ophthalmic administration of corticosteroids could result in sufficient systemic absorption to produce detectable quantities in human milk. Systemically administered corticosteroids appear in human milk and could suppress growth, interfere with endogenous corticosteroid production, or cause other untoward effects. Because of the potential for serious adverse reactions in nursing infants from fluorometholone, a decision should be made whether to discontinue nursing or to discontinue the drug, taking into account the importance of the drug to the mother.

Pediatric Use: Safety and effectiveness in infants below the age of 2 years have not been established.

Geriatric Use: No overall differences in safety or effectiveness have been observed between elderly and younger patients.

Adverse Reactions: Adverse reactions include, in decreasing order of frequency, elevation of intraocular pressure (IOP) with possible development of glaucoma and infrequent optic nerve damage, posterior subcapsular cataract formation, and delayed wound healing.

Although systemic effects are extremely uncommon, there have been rare occurrences of systemic hypercorticoidism after use of topical steroids.

Corticosteroid-containing preparations have also been reported to cause acute anterior uveitis and perforation of the globe. Keratitis, conjunctivitis, corneal ulcers, mydriasis, conjunctival hyperemia, loss of accommodation and ptosis have occasionally been reported following local use of corticosteroids.

The development of secondary ocular infection (bacterial, fungal and viral) has occurred. Fungal and viral infections of the cornea are particularly prone to develop coincidentally with long-term applications of steroids. The possibility of fungal invasion should be considered in any persistent corneal ulceration where steroid treatment has been used (see **Warnings**). Transient burning and stinging upon instillation and other minor symptoms of ocular irritation have been reported with the use of FML® suspension. Other adverse events reported with the use of FML® suspension include: allergic reactions, visual disturbance (blurry vision) and taste perversion.

Dosage and Administration: Instill one drop into the conjunctival sac two to four times daily. During the initial 24 to 48 hours, the dosage may be increased to one application every four hours. Care should be taken not to discontinue therapy prematurely.

If signs and symptoms fail to improve after two days, the patient should be re-evaluated (see **Precautions**).

The dosing of FML® suspension may be reduced, but care should be taken not to discontinue therapy prematurely. In chronic conditions, withdrawal of treatment should be carried out by gradually decreasing the frequency of applications.

How Supplied: FML® (fluorometholone ophthalmic suspension, USP) 0.1% is supplied sterile in opaque white LDPE plastic bottles with droppers with white high impact polystyrene (HIPS) caps as follows:

5 mL in 10 mL bottle – NDC 11980-211-05
10 mL in 15 mL bottle – NDC 11980-211-10
15 mL in 15 mL bottle – NDC 11980-211-15

Note: Store between 2° and 25°C (36°–77°F); protect from freezing. **Shake well before using.**

℞ only
Revised June 2003
©2003 Allergan, Inc.
Irvine, CA 92612
® marks owned by Allergan, Inc.
71598US10M

FML® ℞
(fluorometholone ophthalmic ointment)
0.1%
sterile

Description: FML® (fluorometholone ophthalmic ointment) 0.1% is a topical anti-inflammatory agent for ophthalmic use.

Chemical Name: Fluorometholone: 9-Fluoro-11β, 17-dihydroxy-6α-methylpregna-1,4-diene-3,20-dione.

Contains: Active: fluorometholone 0.1%. **Preservative:** phenylmercuric acetate (0.0008%). **Inactives:** mineral oil; petrolatum (and) lanolin alcohol; and white petrolatum.

Clinical Pharmacology: Corticosteroids inhibit the inflammatory response to a variety of inciting agents and probably delay or slow healing. They inhibit the edema, fibrin deposition, capillary dilation, leukocyte migration, capillary proliferation, fibroblast proliferation, deposition of collagen and scar formation associated with inflammation.

There is no generally accepted explanation for the mechanism of action of ocular corticosteroids. However, corticosteroids are thought to act by the induction of phospholipase A_2 inhibitory proteins, collectively called lipocortins. It is postulated that these proteins control the biosynthesis of potent mediators of inflammation such as prostaglandins and leukotrienes by inhibiting the release of their common precursor arachidonic acid. Arachidonic acid is released from membrane phospholipids by phospholipase A_2.

Corticosteroids are capable of producing a rise in intraocular pressure. In clinical studies of documented steroid-responders, fluorometholone demonstrated a significantly longer average time to produce a rise in intraocular pressure than dexamethasone phosphate; however, in a small percentage of individuals, a significant rise in intraocular pressure occurred within one week. The ultimate magnitude of the rise was equivalent for both drugs.

Indications and Usage: FML® ophthalmic ointment is indicated for the treatment of steroid-responsive inflammation of the palpebral and bulbar conjunctiva, cornea and anterior segment of the globe.

Contraindications: FML® ophthalmic ointment is contraindicated in most viral diseases of the cornea and conjunctiva, including epithelial herpes simplex keratitis (dendritic keratitis), vaccinia, and varicella and also in mycobacterial infection of the eye and fungal diseases of ocular structures. FML® ointment is also contraindicated in individuals with known or suspected hypersensitivity to any of the ingredients of this preparation and to other corticosteroids.

Warnings: Prolonged use of corticosteroids may result in glaucoma with damage to the optic nerve, defects in visual acuity and fields of vision, and in posterior subcapsular cataract formation. Prolonged use may also suppress the host immune response and thus increase the hazard of secondary ocular infections.

Various ocular diseases and long-term use of topical corticosteroids have been known to cause corneal and scleral thinning. Use of topical corticosteroids in the presence of thin corneal or scleral tissue may lead to perforation.

Acute purulent infections of the eye may be masked or activity enhanced by the presence of corticosteroid medication.

If this product is used for 10 days or longer, intraocular pressure should be routinely monitored even though it may be difficult in children and uncooperative patients. Steroids should be used with caution in the presence of glaucoma. Intraocular pressure should be checked frequently.

The use of steroids after cataract surgery may delay healing and increase the incidence of bleb formation.

Use of ocular steroids may prolong the course and may exacerbate the severity of many viral infections of the eye (including herpes simplex). Employment of a corticosteroid medication in the treatment of patients with a history of herpes simplex requires great caution; frequent slit lamp microscopy is recommended.

Corticosteroids are not effective in mustard gas keratitis and Sjögren's keratoconjunctivitis.

Precautions:

General: The initial prescription and renewal of the medication order beyond 8 grams of FML® ophthalmic ointment should be made by a physician only after examination of the patient with the aid of magnification, such as slit lamp biomicroscopy and, where appropriate, fluorescein staining. If signs and symptoms fail to improve after two days, the patient should be re-evaluated.

As fungal infections of the cornea are particularly prone to develop coincidentally with long-term local corticosteroid applications, fungal invasion should be suspected in any persistent

corneal ulceration where a corticosteroid has been used or is in use. Fungal cultures should be taken when appropriate.

If this product is used for 10 days or longer, intraocular pressure should be monitored (see **Warnings**).

Ophthalmic ointments may retard corneal healing.

Information for Patients: If inflammation or pain persists longer than 48 hours or becomes aggravated, the patient should be advised to discontinue use of the medication and consult a physician.

This product is sterile when packaged. To prevent contamination, care should be taken to avoid touching the tube tip to eyelids or to any other surface. The use of this tube by more than one person may spread infection. Keep tube tightly closed when not in use. Keep out of the reach of children.

Carcinogenesis, mutagenesis, impairment of fertility: No studies have been conducted in animals or in humans to evaluate the possibility of these effects with fluorometholone.

Pregnancy: Teratogenic effects. Pregnancy Category C: Fluorometholone has been shown to be embryocidal and teratogenic in rabbits when administered at low multiples of the human ocular dose. Fluorometholone was applied ocularly to rabbits daily on days 6–18 of gestation, and dose-related fetal loss and fetal abnormalities including cleft palate, deformed rib cage, anomalous limbs and neural abnormalities such as encephalocele, craniorachischisis, and spina bifida were observed. There are no adequate and well-controlled studies of fluorometholone in pregnant women, and it is not known whether fluorometholone can cause fetal harm when administered to a pregnant woman. Fluorometholone should be used during pregnancy only if the potential benefit justifies the potential risk to the fetus.

Nursing Mothers: It is not known whether topical ophthalmic administration of corticosteroids could result in sufficient systemic absorption to produce detectable quantities in human milk. Systemically administered corticosteroids appear in human milk and could suppress growth, interfere with endogenous corticosteroid production, or cause other untoward effects. Because of the potential for serious adverse reactions in nursing infants from fluorometholone, a decision should be made whether to discontinue nursing or to discontinue the drug, taking into account the importance of the drug to the mother.

Pediatric Use: Safety and effectiveness in infants below the age of 2 years have not been established.

Geriatric Use: No overall differences in safety and effectiveness have been observed between elderly and younger patients.

Adverse Reactions: Adverse reactions include, in decreasing order of frequency, elevation of intraocular pressure (IOP) with possible development of glaucoma and infrequent optic nerve damage, posterior subcapsular cataract formation, and delayed wound healing.

Although systemic effects are extremely uncommon, there have been rare occurrences of systemic hypercorticoidism after use of topical steroids.

Corticosteroid-containing preparations have also been reported to cause acute anterior uveitis and perforation of the globe. Keratitis, conjunctivitis, corneal ulcers, mydriasis, conjunctival hyperemia, loss of accommodation and ptosis have occasionally been reported following local use of corticosteroids.

The development of secondary ocular infection (bacterial, fungal and viral) has occurred. Fungal and viral infections of the cornea are particularly prone to develop coincidentally with long-term applications of steroids. The possi-

Continued on next page

FML Ointment—Cont.

bility of fungal invasion should be considered in any persistent corneal ulceration where steroid treatment has been used (see **Warnings**).

Dosage and Administration: A small amount (approximately ½ inch ribbon) of ointment should be applied to the conjunctival sac one to three times daily. During the initial 24 to 48 hours, the frequency of dosing may be increased to one application every four hours. Care should be taken not to discontinue therapy prematurely.

If signs and symptoms fail to improve after two days, the patient should be re-evaluated (see **Precautions**).

The dosing of FML® ophthalmic ointment may be reduced, but care should be taken not to discontinue therapy prematurely. In chronic conditions, withdrawal of treatment should be carried out by gradually decreasing the frequency of applications.

How Supplied: FML® (fluorometholone ophthalmic ointment) 0.1% is supplied in a collapsible aluminum tube with a black low density polyethylene screw cap in the following size:

3.5 g in 3.5 g tube—NDC 0023-0316-04

Note: Store at or below 25°C (77°F). Avoid exposure to temperatures above 40°C (104°F).

℞ only

Revised November 2001
©2001 Allergan, Inc.
Irvine, CA 92612, U.S.A.
® marks owned by Allergan, Inc.
71091US11J

Shown in Product Identification Guide, page 103

LUMIGAN®   ℞
(bimatoprost ophthalmic solution) 0.03%

DESCRIPTION LUMIGAN® (bimatoprost ophthalmic solution) 0.03% is a synthetic prostamide analog with ocular hypotensive activity. Its chemical name is (Z)-7-[(1R,2R,3R,5S)-3, 5-Dihydroxy-2-[1E,3S)-3-hydroxy-5-phenyl-1-pentenyl]cyclopentyl]-5-N-ethylheptenamide, and its molecular weight is 415.58. Its molecular formula is $C_{25}H_{37}NO_4$. Its chemical structure is:

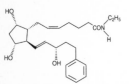

Bimatoprost is a powder, which is very soluble in ethyl alcohol and methyl alcohol and slightly soluble in water. LUMIGAN® is a clear, isotonic, colorless, sterile ophthalmic solution with an osmolality of approximately 290 mOsmol/kg.

Contains: Active: bimatoprost 0.3 mg/mL; **Preservative:** Benzalkonium chloride 0.05 mg/mL; **Inactives:** Sodium chloride; sodium phosphate, dibasic; citric acid; and purified water. Sodium hydroxide and/or hydrochloric acid may be added to adjust pH. The pH during its shelf life ranges from 6.8-7.8.

CLINICAL PHARMACOLOGY

Mechanism of Action: Bimatoprost is a prostamide, a synthetic structural analog of prostaglandin with ocular hypotensive activity. It selectively mimics the effects of naturally occurring substances, prostamides. Bimatoprost is believed to lower intraocular pressure (IOP) in humans by increasing outflow of aqueous humor through both the trabecular meshwork and uveoscleral routes. Elevated IOP presents a major risk factor for glaucomatous field loss. The higher the level of IOP, the greater the

likelihood of optic nerve damage and visual field loss.

Pharmacokinetics

Absorption: After one drop of bimatoprost ophthalmic solution 0.03% was administered once daily to both eyes of 15 healthy subjects for two weeks, blood concentrations peaked within 10 minutes after dosing and were below the lower limit of detection (0.025 ng/mL) in most subjects within 1.5 hours after dosing. Mean C_{max} and AUC_{0-24hr} values were similar on days 7 and 14 at approximately 0.08 ng/mL and 0.09 ng•hr/mL, respectively, indicating that steady state was reached during the first week of ocular dosing. There was no significant systemic drug accumulation over time.

Distribution: Bimatoprost is moderately distributed into body tissues with a steady-state volume of distribution of 0.67 L/kg. In human blood, bimatoprost resides mainly in the plasma. Approximately 12% of bimatoprost remains unbound in human plasma.

Metabolism: Bimatoprost is the major circulating species in the blood once it reaches the systemic circulation following ocular dosing. Bimatoprost then undergoes oxidation, N-deethylation and glucuronidation to form a diverse variety of metabolites.

Elimination: Following an intravenous dose of radiolabeled bimatoprost (3.12 µg/kg) to six healthy subjects, the maximum blood concentration of unchanged drug was 12.2 ng/mL and decreased rapidly with an elimination half-life of approximately 45 minutes. The total blood clearance of bimatoprost was 1.5 L/hr/kg. Up to 67% of the administered dose was excreted in the urine while 25% of the dose was recovered in the feces.

Clinical Studies:

In clinical studies of patients with open angle glaucoma or ocular hypertension with a mean baseline IOP of 26 mmHg, the IOP-lowering effect of LUMIGAN® (bimatoprost ophthalmic solution) 0.03% once daily (in the evening) was 7-8 mmHg.

Results of dosing for up to five years with products in this drug class showed that the onset of noticeable increased iris pigmentation occurred within the first year of treatment for the majority of the patients who developed noticeable iris pigmentation. Patients continued to show sign of increasing iris pigmentation throughout the five years of the study. Observation of increased iris pigmentation did not affect the incidence, nature or severity of adverse events (other than increased iris pigmentation) recorded in the study. IOP reduction was similar regardless of the development of increased iris pigmentation during the study. In patients with a history of liver disease or abnormal ALT, AST and/or bilirubin at baseline, LUMIGAN® had no adverse effect on liver function over 48 months.

INDICATIONS AND USAGE

LUMIGAN® (bimatoprost ophthalmic solution) 0.03% is indicated for the reduction of elevated intraocular pressure in patients with open angle glaucoma or ocular hypertension.

CONTRAINDICATIONS

LUMIGAN® (bimatoprost ophthalmic solution) 0.03% is contraindicated in patients with hypersensitivity to bimatoprost or any other ingredient in this product.

WARNINGS

LUMIGAN® (bimatoprost ophthalmic solution) 0.03% has been reported to cause changes to pigmented tissues. The most frequently reported changes have been increased pigmentation of the iris, periorbital tissue (eyelid) and eyelashes, and growth of eyelashes. Pigmentation is expected to increase as long as LUMIGAN® is administered. After discontinuation of LUMIGAN® pigmentation of the iris is likely to be permanent while pigmentation of the periorbital tissue and eyelash changes have been reported to be reversible in

some patients. Patients who receive treatment should be informed of the possibility of increased pigmentation. The effects of increased pigmentation beyond 5 years are not known.

PRECAUTIONS

General: LUMIGAN® (bimatoprost ophthalmic solution) 0.03% may gradually increase the pigmentation of the iris. The eye color change is due to increased melanin content in the stromal melanocytes of the iris rather than to an increase in the number of melanocytes. This change may not be noticeable for several months to years (see **WARNINGS**).Typically, the brown pigmentation around the pupil spreads concentrically towards the periphery of the iris and the entire iris or parts of the iris become more brownish. Neither nevi nor freckles of the iris appear to be affected by treatment. While treatment with LUMIGAN® can be continued in patients who develop noticeably increased iris pigmentation, these patients should be examined regularly.

During clinical trials, the increase in brown iris pigment has not been shown to progress further upon discontinuation of treatment, but the resultant color change may be permanent. Eyelid skin darkening, which may be reversible upon discontinuation of the treatment has been reported in association with the use of LUMIGAN®.

LUMIGAN® may gradually change eyelashes and vellus hair in the treated eye; these changes include increased length, thickness and number of lashes. Eyelash changes are usually reversible upon discontinuation of treatment.

LUMIGAN® (bimatoprost ophthalmic solution) 0.03% should be used with caution in patients with active intraocular inflammation (e.g., uveitis).

Macular edema, including cystoid macular edema, has been reported during treatment with bimatoprost ophthalmic solution. LUMIGAN® should be used with caution in aphakic patients, in pseudophakic patients with a torn posterior lens capsule, or in patients with known risk factors for macular edema.

LUMIGAN® has not been evaluated for the treatment of angle closure, inflammatory or neovascular glaucoma.

There have been reports of bacterial keratitis associated with the use of multiple-dose containers of topical ophthalmic products. These containers had been inadvertently contaminated by patients who, in most cases, had a concurrent corneal disease or a disruption of the ocular epithelial surface (see **PRECAUTIONS,** Information for Patients).

Contact lenses should be removed prior to instillation of LUMIGAN® and may be reinserted 15 minutes following its administration (see **PRECAUTIONS,** Information for Patients).

Information for Patients: (see **WARNINGS** and **PRECAUTIONS**): Patients should be advised about the potential for increased brown pigmentation of the iris, which may be permanent. Patients should also be informed about the possibility of eyelid skin darkening, which may be reversible after discontinuation of LUMIGAN®.

Patients should also be informed of the possibility of eyelash and vellus hair changes in the treated eye during treatment with LUMIGAN®. These changes may result in a disparity between eyes in length, thickness, pigmentation, number of eyelashes or vellus hairs, and/or direction of eyelash growth. Eyelash changes are usually reversible upon discontinuation of treatment.

Patients should be instructed to avoid allowing the tip of the dispensing container to contact the eye, surrounding structures, fingers, or any other surface in order to avoid contamination of the solution by common bacteria known to cause ocular infections. Serious damage to the eye and subsequent loss of vision may result from using contaminated solutions.

Patients should also be advised that if they develop an intercurrent ocular condition (e.g., trauma or infection) or have ocular surgery, they should immediately seek their physician's advice concerning the continued use of the multidose container.

Patients should be advised that if they develop any ocular reactions, particularly conjunctivitis and eyelid reactions, they should immediately seek their physician's advice.

Patients should be advised that LUMIGAN® contains benzalkonium chloride, which may be absorbed by soft contact lenses. Contact lenses should be removed prior to instillation of LUMIGAN® and may be reinserted 15 minutes following its administration.

If more than one topical ophthalmic drug is being used, the drugs should be administered at least five (5) minutes between applications.

Carcinogenesis, Mutagenesis, Impairment of fertility: Bimatoprost was not carcinogenic in either mice or rats when administered by oral gavage at doses of up to 2 mg/kg/day and 1mg/kg/day respectively (approximately 192 times and 291 times the recommended human exposure based on blood AUC levels respectively) for 104 weeks.

Bimatoprost was not mutagenic or clastogenic in the Ames test, in the mouse lymphoma test, or in the *in vivo* mouse micronucleus tests.

Bimatoprost did not impair fertility in male or female rats up to doses of 0.6 mg/kg/day (approximately 103 times the recommended human exposure based on blood AUC levels).

Pregnancy: Teratogenic effects: *Pregnancy Category C.* In embryo/fetal developmental studies in pregnant mice and rats, abortion was observed at oral doses of bimatoprost which achieved at least 33 or 97 times, respectively, the intended human exposure based on blood AUC levels.

At doses 41 times the intended human exposure based on blood AUC levels, the gestation length was reduced in the dams, the incidence of dead fetuses, late resorptions, peri- and postnatal pup mortality was increased, and pup body weights were reduced.

There are no adequate and well-controlled studies of LUMIGAN® administration in pregnant women. Because animal reproductive studies are not always predictive of human response, LUMIGAN® should be administered during pregnancy only if the potential benefit justifies the potential risk to the fetus.

Nursing mothers: It is not known whether LUMIGAN® is excreted in human milk, although in animal studies, bimatoprost has been shown to be excreted in breast milk. Because many drugs are excreted in human milk, caution should be exercised when LUMIGAN® is administered to a nursing woman.

Pediatric Use: Safety and effectiveness in pediatric patients have not been established.

Geriatric Use: No overall clinical differences in safety or effectiveness have been observed between elderly and other adult patients.

ADVERSE REACTIONS

In clinical trials, the most frequent events associated with the use of LUMIGAN® (bimatoprost ophthalmic solution) 0.03% occurring in approximately 15% to 45% of patients, in descending order of incidence, included conjunctival hyperemia, growth of eyelashes, and ocular pruritus. Approximately 3% of patients discontinued therapy due to conjunctival hyperemia.

Ocular adverse events occurring in approximately 3 to 10% of patients, in descending order of incidence, included ocular dryness, visual disturbance, ocular burning, foreign body sensation, eye pain, pigmentation of the periocular skin, blepharitis, cataract, superficial punctate keratitis, eyelid erythema, ocular ir-

ritation, and eyelash darkening. The following ocular adverse events reported in approximately 1 to 3% of patients, in descending order of incidence, included: eye discharge, tearing, photophobia, allergic conjunctivitis, asthenopia, increases in iris pigmentation, and conjunctival edema. In less than 1% of patients, intraocular inflammation was reported as iritis.

Systemic adverse events reported in approximately 10% of patients were infections (primarily colds and upper respiratory tract infections). The following systemic adverse events reported in approximately 1 to 5% of patients, in descending order of incidence, included headaches, abnormal liver function tests, asthenia and hirsutism.

OVERDOSAGE

No information is available on overdosage in humans. If overdose with LUMIGAN® (bimatoprost ophthalmic solution) 0.03% occurs, treatment should be symptomatic.

In oral (by gavage) mouse and rat studies, doses up to 100 mg/kg/day did not produce any toxicity. This dose expressed as mg/m^2 is at least 70 times higher than the accidental dose of one bottle of LUMIGAN® for a 10 kg child.

DOSAGE AND ADMINISTRATION

The recommended dosage is one drop in the affected eye(s) once daily in the evening. The dosage of LUMIGAN® (bimatoprost ophthalmic solution) 0.03% should not exceed once daily since it has been shown that more frequent administration may decrease the intraocular pressure lowering effect.

Reduction of the intraocular pressure starts approximately 4 hours after the first administration with maximum effect reached within approximately 8 to 12 hours.

LUMIGAN® may be used concomitantly with other topical ophthalmic drug products to lower intraocular pressure. If more than one topical ophthalmic drug is being used, the drugs should be administered at least five (5) minutes apart.

HOW SUPPLIED

LUMIGAN® (bimatoprost ophthalmic solution) 0.03% is supplied sterile in opaque white low density polyethylene ophthalmic dispenser bottles and tips with turquoise polystyrene caps in the following sizes:

2.5 mL fill in 5 mL container - NDC 0023-9187-03
5 mL fill in 10 mL container - NDC 0023-9187-05
7.5 mL fill in 10 mL container - NDC 0023-9187-07

Storage: LUMIGAN® should be stored in the original container at 2° to 25°C (36° to 77°F).

Rx only

Revised September 2006
© 2006 Allergan, Inc.
Irvine, CA 92612
® marks owned by Allergan, Inc.
US Patents 5,688,819 and 6,403,649
9106X
71669US11T

Shown in Product Identification Guide, page 103

OCUFEN®   ℞
(flurbiprofen sodium ophthalmic solution, USP) 0.03%
sterile

Description: OCUFEN® (flurbiprofen sodium ophthalmic solution, USP) 0.03% is a sterile topical nonsteroidal anti-inflammatory product for ophthalmic use.

Chemical Name: Sodium (±)-2-(2-fluoro-4-biphenylyl)-propionate dihydrate.

Contains: Active: flurbiprofen sodium 0.03% (0.3 mg/mL).

Preservative: thimerosal 0.005%.

Inactives: citric acid; edetate disodium; polyvinyl alcohol 1.4%; potassium chloride; purified water; sodium chloride; and sodium citrate. May also contain hydrochloric acid and/ or sodium hydroxide to adjust the pH. The pH of OCUFEN® ophthalmic solution is 6.0 to 7.0. It has an osmolality of 260-330 mOsm/kg.

Clinical Pharmacology: Flurbiprofen sodium is one of a series of phenylalkanoic acids that have shown analgesic, antipyretic, and anti-inflammatory activity in animal inflammatory diseases. Its mechanism of action is believed to be through inhibition of the cyclooxygenase enzyme that is essential in the biosynthesis of prostaglandins.

Prostaglandins have been shown in many animal models to be mediators of certain kinds of intraocular inflammation. In studies performed on animal eyes, prostaglandins have been shown to produce disruption of the blood-aqueous humor barrier, vasodilatation, increased vascular permeability, leukocytosis, and increased intraocular pressure.

Prostaglandins also appear to play a role in the miotic response produced during ocular surgery by constricting the iris sphincter independently of cholinergic mechanisms. In clinical studies, OCUFEN® ophthalmic solution has been shown to inhibit the miosis induced during the course of cataract surgery.

Results from clinical studies indicate that flurbiprofen sodium has no significant effect upon intraocular pressure.

Indications and Usage: OCUFEN® ophthalmic solution is indicated for the inhibition of intraoperative miosis.

Contraindications: OCUFEN® ophthalmic solution is contraindicated in individuals who are hypersensitive to any components of the medication.

Warnings: With nonsteroidal anti-inflammatory drugs, there exists the potential for increased bleeding due to interference with thrombocyte aggregation. There have been reports that OCUFEN® ophthalmic solution may cause increased bleeding of ocular tissues including hyphemas in conjunction with ocular surgery. There exists the potential for cross-sensitivity to acetylsalicylic acid and other nonsteroidal anti-inflammatory drugs. Therefore, caution should be used when treating individuals who have previously exhibited sensitivities to these drugs.

Precautions:

General: Wound healing may be delayed with the use of OCUFEN® ophthalmic solution. It is recommended that OCUFEN® ophthalmic solution be used with caution in surgical patients with known bleeding tendencies or who are receiving other medications which may prolong bleeding time.

Drug Interactions: Interaction of OCUFEN® ophthalmic solution with other topical ophthalmic medications has not been fully investigated. Although clinical studies with acetylcholine chloride and animal studies with acetylcholine chloride or carbachol revealed no interference, and there is no known pharmacological basis for an interaction, there have been reports that acetylcholine chloride and carbachol have been ineffective when used in patients treated with OCUFEN® ophthalmic solution.

Carcinogenesis, Mutagenesis, Impairment of Fertility: Long-term studies in mice and/ or rats have shown no evidence of carcinogenicity with flurbiprofen.

Long-term mutagenicity studies in animals have not been performed.

Pregnancy: Pregnancy Category C. Flurbiprofen has been shown to be embryocidal, delay parturition, prolong gestation, reduce weight, and/or slightly retard growth of fetuses when given to rats in daily oral doses of

Continued on next page

Ocufen—Cont.

0.4 mg/kg (approximately 300 times the human daily topical dose) and above.
There are no adequate and well-controlled studies in pregnant women. OCUFEN® ophthalmic solution should be used during pregnancy only if the potential benefit justifies the potential risk to the fetus.
Nursing Mothers: It is not known whether this drug is excreted in human milk. Because many drugs are excreted in human milk and because of the potential for serious adverse reactions in nursing infants from flurbiprofen sodium, a decision should be made whether to discontinue nursing or to discontinue the drug, taking into account the importance of the drug to the mother.
Pediatric Use: Safety and effectiveness in pediatric patients have not been established.
Geriatric Use: No overall differences in safety or effectiveness have been observed between elderly and younger patients.
Adverse Reactions: Transient burning and stinging upon instillation and other minor symptoms of ocular irritation have been reported with the use of OCUFEN® ophthalmic solution. Other adverse reactions reported with the use of OCUFEN® ophthalmic solution include: fibrosis, miosis, and mydriasis.
Increased bleeding tendency of ocular tissues in conjunction with ocular surgery has also been reported.
Overdosage: Overdosage will not ordinarily cause acute problems. If accidentally ingested, drink fluids to dilute.
Dosage and Administration: A total of four (4) drops of OCUFEN® ophthalmic solution should be administered by instilling 1 drop approximately every ½ hour beginning 2 hours before surgery.
How Supplied: OCUFEN® (flurbiprofen sodium ophthalmic solution, USP) is available for topical ophthalmic administration as a 0.03% sterile solution, and is supplied in the following size:
2.5 mL in 5 mL bottle—NDC 11980-801-03
Note: Store at 15°–25°C (59–77°F)
℞ only
Revised May 2004
©2004 Allergan, Inc.
Irvine, CA 92612, U.S.A.
® marks owned by Allergan, Inc.
71587US12P

OPHTHETIC®   ℞

(proparacaine HCl ophthalmic solution) 0.5% sterile

Description: OPHTHETIC® (proparacaine HCl ophthalmic solution) 0.5% is a topical local anesthetic for ophthalmic use.
Chemical Name:
Benzoic acid, 3-amino-4-propoxy-, 2-(diethylamino)ethyl ester, monohydrochloride.
Contains: **Active:** proparacaine HCl 0.5%
Preservative: benzalkonium chloride (0.01%)
Inactives: glycerin; purified water; sodium chloride; and hydrochloric acid and/or sodium hydroxide to adjust pH (5.0 to 6.0).
Clinical Pharmacology: OPHTHETIC® ophthalmic solution is a rapidly-acting topical anesthetic, with induced anesthesia lasting approximately 10–20 minutes.
Indications and Usage: OPHTHETIC® ophthalmic solution is indicated for procedures in which a topical ophthalmic anesthetic is indicated: corneal anesthesia of short duration, e.g., tonometry, gonioscopy, removal of corneal for-

eign bodies, and for short corneal and conjunctival procedures.
Contraindications: OPHTHETIC® ophthalmic solution should be considered contraindicated in patients with known hypersensitivity to any of the ingredients of this preparation.
Warnings: Prolonged use of a topical ocular anesthetic is not recommended. It may produce permanent corneal opacification with accompanying visual loss.
Precautions: Carcinogenesis, Mutagenesis, Impairment of Fertility: Long-term studies in animals have not been performed to evaluate carcinogenic potential, mutagenicity, or possible impairment of fertility in males or females.
Pregnancy: Pregnancy Category C: Animal reproduction studies have not been conducted with OPHTHETIC® (proparacaine hydrochloride ophthalmic solution) 0.5%. It is also not known whether proparacaine hydrochloride can cause fetal harm when administered to a pregnant woman or can affect reproduction capacity. Proparacaine hydrochloride should be administered to a pregnant woman only if clearly needed.
Nursing Mothers: It is not known whether this drug is excreted in human milk. Because many drugs are excreted in human milk, caution should be exercised when proparacaine hydrochloride is administered to a nursing mother.
Pediatric Use: Safety and effectiveness of proparacaine HCl ophthalmic solution in pediatric patients have not been established. Use of proparacaine HCl is supported by evidence from adequate and well-controlled studies in adults and children over the age of twelve, and safety information in neonates and other pediatric patients.
Geriatric Use: No overall clinical differences in safety or effectiveness have been observed between the elderly and other adult patients.
Adverse Reactions: Occasional temporary stinging, burning, and conjunctival redness may occur with the use of proparacaine. A rare, severe, immediate-type, apparently hyperallergic corneal reaction, characterized by acute, intense and diffuse epithelial keratitis, a gray, ground glass appearance, sloughing of large areas of necrotic epithelium, corneal filaments and sometimes, iritis with descemetitis has been reported.
Allergic contact dermatitis from proparacaine with drying and fissuring of the fingertips has also been reported.
Dosage and Administration:
Usual Dosage: Removal of foreign bodies and sutures, and for tonometry: 1 to 2 drops (in single instillations) in each eye before operating.
Short corneal and conjunctival procedures: 1 drop in each eye every 5 to 10 minutes for 5–7 doses.
Note: OPHTHETIC® should be clear to straw-color. If the solution becomes darker, discard the solution.
How Supplied:
OPHTHETIC® (proparacaine HCl ophthalmic solution) 0.5% is supplied sterile in opaque natural LDPE plastic bottles with dropper tips and white high impact polystyrene (HIPS) caps as follows:
15 mL in 15 mL bottle—NDC 11980-048-15
Bottle must be stored in unit carton to protect contents from light. Store bottles under refrigeration at 2°C to 8°C (36°F to 46°F).
℞ only
Revised July 2002
©2004 Allergan, Inc
Irvine, CA 92612, U.S.A.
® marks owned by Allergan, Inc.
71742US10P

OPTIVE™   OTC

OPTIVE™ Lubricant Eye Drops advances dry eye relief by providing a **dual-action formula** that moisturizes the surface of your eye while also hydrating the areas where dry-eye starts, giving your eyes long-lasting moisturizing protection. It's the evolution of eye-drops, optimistically formulated for the way you see the world – it's OPTIVE™.
Drug Facts

Active ingredients	Purpose
Carboxymethylcellulose sodium 0.5%	Eye lubricant
Glycerin 0.9%	Eye lubricant

Uses
- For the temporary relief of burning, irritation, and discomfort due to dryness of the eye or exposure to wind or sun.
- May be used as a protectant against further irritation.

Warnings
- **For external use only.**
- **To avoid contamination, do not touch tip of container to any surface. Replace cap after using.**
- **Do not use if solution changes color.**

Stop use and ask a doctor if you experience eye pain, changes in vision, continued redness, or irritation of the eye, or if the condition worsens or persists for more than 72 hours.
Keep out of reach of children. If swallowed, get medical help or contact a Poison Control Center right away.
Directions: Instill 1 or 2 drops in the affected eye(s) as needed.
Other information
- **Use only if printed tape seals on top and bottom flaps are intact and clearly legible.**
- **RETAIN THIS CARTON FOR FUTURE REFERENCE.**

Inactive ingredients:
Boric acid, calcium chloride dihydrate, erythritol, levocarnitine, magnesium chloride hexahydrate, potassium chloride, purified water, PURITE® (stabilized oxychloro complex), sodium borate decahydrate, and sodium citrate dihydrate.
How supplied: OPTIVE™ Lubricant Eye Drops are supplied in the following sizes:
15 mL bottle – NDC 0023-3240-15
30 mL bottle – NDC 0023-3240-30
Allergan, Inc
Irvine, CA 92612, U.S.A.
©2007 Allergan, Inc
® and ™ marks owned by Allergan, Inc.
U.S. Patent 5,424,078
Revised June 2007
Shown in Product Identification Guide, page 103

POLY-PRED®   ℞

[pole̅-pred]
(prednisolone acetate, neomycin sulfate, polymyxin B sulfate ophthalmic suspension, USP)
sterile

Description: POLY-PRED® (prednisolone acetate, neomycin sulfate, polymyxin B sulfate ophthalmic suspension, USP) is a topical anti-inflammatory/anti-infective combination product for ophthalmic use with a pH of 5.0 - 7.0 and an osmolality of 260-340 mOsm/kg.
Chemical Name: Prednisolone acetate: 11b, 17, 21-Trihydroxypregna-1, 4-diene-3, 20-dione 21-acetate.
Neomycin sulfate is the sulfate salt of neomycin B and neomycin C which are produced by the growth of *Streptomyces fradiae* (Fam. *Streptomycetaceae*). It has a potency

equivalent to not less than 600 micrograms per milligram of neomycin base, calculated on an anhydrous basis.

Polymyxin B sulfate is the sulfate salt of polymyxin B$_1$ and polymyxin B$_2$ which are produced by the growth of *Bacillus polymyxa* (Prazmowski) Migula (Fam. *Bacillaceae*). It has a potency of not less than 6,000 polymyxin B units per milligram, calculated on an anhydrous basis.

Contains: Actives: prednisolone acetate (microfine suspension) 0.5%, neomycin sulfate equivalent to 0.35% neomycin base, polymyxin B sulfate 10,000 units/mL. Inactives: polysorbate 80; polyvinyl alcohol; propylene glycol; purified water; sodium acetate; and thimerosal 0.001% (preservative). The pH range is 5.0 - 7.0.

Clinical Pharmacology: Corticosteroids suppress the inflammatory response to a variety of agents and they probably delay or slow healing. Since corticosteroids may inhibit the body's defense mechanism against infection, a concomitant antimicrobial drug may be used when this inhibition is considered to be clinically significant in a particular case.

The anti-infective components in POLY-PRED® ophthalmic suspension are included to provide action against specific organisms susceptible to them. Neomycin sulfate and polymyxin B sulfate are considered active against the following microorganisms: *Staphylococcus aureus; Escherichia coli; Hemophilus influenzae; Klebsiella / Enterobacter* species; *Neisseria* species; and *Pseudomonas aeruginosa*.

When a decision to administer both a corticosteroid and an antimicrobial is made, the administration of such drugs in combination has the advantage of greater patient compliance and convenience, with the added assurance that the appropriate dosage of both drugs is administered. When both types of drugs are in the same formulation, compatibility of ingredients is assured and the correct volume of drug is delivered and retained.

The relative potency of corticosteroids depends on the molecular structure, concentration and release from the vehicle.

Indications and Usage: A steroid/anti-infective combination is indicated for steroid-responsive inflammatory ocular conditions for which a corticosteroid is indicated and where bacterial infection or a risk of bacterial ocular infection exists.

Ocular steroids are indicated in inflammatory conditions of the palpebral and bulbar conjunctiva, cornea, and anterior segment of the globe where the inherent risk of steroid use in certain infective conjunctivitides is accepted to obtain a diminution in edema and inflammation. They are also indicated in chronic anterior uveitis and corneal injury from chemical, radiation, or thermal burns or penetration of foreign bodies.

The use of a combination drug with an anti-infective component is indicated where the risk of infection is high or where there is an expectation that potentially dangerous numbers of bacteria will be present in the eye.

The particular anti-infective drugs in this product are active against the following common bacterial eye pathogens: *Staphylococcus aureus; Escherichia coli; Hemophilus influenzae; Klebsiella / Enterobacter* species; *Neisseria* species; and *Pseudomonas aeruginosa*.

The product does not provide adequate coverage against: *Serratia marcescens; Streptococci*, including *Streptococcus pneumoniae*.

Contraindications: Epithelial herpes simplex keratitis (dendritic keratitis), vaccinia, varicella, and many other viral diseases of the cornea and conjunctiva. Mycobacterial infection of the eye. Fungal diseases of the ocular structures. Hypersensitivity to a component of the medication. (Hypersensitivity to the antibiotic component occurs at a higher rate than for other components.)

The use of these combinations is always contraindicated after uncomplicated removal of a corneal foreign body.

Warnings:
NOT FOR INJECTION INTO THE EYE.
Prolonged use may result in glaucoma, with damage to the optic nerve, defects in visual acuity and fields of vision, and in posterior subcapsular cataract formation. Prolonged use may suppress the host response and thus increase the hazard of secondary ocular infections. In those diseases causing thinning of the cornea or sclera, perforations have been known to occur with the use of topical steroids. In acute purulent conditions of the eye, steroids may mask infection or enhance existing infection. If these products are used for 10 days or longer, intraocular pressure should be routinely monitored even though it may be difficult in children and uncooperative patients.

Employment of a steroid medication in the treatment of herpes simplex requires great caution.

There exists a potential for neomycin sulfate to cause cutaneous sensitization. The exact incidence of this reaction is unknown. The manifestations of sensitization to topical antibiotics are usually itching, reddening, and edema of the conjunctiva and eyelid. A sensitization reaction may manifest simply as a failure to heal. During long-term use of topical antibiotic products, periodic examination for such signs is advisable, and the patient should be told to discontinue the product if they are observed. Symptoms usually subside quickly on withdrawing the medication. Application of products containing these ingredients should be avoided for the patient thereafter (see PRECAUTIONS: **General**).

Precautions:
General: The initial prescription and renewal of the medication order beyond 20 milliliters should be made by a physician only after examination of the patient with the aid of magnification, such as slit lamp biomicroscopy and, where appropriate, fluorescein staining.

The possibility of persistent fungal infections of the cornea should be considered after prolonged steroid dosing.

As with other antimicrobial preparations, prolonged use may result in overgrowth of non-susceptible organisms, including fungi. If superinfection occurs, appropriate therapy should be initiated.

Bacterial resistance to POLY-PRED® ophthalmic suspension may also develop. If purulent discharge, inflammation, or pain becomes aggravated, the patient should discontinue use of the medication and consult a physician.

Allergic cross-reactions may occur which could prevent the use of any or all of the following antibiotics for the treatment of future infections: kanamycin, paromomycin, streptomycin, and possibly gentamicin.

Information for Patients: If inflammation or pain persists longer than 48 hours or becomes aggravated, the patient should be advised to discontinue use of the medication and consult a physician (See WARNINGS).

This product is sterile when packaged. To prevent contamination, care should be taken to avoid touching the applicator tip to eyelids or to any other surface. The use of this bottle by more than one person may spread infection. Keep bottle tightly closed when not in use. Keep out of the reach of children.

Patients should be advised not to wear contact lenses if they have signs and symptoms of ocular bacterial infections.

Carcinogenesis, Mutagenesis, Impairment of Fertility: No studies have been conducted in animals or in humans to evaluate the potential of these effects due to prednisolone.

Treatment of human lymphocytes *in vitro* with neomycin increased the frequency of chromosome aberrations at the highest concentration (80 µg/mL) tested; however, the effects of neomycin on carcinogenesis and mutagenesis in humans are unknown.

No studies have been conducted with polymyxin B sulfate to evaluate carcinogenic or mutagenic potential. Polymyxin B has been reported to impair the motility of equine sperm, but its effects on male or female fertility are unknown.

Pregnancy: Teratogenic Effects: Pregnancy Category C. Prednisolone has been shown to be teratogenic in rabbits, hamsters, and mice. In mice, prednisolone has been shown to be teratogenic when given in doses 1 to 10 times the human ocular dose. Dexamethasone, hydrocortisone and prednisolone were applied to both eyes of pregnant mice five times per day on days 10 through 13 of gestation. A significant increase in the incidence of cleft palate was observed in the fetuses of the treated mice. There are no adequate well-controlled studies in pregnant women dosed with corticosteroids.

Animal reproduction studies have not been conducted with polymyxin B sulfate or neomycin sulfate. It is also not known whether polymyxin B sulfate or neomycin sulfate can cause fetal harm when administered to a pregnant woman or can affect reproduction capacity.

POLY-PRED® ophthalmic suspension should be used during pregnancy only if the potential benefit justifies the potential risk to the fetus.

Nursing Mothers: This drug is excreted in human milk. Caution should be exercised when POLY-PRED® ophthalmic suspension is administered to a nursing woman.

Pediatric Use: Safety and effectiveness in pediatric patients have not been established.

Geriatric Use: No overall differences in safety or effectiveness have been observed between elderly and younger patients.

Adverse Reactions: Adverse reactions have occurred with steroid/anti-infective combination drugs which can be attributed to the steroid component, the anti-infective component, or the combination. Exact incidence figures are not available since no denominator of treated patients is available.

Reactions occurring most often from the presence of the anti-infective ingredients are allergic sensitizations including itching, swelling, and conjunctival erythema (see WARNINGS). More serious hypersensitivity reactions, including anaphylaxis, have been reported rarely. The reactions due to the steroid component in decreasing order of frequency are: elevation of intraocular pressure (IOP) with possible development of glaucoma, and infrequent optic nerve damage; posterior subcapsular cataract formation; and delayed wound healing.

Although systemic effects are extremely uncommon, there have been rare occurences of systemic hypercorticoidism after use of topical steroids.

Corticosteroid-containing preparations have also been reported to cause perforation of the globe. Keratitis, conjunctivitis, corneal ulcers, and conjunctival hyperemia have occasionally been reported following local use of steroids.

Secondary infection: The development of secondary infection has occurred after use of combinations containing steroids and antimicrobials. Fungal infections of the cornea are particularly prone to develop coincidentally with long-term applications of steroids. The possibility of fungal invasion must be considered in any persistent corneal ulceration where steroid treatment has been used.

Secondary bacterial ocular infection following suppression of host responses also occurs.

Continued on next page

Poly-Pred—Cont.

Dosage and Administration: TO TREAT THE EYE: Instill 1 or 2 drops every 3 or 4 hours, or more frequently as required. Acute infections may require administration every 30 minutes, with frequency of administration reduced as the infection is brought under control. TO TREAT THE LIDS: Instill 1 or 2 drops in the eye every 3 to 4 hours, close the eye and rub the excess on the lids and lid margins.

Not more than 20 milliliters should be prescribed initially and the prescription should not be refilled without further evaluation as outlined in the PRECAUTIONS section above.

How Supplied: POLY-PRED® (prednisolone acetate, neomycin sulfate, polymyxin B sulfate ophthalmic suspension, USP) is supplied sterile in opaque white LDPE plastic bottles with droppers with white high impact polystyrene (HIPS) caps as follows:

5 mL in 10 mL bottle – NDC 0023-0028-05

Note: Store at 15 - 25°C (59 - 77°F). Protect from freezing. Shake well before using. Store in an upright position.

Rx Only

Revised December 2004

© 2004 Allergan, Inc.

Irvine, CA 92612, U.S.A.

® marks owned by Allergan, Inc.

71746US10P

POLYTRIM®   ℞
(polymyxin B sulfate and trimethoprim ophthalmic solution, USP) Sterile

Description: POLYTRIM® (polymyxin B sulfate and trimethoprim ophthalmic solution, USP) is a sterile antimicrobial solution for topical ophthalmic use. It has pH of 4.0 to 6.2 and osmolality of 270 to 310 mOsm/kg.

Chemical Names: Trimethoprim sulfate, 2, 4-Diamino-5-(3,4,5-trimethoxybenzyl) pyrimidine sulfate, is a white, odorless, crystalline powder with a molecular weight of 678.72. Polymyxin B sulfate is the sulfate salt of polymyxin B_1 and B_2 which are produced by the growth of *Bacillus polymyxa* (Prazmowski) Migula (Fam. Bacillaceae). It has a potency of not less than 6,000 polymyxin B units per mg, calculated on an anhydrous basis.

Contains: Actives: polymyxin B sulfate 10,000 units/mL; trimethoprim sulfate equivalent to 1 mg/mL. Preservative: benzalkonium chloride 0.04 mg/mL. Inactives: purified water; sodium chloride; and sulfuric acid. May also contain sodium hydroxide to adjust the pH.

Clinical Pharmacology: Trimethoprim is a synthetic antibacterial drug active against a wide variety of aerobic gram-positive and gram-negative ophthalmic pathogens. Trimethoprim blocks the production of tetrahydrofolic acid from dihydrofolic acid by binding to and reversibly inhibiting the enzyme dihydrofolate reductase. This binding is stronger for the bacterial enzyme than for the corresponding mammalian enzyme and therefore selectively interferes with bacterial biosynthesis of nucleic acids and proteins.

Polymyxin B, a cyclic lipopeptide antibiotic, is bactericidal for a variety of gram-negative organisms, especially *Pseudomonas aeruginosa*. It increases the permeability of the bacterial cell membrane by interacting with the phospholipid components of the membrane.

Blood samples were obtained from 11 human volunteers at 20 minutes, 1 hour and 3 hours following instillation in the eye of 2 drops of ophthalmic solution containing 1 mg trimethoprim and 10,000 units polymyxin B per mL. Peak serum concentrations were approximately 0.03 µg/mL trimethoprim and 1 unit/ mL polymyxin B.

Microbiology: *In vitro* studies have demonstrated that the anti-infective components of POLYTRIM® are active against the following bacterial pathogens that are capable of causing external infections of the eye:

Trimethoprim: Staphylococcus aureus and *Staphylococcus epidermidis, Streptococcus pyogenes, Streptococcus faecalis, Streptococcus pneumoniae, Haemophilus influenzae, Haemophilus aegyptius, Escherichia coli, Klebsiella pneumoniae, Proteus mirabilis* (indole-negative), *Proteus vulgaris* (indole-positive), *Enterobacter aerogenes,* and *Serratia marcescens.*

Polymyxin B: Pseudomonas aeruginosa, Escherichia coli, Klebsiella pneumoniae, Enterobacter aerogenes and *Haemophilus influenzae.*

Indications and Usage: POLYTRIM® Ophthalmic Solution is indicated in the treatment of surface ocular bacterial infections, including acute bacterial conjunctivitis, and blepharoconjunctivitis, caused by susceptible strains of the following microorganisms: *Staphylococcus aureus, Staphylococcus epidermidis, Streptococcus pneumoniae, Streptococcus viridans, Haemophilus influenzae* and *Pseudomonas aeruginosa.* *

---

*Efficacy for this organism in this organ system was studied in fewer than 10 infections.

Contraindications: POLYTRIM® Ophthalmic Solution is contraindicated in patients with known hypersensitivity to any of its components.

Warnings: NOT FOR INJECTION INTO THE EYE.

If a sensitivity reaction to POLYTRIM® occurs, discontinue use. POLYTRIM® Ophthalmic Solution is not indicated for the prophylaxis or treatment of ophthalmia neonatorum.

Precautions:

General: As with other antimicrobial preparations, prolonged use may result in overgrowth of nonsusceptible organisms, including fungi. If superinfection occurs, appropriate therapy should be initiated.

Information for Patients: Avoid contaminating the applicator tip with material from the eye, fingers, or other source. This precaution is necessary if the sterility of the drops is to be maintained.

If redness, irritation, swelling or pain persists or increases, discontinue use immediately and contact your physician. Patients should be advised not to wear contact lenses if they have signs and symptoms of ocular bacterial infections.

Carcinogenesis, Mutagenesis, Impairment of Fertility:

Carcinogenesis: Long-term studies in animals to evaluate carcinogenic potential have not been conducted with polymyxin B sulfate or trimethoprim.

Mutagenesis: Trimethoprim was demonstrated to be non-mutagenic in the Ames assay. In studies at two laboratories no chromosomal damage was detected in cultured Chinese hamster ovary cells at concentrations approximately 500 times human plasma levels after oral administration; at concentrations approximately 1000 times human plasma levels after oral administration in these same cells, a low level of chromosomal damage was induced at one of the laboratories. Studies to evaluate mutagenic potential have not been conducted with polymyxin B sulfate.

Impairment of Fertility: Polymyxin B sulfate has been reported to impair the motility of equine sperm, but its effects on male or female fertility are unknown.

No adverse effects on fertility or general reproductive performance were observed in rats given trimethoprim in oral dosages as high as 70 mg/kg/day for males and 14 mg/kg/day for females.

Pregnancy: Teratogenic Effects: Pregnancy Category C. Animal reproduction studies have not been conducted with polymyxin B sulfate. It is not known whether polymyxin B sulfate can cause fetal harm when administered to a pregnant woman or can affect reproduction capacity.

Trimethoprim has been shown to be teratogenic in the rat when given in oral doses 40 times the human dose. In some rabbit studies, the overall increase in fetal loss (dead and resorbed and malformed conceptuses) was associated with oral doses 6 times the human therapeutic dose.

While there are no large well-controlled studies on the use of trimethoprim in pregnant women, Brumfitt and Pursell, in a retrospective study, reported the outcome of 186 pregnancies during which the mother received either placebo or oral trimethoprim in combination with sulfamethoxazole. The incidence of congenital abnormalities was 4.5% (3 of 66) in those who received placebo and 3.3% (4 of 120) in those receiving trimethoprim and sulfamethoxazole. There were no abnormalities in the 10 children whose mothers received the drug during the first trimester. In a separate survey, Brumfitt and Pursell also found no congenital abnormalities in 35 children whose mothers had received oral trimethoprim and sulfamethoxazole at the time of conception or shortly thereafter.

Because trimethoprim may interfere with folic acid metabolism, trimethoprim should be used during pregnancy only if the potential benefit justifies the potential risk to the fetus.

Nonteratogenic Effects: The oral administration of trimethoprim to rats at a dose of 70 mg/kg/day commencing with the last third of gestation and continuing through parturition and lactation caused no deleterious effects on gestation or pup growth and survival.

Nursing Mothers: It is not known whether this drug is excreted in human milk. Because many drugs are excreted in human milk, caution should be exercised when POLYTRIM® Ophthalmic Solution is administered to a nursing woman.

Pediatric Use: Safety and effectiveness in children below the age of 2 months have not been established (see **Warnings**).

Geriatric Use: No overall differences in safety or effectiveness have been observed between elderly and other adult patients.

Adverse Reactions: The most frequent adverse reaction to POLYTRIM® Ophthalmic Solution is local irritation consisting of increased redness, burning, stinging, and/or itching. This may occur on instillation, within 48 hours, or at any time with extended use. There are also multiple reports of hypersensitivity reactions consisting of lid edema, itching, increased redness, tearing, and/or circumocular rash. Photosensitivity has been reported in patients taking oral trimethoprim.

Dosage and Administration: In mild to moderate infections, instill one drop in the affected eye(s) every three hours (maximum of 6 doses per day) for a period of 7 to 10 days.

How Supplied: Polytrim® (polymyxin B sulfate and trimethoprim ophthalmic solution, USP) is supplied sterile in opaque white low density polyethylene ophthalmic dispenser bottles and tips with white high impact polystyrene (HIPS) caps as follows: 10 mL in 10 mL bottle—NDC 0023-7824-10.

Note: Store at 15°–25°C (59°–77°F) and protect from light.

℞ only

Revised August 2004

©2004 Allergan, Inc.

Irvine, CA 92612, U.S.A.

® marks owned by Allergan, Inc.

71756US10P

PRED FORTE® Rx
(prednisolone acetate ophthalmic suspension, USP) 1% sterile

Description: PRED FORTE® (prednisolone acetate ophthalmic suspension, USP) 1% is a topical anti-inflammatory agent for ophthalmic use.

Chemical Name: 11β, 17, 21-Trihydroxy-pregna-1, 4-diene-3,20-dione 21-acetate.

Contains: Active: prednisolone acetate (microfine suspension) 1.0%. **Preservative:** benzalkonium chloride. **Inactives:** boric acid; edetate disodium; hypromellose; polysorbate 80; purified water; sodium bisulfite; sodium chloride; and sodium citrate. The pH during its shelf life ranges from 5.0 to 6.0.

Clinical Pharmacology: Prednisolone acetate is a glucocorticoid that, on the basis of weight, has 3 to 5 times the anti-inflammatory potency of hydrocortisone. Glucocorticoids inhibit the edema, fibrin deposition, capillary dilation and phagocytic migration of the acute inflammatory response, as well as capillary proliferation, deposition of collagen, and scar formation.

Indications and Usage: PRED FORTE® is indicated for the treatment of steroid-responsive inflammation of the palpebral and bulbar conjunctiva, cornea and anterior segment of the globe.

Contraindications: PRED FORTE® suspension is contraindicated in most viral diseases of the cornea and conjunctiva including epithelial herpes simplex keratitis (dendritic keratitis), vaccinia, and varicella, and also in mycobacterial infection of the eye and fungal diseases of ocular structures. PRED FORTE® suspension is also contraindicated in individuals with known or suspected hypersensitivity to any of the ingredients of this preparation and to other corticosteroids.

Warnings: Prolonged use of corticosteroids may result in glaucoma with damage to the optic nerve, defects in visual acuity and fields of vision, and in posterior subcapsular cataract formation. Prolonged use may also suppress the host immune response and thus increase the hazard of secondary ocular infections.

Various ocular diseases and long-term use of topical corticosteroids have been known to cause corneal and scleral thinning. Use of topical corticosteroids in the presence of thin corneal or scleral tissue may lead to perforation.

Acute purulent infections of the eye may be masked or activity enhanced by the presence of corticosteroid medication.

If this product is used for 10 days or longer, intraocular pressure should be routinely monitored even though it may be difficult in children and uncooperative patients. Steroids should be used with caution in the presence of glaucoma. Intraocular pressure should be checked frequently.

The use of steroids after cataract surgery may delay healing and increase the incidence of bleb formation.

Use of ocular steroids may prolong the course and may exacerbate the severity of many viral infections of the eye (including herpes simplex). Employment of a corticosteroid medication in the treatment of patients with a history of herpes simplex requires great caution; frequent slit lamp microscopy is recommended.

Corticosteroids are not effective in mustard gas keratitis and Sjögren's keratoconjunctivitis.

Contains sodium bisulfite, a sulfite that may cause allergic-type reactions, including anaphylactic symptoms and life-threatening or less severe asthmatic episodes in certain susceptible people. The overall prevalence of sulfite sensitivity in the general population is unknown and probably low. Sulfite sensitivity is seen more frequently in asthmatic than in nonasthmatic people.

Precautions:
General: The initial prescription and renewal of the medication order beyond 20 milliliters of PRED FORTE® suspension should be made by a physician only after examination of the patient with the aid of magnification, such as slitlamp biomicroscopy, and, where appropriate, fluorescein staining. If signs and symptoms fail to improve after 2 days, the patient should be re-evaluated.

As fungal infections of the cornea are particularly prone to develop coincidentally with long-term local corticosteroid applications, fungal invasion should be suspected in any persistent corneal ulceration where a corticosteroid has been used or is in use. Fungal cultures should be taken when appropriate.

If this product is used for 10 days or longer, intraocular pressure should be monitored (see **Warnings**).

Information for Patients: If inflammation or pain persists longer than 48 hours or becomes aggravated, the patient should be advised to discontinue use of the medication and consult a physician.

This product is sterile when packaged. To prevent contamination, care should be taken to avoid touching the bottle tip to eyelids or to any other surface. The use of this bottle by more than one person may spread infection. Keep bottle tightly closed when not in use. Keep out of the reach of children.

Carcinogenesis, Mutagenesis, Impairment of Fertility: No studies have been conducted in animals or in humans to evaluate the potential of these effects.

Pregnancy Category C: Prednisolone has been shown to be teratogenic in mice when given in doses 1–10 times the human dose. There are no adequate well-controlled studies in pregnant women. Prednisolone should be used during pregnancy only if the potential benefit justifies the potential risk to the fetus. Dexamethasone, hydrocortisone and prednisolone were ocularly applied to both eyes of pregnant mice five times per day on days 10 through 13 of gestation. A significant increase in the incidence of cleft palate was observed in the fetuses of the treated mice.

Nursing Mothers: It is not known whether topical ophthalmic administration of corticosteroids could result in sufficient systemic absorption to produce detectable quantities in breast milk. Systemically administered corticosteroids appear in human milk and could suppress growth, interfere with endogenous corticosteroid production, or cause other untoward effects. Because of the potential for serious adverse reactions in nursing infants from prednisolone, a decision should be made whether to discontinue nursing or discontinue the drug, taking into account the importance of the drug to the mother.

Pediatric Use: Safety and effectiveness in pediatric patients have not been established.

Geriatric Use: No overall differences in safety or effectiveness have been observed between elderly and younger patients.

Adverse Reactions: Adverse reactions include, in decreasing order of frequency, elevation of intraocular pressure (IOP) with possible development of glaucoma and infrequent optic nerve damage, posterior subcapsular cataract formation, and delayed wound healing.

Although systemic effects are extremely uncommon, there have been rare occurrences of systemic hypercorticoidism after use of topical steroids.

Corticosteroid-containing preparations have also been reported to cause acute anterior uveitis and perforation of the globe. Keratitis, conjunctivitis, corneal ulcers, mydriasis, conjunctival hyperemia, loss of accommodation and ptosis have occasionally been reported following local use of corticosteroids.

The development of secondary ocular infection (bacterial, fungal, and viral) have occurred. Fungal and viral infections of the cornea are particularly prone to develop coincidentally with long-term applications of steroid. The possibility of fungal invasion should be considered in any persistent corneal ulceration where steroid treatment has been used (see **Warnings**).

Transient burning and stinging upon instillation and other minor symptoms of ocular irritation have been reported with the use of PRED FORTE® suspension. Other adverse events reported with the use of PRED FORTE® suspension include: visual disturbance (blurry vision) and allergic reactions.

Overdosage: Overdosage will not ordinarily cause acute problems. If accidentally ingested, drink fluids to dilute.

Dosage and Administration: Shake well before using. Instill one to two drops into the conjunctival sac two to four times daily. During the initial 24 to 48 hours, the dosing frequency may be increased if necessary. Care should be taken not to discontinue therapy prematurely. If signs and symptoms fail to improve after 2 days, the patient should be re-evaluated (see **Precautions**).

How Supplied: PRED FORTE® (prednisolone acetate ophthalmic suspension, USP) 1% is supplied sterile in opaque white LDPE plastic bottles with droppers with white high impact polystyrene (HIPS) caps as follows:
1 mL in 5 mL bottle – NDC 11980-180-01
5 mL in 10 mL bottle – NDC 11980-180-05
10 mL in 15 mL bottle – NDC 11980-180-10
15 mL in 15 mL bottle – NDC 11980-180-15
Note: Store at temperatures up to 25°C (77°F). Protect from freezing. Store in an upright position.

Rx only
Revised March 2004
©2004 Allergan, Inc.
Irvine, CA 92612, U.S.A.
® marks owned by Allergan, Inc.
71592US10M
Shown in Product Identification Guide, page 103

PRED–G® Rx
(gentamicin and prednisolone acetate ophthalmic suspension, USP) 0.3%/1% sterile

Description: PRED-G® sterile ophthalmic suspension is a topical anti-inflammatory/anti-infective combination product for ophthalmic use.

Chemical Names: Prednisolone acetate: 11β, 17,21-Trihydroxypregna-1, 4-diene-3,20-dione 21-acetate.

Gentamicin sulfate is the sulfate salt of gentamicin C_1, gentamicin C_2, and gentamicin C_{1A} which are produced by the growth of *Micromonospora purpurea*.

Contains: Actives: Gentamicin sulfate equivalent to 0.3% gentamicin base; prednisolone acetate (microfine suspension) 1.0%. **Preservative:** Benzalkonium chloride 0.005%. **Inactives:** Edetate disodium; hypromellose; polyvinyl alcohol 1.4%; polysorbate 80; purified water; sodium chloride; and sodium citrate, dihydrate. May contain sodium hydroxide and/ or hydrochloric acid to adjust the pH (5.4 to 6.6).
PRED-G® suspension is formulated with a pH from 5.4 to 6.6 and its osmolality ranges from 260 to 340 mOsm/kg.

Clinical Pharmacology: Corticosteroids suppress the inflammatory response to a variety of agents and they probably delay or slow healing. Since corticosteroids may inhibit the body's defense mechanism against infection, a concom-

Continued on next page

Pred-G Suspension—Cont.

itant antimicrobial drug may be used when this inhibition is considered to be clinically significant in a particular case.

The anti-infective component in PRED-G® is included to provide action against specific organisms susceptible to it. Gentamicin sulfate is active *in vitro* against susceptible strains of the following microorganisms: *Staphylococcus aureus, Streptococcus pyogenes, Streptococcus pneumoniae, Enterobacter aerogenes, Escherichia coli, Haemophilus influenzae, Klebsiella pneumoniae, Neisseria gonorrhoeae, Pseudomonas aeruginosa,* and *Serratia marcescens.*

When a decision to administer both a corticosteroid and an antimicrobial is made, the administration of such drugs in combination has the advantage of greater patient compliance and convenience, with the added assurance that the appropriate dosage of both drugs is administered. When both types of drugs are in the same formulation, compatibility of ingredients is assured and the correct volume of drug is delivered and retained.

The relative potency of corticosteroids depends on the molecular structure, concentration, and release from the vehicle.

Indications and Usage: PRED-G® suspension is indicated for steroid-responsive inflammatory ocular conditions for which a corticosteroid is indicated and where superficial bacterial ocular infection or a risk of bacterial ocular infection exists.

Ocular steroids are indicated in inflammatory conditions of the palpebral and bulbar conjunctiva, cornea, and anterior segment of the globe where the inherent risk of steroid use in certain infective conjunctivitides is accepted to obtain a diminution in edema and inflammation. They are also indicated in chronic anterior uveitis and corneal injury from chemical, radiation, or thermal burns or penetration of foreign bodies.

The use of a combination drug with an anti-infective component is indicated where the risk of superficial ocular infection is high or where there is an expectation that potentially dangerous numbers of bacteria will be present in the eye.

The particular anti-infective drug in this product is active against the following common bacterial eye pathogens: *Staphylococcus aureus, Streptococcus pyogenes, Streptococcus pneumoniae, Enterobacter aerogenes, Escherichia coli, Haemophilus influenzae, Klebsiella pneumoniae, Neisseria gonorrhoeae, Pseudomonas aeruginosa,* and *Serratia marcescens.*

Contraindications: PRED-G® suspension is contraindicated in most viral diseases of the cornea and conjunctiva including epithelial herpes simplex keratitis (dendritic keratitis), vaccinia, and varicella, and also in mycobacterial infection of the eye and fungal diseases of the ocular structures. PRED-G® suspension is also contraindicated in individuals with known or suspected hypersensitivity to any of the ingredients of this preparation or to other corticosteroids.

Warnings: Prolonged use of corticosteroids may result in glaucoma with damage to the optic nerve, defects in visual acuity and fields of vision, and in posterior subcapsular cataract formation. Prolonged use of corticosteroids may suppress the host response and thus increase the hazard of secondary ocular infections.

Various ocular diseases and long-term use of topical corticosteroids have been known to cause corneal and scleral thinning. Use of topical corticosteroids in the presence of thin corneal or scleral tissue may lead to perforation.

Acute purulent infections of the eye may be masked or enhanced by the presence of corticosteroid medication.

If this product is used for 10 days or longer, intraocular pressure should be routinely mon-

itored even though it may be difficult in children and uncooperative patients. Steroids should be used with caution in the presence of glaucoma. Intraocular pressure should be checked frequently.

The use of steroids after cataract surgery may delay healing and increase the incidence of bleb formation.

Use of ocular steroids may prolong the course and may exacerbate the severity of many viral infections of the eye (including herpes simplex). Employment of a corticosteroid medication in the treatment of patients with a history of herpes simplex requires great caution; frequent slit lamp microscopy is recommended.

PRED-G® sterile ophthalmic suspension is not for injection. It should never be injected subconjunctivally, nor should it be directly introduced into the anterior chamber of the eye.

Precautions:

General: Ocular irritation and punctate keratitis have been associated with the use of PRED-G® suspension. The initial prescription and renewal of the medication order beyond 20 milliliters should be made by a physician only after examination of the patient's intraocular pressure, examination of the patient with the aid of magnification such as slit lamp biomicroscopy and, where appropriate, fluorescein staining.

As fungal infections of the cornea are particularly prone to develop coincidentally with long-term corticosteroid applications, fungal invasion should be suspected in any persistent corneal ulceration where a corticosteroid has been used or is in use. Fungal cultures should be taken when appropriate.

Information for Patients: If inflammation or pain persists longer than 48 hours or becomes aggravated, the patient should be advised to discontinue use of the medication and consult a physician.

This product is sterile when packaged. To prevent contamination, care should be taken to avoid touching the bottle tip to eyelids or to any other surface. The use of this bottle by more than one person may spread infection. Store at 15°–25°C (59°–77°F). Protect from freezing and from heat of 40°C (104°F) and above. Keep out of the reach of children. Shake well before using.

Carcinogenesis, mutagenesis, impairment of fertility: There are no published carcinogenicity or impairment of fertility studies on gentamicin. Aminoglycoside antibiotics have been found to be non-mutagenic.

There are no published mutagenicity or impairment of fertility studies on prednisolone. Prednisolone has been reported to be noncarcinogenic.

Pregnancy: Pregnancy Category C. Gentamicin has been shown to depress body weight, kidney weight, and median glomerular counts in newborn rats when administered systemically to pregnant rats in daily doses approximately 500 times the maximum recommended ophthalmic human dose. There are no adequate and well-controlled studies in pregnant women. Gentamicin should be used during pregnancy only if the potential benefit justifies the potential risk to the fetus.

Prednisolone has been shown to be teratogenic in mice when given in doses 1–10 times the human ocular dose. Dexamethasone, hydrocortisone and prednisolone were applied to both eyes of pregnant mice five times per day on days 10 through 13 of gestation. A significant increase in the incidence of cleft palate was observed in the fetuses of the treated mice. There are no adequate well-controlled studies in pregnant women. PRED-G® suspension should be used during pregnancy only if the potential benefit justifies the potential risk to the fetus.

Nursing Mothers: It is not known whether topical administration of corticosteroids could result in sufficient systemic absorption to produce detectable quantities in human milk. Systemically administered corticosteroids appear in human milk and could suppress growth, interfere with endogenous corticosteroid production, or cause other untoward effects. Because of the potential for serious adverse reactions in nursing infants from PRED-G® suspension, a decision should be made whether to discontinue nursing while the drug is being administered or to discontinue the medication.

Pediatric Use: Safety and effectiveness in pediatric patients have not been established.

Geriatric Use: No overall differences in safety or effectiveness have been observed between elderly and younger patients.

Adverse Reactions: Adverse reactions have occurred with steroid/anti-infective combination drugs which can be attributed to the steroid component, the anti-infective component, or the combination. Exact incidence figures are not available since no denominator of treated patients is available.

Reactions occurring most often from the presence of the anti-infective ingredient are allergic sensitizations. The reactions due to the steroid component in decreasing order of frequency are: elevation of intraocular pressure (IOP) with possible development of glaucoma, and infrequent optic nerve damage; posterior subcapsular cataract formation; and delayed wound healing.

Burning, stinging and other symptoms of irritation have been reported with PRED-G®. Superficial punctate keratitis has been reported occasionally with onset occurring typically after several days of use.

Secondary Infection: The development of secondary infection has occurred after use of combinations containing steroids and antimicrobials. Fungal and viral infections of the cornea are particularly prone to develop coincidentally with long-term applications of steroid. The possibility of fungal invasion should be considered in any persistent corneal ulceration where steroid treatment has been used. (See **Warnings**).

Secondary bacterial ocular infection following suppression of host responses also occurs.

Dosage and Administration: Instill one drop into the conjunctival sac two to four times daily. During the initial 24 to 48 hours, the dosing frequency may be increased, if necessary, up to 1 drop every hour. Care should be taken not to discontinue therapy prematurely. If signs and symptoms fail to improve after two days, the patient should be re-evaluated. (See **Precautions**)

Not more than 20 milliliters should be prescribed initially and the prescription should not be refilled without further evaluation as outlined in **Precautions** above.

How Supplied: PRED-G® (gentamicin and prednisolone acetate ophthalmic suspension, USP) 0.3%/1.0% is supplied sterile in opaque white LDPE plastic bottles with droppers with white high impact polystyrene (HIPS) caps as follows:

5 mL in 10 mL bottle – NDC 0023-0106-05
10 mL in 15 mL bottle – NDC 0023-0106-10

Note: Store at 15°–25°C (59°–77°F). Avoid excessive heat, 40° C (104° F) and above. Protect from freezing. **Shake well before using.**

℞ only

Revised December 2005
© 2006 Allergan, Inc.
Irvine, CA 92612, U.S.A.
® marks owned by Allergan, Inc.
71591US12T

PRED-G® ℞
(gentamicin and prednisolone acetate ophthalmic ointment, USP) 0.3%/0.6% sterile

Description: PRED-G® sterile ophthalmic ointment is a topical anti-inflammatory/anti-infective combination product for ophthalmic use.

Chemical Names: Prednisolone acetate: 11β,17,21-Trihydroxypregna-1, 4-diene-3, 20-dione 21-acetate.

Gentamicin sulfate is the sulfate salt of gentamicin C_1, gentamicin C_2, and gentamicin C_{1A} which are produced by the growth of *Micromonospora purpurea*.

Contains: Actives: gentamicin sulfate equivalent to 0.3% gentamicin base, prednisolone acetate 0.6%. **Preservative:** chlorobutanol (chloral derivative) 0.5%. **Inactives:** mineral oil; petrolatum (and) lanolin alcohol; purified water; and white petrolatum.

Clinical Pharmacology: Corticosteroids suppress the inflammatory response to a variety of agents and they probably delay or slow healing. Since corticosteroids may inhibit the body's defense mechanism against infection, a concomitant antimicrobial drug may be used when this inhibition is considered to be clinically significant in a particular case.

The anti-infective component in PRED-G® ophthalmic ointment is included to provide action against specific organisms susceptible to it. Gentamicin sulfate is active *in vitro* against susceptible strains of the following microorganisms: *Staphylococcus aureus, Streptococcus pyogenes, Streptococcus pneumoniae, Enterobacter aerogenes, Escherichia coli, Haemophilus influenzae, Klebsiella pneumoniae, Neisseria gonorrhoeae, Pseudomonas aeruginosa,* and *Serratia marcescens.*

When a decision to administer both a corticosteroid and an antimicrobial is made, the administration of such drugs in combination has the advantage of greater patient compliance and convenience, with the added assurance that the appropriate dosage of both drugs is administered. When both types of drugs are in the same formulation, compatibility of ingredients is assured and the correct volume of drug is delivered and retained.

The relative potency of corticosteroids depends on the molecular structure, concentration, and release from the vehicle.

Indications and Usage: PRED-G® ophthalmic ointment is indicated for steroid-responsive inflammatory ocular conditions for which a corticosteroid is indicated and where superficial bacterial ocular infection or a risk of bacterial ocular infection exists.

Ocular steroids are indicated in inflammatory conditions of the palpebral and bulbar conjunctiva, cornea, and anterior segment of the globe where the inherent risk of steroid use in certain infective conjunctivitides is accepted to obtain a diminution in edema and inflammation. They are also indicated in chronic anterior uveitis and corneal injury from chemical, radiation, or thermal burns or penetration of foreign bodies.

The use of a combination drug with an anti-infective component is indicated where the risk of superficial ocular infection is high or where there is an expectation that potentially dangerous numbers of bacteria will be present in the eye.

The particular anti-infective drug in this product is active against the following common bacterial eye pathogens: *Staphylococcus aureus, Streptococcus pyogenes, Streptococcus pneumoniae, Enterobacter aerogenes, Escherichia coli, Hemophilus influenzae, Klebsiella pneumoniae, Neisseria gonorrhoeae, Pseudomonas aeruginosa,* and *Serratia marcescens.*

Contraindications: PRED-G® ophthalmic ointment is contraindicated in most viral diseases of the cornea and conjunctiva including epithelial herpes simplex keratitis (dendritic keratitis), vaccinia and varicella, and also in mycobacterial infection of the eye and fungal diseases of ocular structures. PRED-G® ointment is also contraindicated in individuals with known or suspected hypersensitivity to any of the ingredients of this preparation or to other corticosteroids.

Warnings: Prolonged use of corticosteroids may result in glaucoma, with damage to the optic nerve, defects in visual acuity and fields of vision, and in posterior subcapsular cataract formation. Prolonged use of corticosteroids may suppress the host immune response and thus increase the hazard of secondary ocular infections. Various ocular diseases and long term use of topical corticosteroids have been known to cause corneal and scleral thinning. Use of topical corticosteroids in the presence of thin corneal or scleral tissue may lead to perforation. Acute purulent infections of the eye may be masked or enhanced by the presence of corticosteroid medication.

If these products are used for 10 days or longer, intraocular pressure should be routinely monitored even though it may be difficult in children and uncooperative patients. Steroids should be used with caution in the presence of glaucoma. Intraocular pressure should be checked frequently.

The use of steroids after cataract surgery may delay healing and increase the incidence of bleb formation.

Use of ocular steroids may prolong the course and may exacerbate the severity of many viral infections of the eye (including herpes simplex). Employment of a corticosteroid medication in the treatment of patients with a history of herpes simplex requires great caution, frequent slit lamp microscopy is recommended.

Precautions:

General: Ocular irritation and punctate keratitis have been associated with the use of PRED-G® ophthalmic ointment. The initial prescription and renewal of the medication order beyond 8 grams should be made by a physician only after examination of the patient's intraocular pressure, examination of the patient with the aid of magnification, such as slit lamp biomicroscopy and, where appropriate, fluorescein staining. As fungal infections of the cornea are particularly prone to develop coincidentally with long term corticosteroid applications, fungal invasion should be suspected in any persistent corneal ulceration where a corticosteroid has been used or is in use. Fungal cultures should be taken when appropriate.

Information for Patients: If inflammation or pain persists longer than 48 hours or becomes aggravated the patient should be advised to discontinue use of the medication and consult a physician.

This product is sterile when packaged. To prevent contamination care should be taken to avoid touching the tip of the tube to eyelids or to any other surface. The use of this tube by more than one person may spread infection. Keep out of reach of children.

Carcinogenesis, mutagenesis, impairment of fertility: There are no published carcinogenicity or impairment of fertility studies on gentamicin. Aminoglycoside antibiotics have been found to be non-mutagenic.

There are no published mutagenicity or impairment of fertility studies on prednisolone. Prednisolone has been reported to be non-carcinogenic.

Pregnancy: Pregnancy Category C: Gentamicin has been shown to depress newborn body weights, kidney weights and median glomerular counts in newborn rats when administered systemically to pregnant rats in daily doses of approximately 500 times the maximum recommended ophthalmic dose in humans. There are no adequate and well-controlled studies in pregnant women. Gentamicin should be used during pregnancy only if the potential benefit justifies the potential risk to the fetus. Prednisolone has been shown to be teratogenic in mice when given in doses 1–10 times the human ocular dose. Dexamethasone, hydrocortisone and prednisolone were ocularly applied to both eyes of pregnant mice five times per day on days 10 through 13 of gestation. A significant increase in the incidence of cleft palate was observed in the fetuses of the treated mice. There are no adequate well-controlled studies in pregnant women. PRED-G® should be used during pregnancy only if the potential benefit justifies the potential risk to the fetus.

Nursing Mothers: It is not known whether topical administration of corticosteroids could result in sufficient systemic absorption to produce detectable quantities in breast milk. Systemically administered corticosteroids appear in breast milk and could suppress growth, interfere with endogenous corticosteroid production, or cause untoward effects. Because of the potential for serious adverse reactions in nursing infants from PRED-G® a decision should be made whether to discontinue nursing while the drug is being administered or to discontinue the medication.

Pediatric Use: Safety and effectiveness in pediatric patients have not been established.

Geriatric Use: No overall differences in safety or effectiveness have been observed between elderly and young patients.

Adverse Reactions: Adverse reactions have occurred with steroid/anti-infective combination drugs which can be attributed to the steroid component, the anti-infective component, or the combination. Exact incidence figures are not available since no denominator of treated patients is available.

The most frequent reactions observed include ocular discomfort, irritation upon instillation of the medication and punctate keratitis. These reactions have resolved upon discontinuation of the medication.

Reactions occurring most often from the presence of the anti-infective ingredient are allergic sensitizations. The reactions due to the steroid component in decreasing order of frequency are: elevation of intraocular pressure (IOP) with possible development of glaucoma, and infrequent optic nerve damage; posterior subcapsular cataract formation; and delayed wound healing.

Secondary Infection: The development of secondary infection has occurred after use of combinations containing steroids and antimicrobials. Fungal and viral infections of the cornea are particularly prone to develop coincidentally with long-term applications of steroid. The possibility of fungal invasion must be considered in any persistent corneal ulceration where steroid treatment has been used. (See **Warnings**)

Secondary bacterial ocular infection following suppression of host responses also occurs.

Dosage and Administration: A small amount (½ inch ribbon) of ointment should be applied in the conjunctival sac one to three times daily. Care should be taken not to discontinue therapy prematurely.

Not more than 8 grams should be prescribed initially and the prescription should not be refilled without further evaluation as outlined in Precautions above. If signs and symptoms fail to improve after two days, the patient should be re-evaluated (see **Precautions**).

How Supplied: PRED-G® (gentamicin and prednisolone acetate ophthalmic ointment, USP) 0.3%/0.6% is supplied sterile in collapsible aluminum tubes with epoxy-phenolic liners with tips with black LDPE caps of the following size:

3.5 g—NDC 0023-0066-04

Continued on next page

Pred-G Ointment—Cont.

Note: Store at 15°–25°C (59°–77°F).
℞ only
Revised January 2004
© 2004 Allergan, Inc.
Irvine, CA 92612, U.S.A.
® marks owned by Allergan, Inc.
71725US10P

PRED MILD®   ℞
(prednisolone acetate
ophthalmic suspension, USP) 0.12%
sterile

Description: PRED MILD® (prednisolone acetate ophthalmic suspension, USP) 0.12% is a topical anti-inflammatory agent for ophthalmic use.
Chemical Name: 11β,17,21-Trihydroxypregna-1, 4-diene-3,20-dione 21-acetate.
Contains: Active: prednisolone acetate (microfine suspension) 0.12%. **Preservative:** benzalkonium chloride. **Inactives:** boric acid; edetate disodium; hypromellose; polysorbate 80; purified water; sodium bisulfite; sodium chloride; and sodium citrate. The pH during its shelf life ranges from 5.0 to 6.0.
Clinical Pharmacology: Prednisolone acetate is a glucocorticoid that, on the basis of weight, has 3 to 5 times the anti-inflammatory potency of hydrocortisone. Glucocorticoids inhibit the edema, fibrin deposition, capillary dilation and phagocytic migration of the acute inflammatory response as well as capillary proliferation, deposition of collagen and scar formation.
Indications and Usage: PRED MILD® is indicated for the treatment of mild to moderate noninfectious allergic and inflammatory disorders of the lid, conjunctiva, cornea and sclera (including chemical and thermal burns).
Contraindications: PRED MILD® suspension is contraindicated in acute untreated purulent ocular infections, in most viral diseases of the cornea and conjunctiva including epithelial herpes simplex keratitis (dendritic keratitis), vaccinia, and varicella, and also in mycobacterial infection of the eye and fungal diseases of ocular structures. PRED MILD® suspension is also contraindicated in individuals with known or suspected hypersensitivity to any of the ingredients of this preparation and to other corticosteroids.
Warnings: Prolonged use of corticosteroids may result in glaucoma with damage to the optic nerve, defects in visual acuity and fields of vision, and in posterior subcapsular cataract formation. Prolonged use may also suppress the host immune response and thus increase the hazard of secondary ocular infections.
Various ocular diseases and long-term use of topical corticosteroids have been known to cause corneal and scleral thinning. Use of topical corticosteroids in the presence of thin corneal or scleral tissue may lead to perforation.
Acute purulent infections of the eye may be masked or activity enhanced by the presence of corticosteroid medication.
If this product is used for 10 days or longer, intraocular pressure should be routinely monitored even though it may be difficult in children and uncooperative patients. Steroids should be used with caution in the presence of glaucoma. Intraocular pressure should be checked frequently.
The use of steroids after cataract surgery may delay healing and increase the incidence of bleb formation.
Use of ocular steroids may prolong the course and may exacerbate the severity of many viral infections of the eye (including herpes simplex). Employment of a corticosteroid medication in the treatment of patients with a history

of herpes simplex requires great caution; frequent slit lamp microscopy is recommended.
Corticosteroids are not effective in mustard gas keratitis and Sjögren's keratoconjunctivitis.
Contains sodium bisulfite, a sulfite that may cause allergic-type reactions, including anaphylactic symptoms and life-threatening or less severe asthmatic episodes in certain susceptible people. The overall prevalence of sulfite sensitivity in the general population is unknown and probably low. Sulfite sensitivity is seen more frequently in asthmatic than in nonasthmatic people.
Precautions:
General: The initial prescription and renewal of the medication order beyond 20 milliliters of PRED MILD® should be made by a physician only after examination of the patient with the aid of magnification, such as slit lamp biomicroscopy, and, where appropriate, fluorescein staining. If signs and symptoms fail to improve after 2 days, the patient should be re-evaluated.
As fungal infections of the cornea are particularly prone to develop coincidentally with long-term local corticosteroid applications, fungal invasion should be suspected in any persistent corneal ulceration where a corticosteroid has been used or is in use. Fungal cultures should be taken when appropriate.
If this product is used for 10 days or longer, intraocular pressure should be monitored (see **Warnings**).
Information for patients: If inflammation or pain persists longer than 48 hours or becomes aggravated, the patient should be advised to discontinue use of the medication and consult a physician.
This product is sterile when packaged. To prevent contamination, care should be taken to avoid touching the bottle tip to eyelids or to any other surface. The use of this bottle by more than one person may spread infection. Keep bottle tightly closed when not in use. Keep out of the reach of children.
Carcinogenesis, Mutagenesis, Impairment of Fertility: No studies have been conducted in animals or in humans to evaluate the potential of these effects.
Pregnancy Category C: Prednisolone has been shown to be teratogenic in mice when given in doses 1–10 times the human dose. There are no adequate well-controlled studies in pregnant women. Prednisolone should be used during pregnancy only if the potential benefit justifies the potential risk to the fetus. Dexamethasone, hydrocortisone and prednisolone were ocularly applied to both eyes of pregnant mice five times per day on days 10 through 13 of gestation. A significant increase in the incidence of cleft palate was observed in the fetuses of the treated mice.
Nursing Mothers: It is not known whether topical ophthalmic administration of corticosteroids could result in sufficient systemic absorption to produce detectable quantities in breast milk. Systemically administered corticosteroids appear in human milk and could suppress growth, interfere with endogenous corticosteroid production, or cause other untoward effects. Because of the potential for serious adverse reactions in nursing infants from prednisolone, a decision should be made whether to discontinue nursing or to discontinue the drug, taking into account the importance of the drug to the mother.
Pediatric Use: Safety and effectiveness in pediatric patients have not been established.
Geriatric Use: No overall differences in safety or effectiveness have been observed between elderly and younger patients.
Adverse Reactions: Adverse reactions include, in decreasing order of frequency, elevation of intraocular pressure (IOP) with possible

development of glaucoma and infrequent optic nerve damage, posterior subcapsular cataract formation, and delayed wound healing.
Although systemic effects are extremely uncommon, there have been rare occurrences of systemic hypercorticoidism after use of topical steroids.
Corticosteroid-containing preparations have also been reported to cause acute anterior uveitis and perforation of the globe. Keratitis, conjunctivitis, corneal ulcers, mydriasis, conjunctival hyperemia, loss of accommodation and ptosis have occasionally been reported following local use of corticosteroids.
The development of secondary ocular infection (bacterial, fungal, and viral) has occurred. Fungal and viral infections of the cornea are particularly prone to develop coincidentally with long-term applications of steroids. The possibility of fungal invasion should be considered in any persistent corneal ulceration where steroid treatment has been used (see **Warnings**).
Transient burning and stinging upon instillation and other minor symptoms of ocular irritation have been reported with the use of PRED MILD® suspension.
Overdosage: Overdosage will not ordinarily cause acute problems. If accidentally ingested, drink fluids to dilute.
Dosage and Administration: **Shake well before using.** Instill one to two drops into the conjunctival sac two to four times daily. During the initial 24 to 48 hours, the dosing frequency may be increased if necessary. Care should be taken not to discontinue therapy prematurely. If signs and symptoms fail to improve after 2 days, the patient should be re-evaluated (see **Precautions**).
How Supplied: PRED MILD® (prednisolone acetate ophthalmic suspension, USP) 0.12% is supplied sterile in opaque white LDPE plastic bottles with droppers with white high impact polystyrene (HIPS) caps as follows:
5 mL in 10 mL bottle – NDC 11980-174-05
10 mL in 15 mL bottle – NDC 11980-174-10
Note: Store at 15°C–30°C (59°F–86°F). Protect from freezing. Store in an upright position.
Rx only
Revised June 2004
©2004 Allergan, Inc.
Irvine, CA 92612, U.S.A.
® marks owned by Allergan, Inc.
71739US10P

PROPINE®   ℞
(dipivefrin hydrochloride)
ophthalmic solution, USP, 0.1% sterile
Description: PROPINE® contains dipivefrin hydrochloride in a sterile, isotonic solution. Dipivefrin HCl is a white, crystalline powder, freely soluble in water with an osmolality of approx. 250–330 mOsmol/kg.
Empirical Formula: $C_{19}H_{29}O_5N \cdot HCl$
Chemical Name: (±)-3,4-Dihydroxy-α-[(methylamino)methyl]benzyl alcohol 3,4-dipivalate hydrochloride.
Contains:
Active: dipivefrin HCl 0.1%
Preservative: benzalkonium chloride
Inactives: edetate disodium; sodium chloride; hydrochloric acid to adjust pH; and purified water. The pH during its shelf life ranges from 2.5–3.5.
Clinical Pharmacology: PROPINE® (dipivefrin HCl ophthalmic solution, USP) is a member of a class of drugs known as prodrugs. Prodrugs are usually not active in themselves and require biotransformation to the parent compound before therapeutic activity is seen. These modifications are undertaken to enhance absorption, decrease side effects and enhance stability and comfort, thus making the parent compound a more useful drug. Enhanced ab-

sorption makes the prodrug a more efficient delivery system for the parent drug because less drug will be needed to produce the desired therapeutic response.

PROPINE® ophthalmic solution is a prodrug of epinephrine formed by the diesterification of epinephrine and pivalic acid. The addition of pivaloyl groups to the epinephrine molecule enhances its lipophilic character and, as a consequence, its penetration into the anterior chamber.

PROPINE® is converted to epinephrine inside the human eye by enzyme hydrolysis. The liberated epinephrine, an adrenergic agonist, appears to exert its action by decreasing aqueous production and by enhancing outflow facility. The PROPINE® prodrug delivery system is a more efficient way of delivering the therapeutic effects of epinephrine, with fewer side effects than are associated with conventional epinephrine therapy.

The onset of action with one drop of PROPINE® occurs about 30 minutes after treatment, with maximum effect seen at about one hour.

Using a prodrug means that less drug is needed for therapeutic effect since absorption is enhanced with the prodrug. PROPINE® ophthalmic solution at 0.1% dipivefrin was judged less irritating than a 1% solution of epinephrine hydrochloride or bitartrate. In addition, only 8 of 455 patients (1.8%) treated with PROPINE® reported discomfort due to photophobia, glare or light sensitivity.

Indications: PROPINE® (dipivefrin HCl ophthalmic solution, USP) is indicated as initial therapy for the control of intraocular pressure in chronic open-angle glaucoma. Patients responding inadequately to other antiglaucoma therapy may respond to addition of PROPINE®. In controlled and open-label studies of glaucoma, PROPINE® ophthalmic solution demonstrated a statistically significant intraocular pressure-lowering effect. Patients using PROPINE® twice daily in studies with mean durations of 76–146 days experienced mean pressure reductions ranging from 20–24%.

Therapeutic response to PROPINE® ophthalmic solution twice daily is somewhat less than 2% epinephrine twice daily. Controlled studies showed statistically significant differences in lowering of intraocular pressure between PROPINE® and 2% epinephrine. In controlled studies in patients with a history of epinephrine intolerance, only 3% of patients treated with PROPINE® ophthalmic solution exhibited intolerance, while 55% of those treated with epinephrine again developed intolerance. Therapeutic response to PROPINE® twice daily therapy is comparable to 2% pilocarpine 4 times daily. In controlled clinical studies comparing PROPINE® ophthalmic solution and 2% pilocarpine, there were no statistically significant differences in the maintenance of IOP levels for the two medications. PROPINE® does not produce miosis or accommodative spasm which cholinergic agents are known to produce. Night blindness often associated with miotic agents is not present with PROPINE® therapy. Patients with cataracts avoid the inability to see around lenticular opacities caused by constricted pupil.

Contraindications: PROPINE® should not be used in patients with narrow angles since any dilation of the pupil may predispose the patient to an attack of angle-closure glaucoma. This product is contraindicated in patients who are hypersensitive to any of its components.

Precautions: Aphakic Patients. Macular edema has been shown to occur in up to 30% of aphakic patients treated with epinephrine. Discontinuation of epinephrine generally results in reversal of the maculopathy.

Pregnancy: Pregnancy Category B. Reproduction studies have been performed in rats and rabbits at daily oral doses up to 10 mg/kg body weight (5 mg/kg in teratogenicity studies), and have revealed no evidence of impaired fertility or harm to the fetus due to dipivefrin HCl. There are, however, no adequate and well-controlled studies in pregnant women. Because animal reproduction studies are not always predictive of human response, this drug should be used during pregnancy only if clearly needed.

Nursing Mothers. It is not known whether this drug is excreted in human milk. Because many drugs are excreted in human milk, caution should be exercised when PROPINE® ophthalmic solution is administered to a nursing woman.

Pediatric Use: Safety and effectiveness in pediatric patients have not been established.

Geriatric Use. No overall clinical differences in safety or effectiveness have been observed between elderly and other adult patients.

Animal Studies. Rabbit studies indicated a dose-related incidence of meibomian gland retention cysts following topical administration of both dipivefrin hydrochloride and epinephrine.

Adverse Reactions:

Cardiovascular Effects. Tachycardia, arrhythmias and hypertension have been reported with ocular administration of epinephrine.

Local Effects. The most frequent side effects reported with PROPINE® alone were injection in 6.5% of patients and burning and stinging in 6%. Follicular conjunctivitis, eye pain, mydriasis, blurry vision, eye pruritus, headache, and allergic reaction to PROPINE® ophthalmic solution have been reported. Epinephrine therapy can lead to adrenochrome deposits in the conjunctiva and cornea.

Dosage and Administration:

Initial Glaucoma Therapy. The usual dosage of PROPINE® is one drop in the eye(s) every 12 hours.

Replacement with PROPINE®. When patients are being transferred to PROPINE® from antiglaucoma agents other than epinephrine, on the first day continue the previous medication and add one drop of PROPINE® ophthalmic solution in each eye every 12 hours. On the following day, discontinue the previously used antiglaucoma agent and continue with PROPINE®.

In transferring patients from conventional epinephrine therapy to PROPINE® ophthalmic solution, simply discontinue the epinephrine medication and institute the PROPINE® regimen.

Addition of PROPINE®. When patients on other antiglaucoma agents require additional therapy, add one drop of PROPINE® every 12 hours.

Concomitant Therapy. For difficult to control patients, the addition of PROPINE® ophthalmic solution to other agents such as pilocarpine, carbachol, echothiophate iodide or acetazolamide has been shown to be effective.

Note: Not for injection.

How Supplied: PROPINE® (dipivefrin HCl ophthalmic solution, USP) 0.1%, is supplied sterile in opaque white low density polyethylene ophthalmic dispenser bottles and tips with purple polystyrene caps as follows:

10 mL in 10 mL bottle—NDC 0023-9208-10
15 mL in 15 mL bottle—NDC 0023-9208-15

Note: Store in a tight, light-resistant container at 15° to 25°C (59° to 77°F).

℞ only
Revised December 2005
©2006 Allergan, Inc.
Irvine, CA 92612, U.S.A.
® marks owned by Allergan, Inc.
71738US11T

REFRESH® CELLUVISC®   OTC
(carboxymethylcellulose sodium) 1%
Lubricant Eye Drops
Preservative-Free

Soothing Relief For Dry, Irritated Eyes.

Due to its thicker formula, REFRESH® CELLUVISC® Lubricant Eye Drops is an ideal eye drop, for persistent dry eye conditions. REFRESH® CELLUVISC® restores the moisture your eyes crave, with a gentle protecting and lubricating formula that has some of the same healthy qualities as natural tears. So, you can enjoy long-lasting relief, from the irritating, scratchy feeling of dry, irritated eyes.

To avoid the use of potentially irritating preservatives found in some bottled eye drops, REFRESH® CELLUVISC® Lubricant Eye Drops comes in preservative-free, air-tight, single-use containers. So, you can apply REFRESH® CELLUVISC® as often as necessary, to provide 24-hour comfort.

Drug Facts

Active Ingredient: **Purpose:**
Carboxymethylcellulose .... Eye Lubricant sodium (CMC) 1.0%

Uses
• For the temporary relief of burning, irritation, and discomfort due to dryness of the eye or to exposure to wind or sun.
• May be used as a protectant against further irritation.

Warnings:
• For external use only.
• To avoid contamination, do not touch tip of container to any surface. Do not reuse. Once opened, discard.
• Do not touch unit-dose tip to eye.
• Do not use if solution changes color or becomes cloudy.

Stop use and ask a doctor if you experience eye pain, changes in vision, continued redness or irritation of the eye, or if the condition worsens or persists, for more than 72 hrs.

Keep out of reach of children. If swallowed, get medical help, or contact a Poison Control Center right away.

Directions to open, twist and pull tab to remove. Instill 1 or 2 drops in the affected eye(s) as needed and discard container.

Other Information:
• Use only if single-use container is intact.
• REFRESH® CELLUVISC® may cause temporary blurring due to its viscosity.
• RETAIN CARTON FOR FUTURE REFERENCE.

Inactive ingredients:
Calcium chloride, potassium chloride, purified water, sodium chloride, and sodium lactate.

How Supplied: REFRESH® CELLUVISC® (carboxymethylcellulose sodium) 1.0% Lubricant Eye Drops are supplied in sterile, preservative-free, disposable, single-use containers of 0.4 mL (0.01 fl oz) each, in the following size:

30 Sterile Single-Use Containers
NDC 0023-4554-30
® marks owned by Allergan, Inc.
©2006 Allergan, Inc.
Irvine, CA 92612, U.S.A.
Shown in Product Identification Guide, page 103

REFRESH ENDURA®   OTC
Lubricant Eye Drops

Breakthrough technology, for complete relief plus protection. With its unique formulation,

Continued on next page

Refresh Endura—Cont.

REFRESH ENDURA® does more than wet the eye. It is the first eye drop, which benefits all three layers of the tear film.

REFRESH ENDURA® Lubricant Eye Drops create a soothing shield, with a long lasting layer of moisture, for sustained relief of persistent dry eye symptoms.

The unique formulation of REFRESH ENDURA® appears as a light milky eye drop. It looks and feels different, because it is different.

Technologically advanced REFRESH ENDURA® Lubricant Eye Drops are safe to use, as often as necessary and provides 24-hour comfort for dry, irritated eyes.

Drug Facts

Active Ingredients:	Purpose:
Glycerin 1%	Eye lubricant
Polysorbate 80 1%	Eye lubricant

Uses:
- For the temporary relief of burning, irritation, and discomfort due to the dryness of the eye or exposure to wind or sun.
- May be used as a protectant against further irritation.

Warnings:
- **For external use only.**
- **To avoid contamination, do not touch tip of container to any surface. Do not reuse. Once opened, discard.**
- **Do not touch unit-dose tip to eye.**
- **Do not use if solution changes color.**

Stop use and ask a doctor if you experience eye pain, changes in vision, continued redness, or irritation of the eye, or if the condition worsens or persists for more than 72 hours.

Keep out of reach of children. If swallowed, get medical help, or contact a Poison Control Center right away.

Directions: To open, **TWIST AND PULL TAB TO REMOVE.** Instill 1 or 2 drops in the affected eye(s) as needed and discard container.

Other Information
- **Use only if single-use container is intact.**
- **RETAIN CARTON FOR FUTURE REFERENCE.**

Inactive Ingredients:
Carbomer; castor oil; mannitol; purified water; and sodium hydroxide.

How Supplied: In sterile, preservative-free, disposable, single-use containers of 0.01 fluid ounces each in the following size:
20 sterile single-use containers—NDC 0023-9235-20

® marks owned by Allergan, Inc.
©2007 Allergan, Inc.
Irvine, CA 92612, U.S.A.
U.S. Patent 5,981,607

Shown in Product Identification Guide, page 103

REFRESH LIQUIGEL®   OTC
(carboxymethylcellulose sodium) 1%
Lubricant Eye Drops

REFRESH LIQUIGEL® Lubricant Eye Drops is a unique, extra-strength eye drop, specially formulated to provide added moisture, for immediate relief of moderate-to-severe dry eye symptoms. REFRESH LIQUIGEL® works like your own natural tears. It is safe to use as often as needed.

Drug Facts

Active Ingredients:	Purpose:
Carboxymethylcellulose sodium 1.0%	Eye Lubricant

Uses:
- For the temporary relief of burning, irritation, and discomfort, due to the dryness of the eye or exposure to the wind or sun.
- May be used as a protectant against further irritation.

Warnings:
- **For external use only.**
- **To avoid contamination, do not touch tip of the container to any surface. Replace cap after using.**

Stop use and ask a doctor if you experience eye pain, changes in vision, continued redness, or irritation of the eye, or if the condition worsens or persists for more than 72 hours.

Keep out of reach of children. If swallowed, get medical help, or contact a Poison Control Center right away.

Directions: Instill 1 or 2 drops in the affected eye(s), as needed.

Other Information:
- **Use only if imprinted tape seals on top and bottom flaps are intact and clearly legible.**
- **RETAIN CARTON FOR FUTURE REFERENCE.**

Inactive Ingredients:
Boric acid, calcium chloride, magnesium chloride, potassium chloride, purified water, PURITE® (stabilized oxychloro complex), sodium borate, and sodium chloride.

How Supplied: REFRESH LIQUIGEL® (carboxymethylcellulose sodium) 1.0% Lubricant Eye Drops are supplied in the following sizes:
15 mL bottle — NDC 0023-9205-15
30 mL bottle — NDC 0023-9205-30
® marks owned by Allergan, Inc.
©2007 Allergan, Inc.
Irvine, CA 92612, U.S.A.
U.S. Patents 5,424,078; 5,736,165; 5,858,346; and 6,024,954

Shown in Product Identification Guide, page 103

REFRESH PLUS®   OTC
(carboxymethylcellulose sodium) 0.5%
Lubricant Eye Drops
Preservative-Free

Immediate, Long-Lasting Relief Plus Protection.

Many things can make your eyes feel dry, scratchy, burning, or uncomfortable: Air conditioners, heaters, computer use, reading, some medications, wind, LASIK procedures,* or a reduction in the amount of tears your body produces, which help to lubricate and nourish your eyes. REFRESH PLUS® Lubricant Eye Drops restore the moisture your eyes crave, with a special formula that has some of the same healthy qualities as natural tears.

Since REFRESH PLUS® is preservative-free, it also avoids the potential irritation to your eyes caused by some preservatives found in bottled eye drops. REFRESH PLUS® is formulated for the mild-to-moderate dry eye, and can be used as often as needed, to provide 24-hour comfort.

Drug Facts

Active Ingredient:	Purpose:
Carboxymethylcellulose sodium (CMC) 0.5%	Eye lubricant

Uses:
- For the temporary relief of burning, irritation, and discomfort, due to dryness of the eye, or exposure to wind or sun
- May be used as a protectant against further irritation.

Warnings:
- **For external use only.**
- **To avoid contamination, do not touch tip of container to any surface. Do not reuse. Once opened, discard.**
- **Do not touch unit-dose tip to eye.**
- **Do not use, if solution changes color or becomes cloudy.**

Stop use and ask a doctor if you experience eye pain, changes in vision, continued redness or irritation of the eye, or if the condition worsens or persists for more than 72 hours.

Keep out of reach of children. If swallowed, get medical help, or contact a Poison Control Center right away.

*If used for post-operative (e.g., LASIK) dryness and discomfort, follow your eye doctor's instructions.

Other Information:
- **Use only if single-use container is intact.**
- **RETAIN CARTON FOR FUTURE REFERENCE.**

Inactive Ingredients: Calcium chloride, magnesium chloride, potassium chloride, purified water, sodium chloride, and sodium lactate. May also contain hydrochloric acid and/or sodium hydroxide to adjust pH.

How Supplied: In sterile, preservative- free, disposable, single-use containers of 0.01 fluid ounces each in the following sizes:
30 single-use containers—NDC 0023-0403-30.
50 single-use containers—NDC 0023-0403-50.
70 single-use containers—NDC 0023-0403-70.
100 single-use containers—NDC 0023-0403-10.
® marks owned by Allergan, Inc.
©2007 Allergan, Inc.
Irvine, CA 92612, U.S.A.

Shown in Product Identification Guide, page 103

REFRESH P.M.®   OTC
Lubricant Eye Ointment
Preservative-Free Formula

Nighttime relief and protection for dry eyes. Strong relief for dry, irritated eyes.

REFRESH P.M.® has been specially formulated to soothe, moisturize, and protect dry, irritated eyes. REFRESH P.M.® is ideal for use at bedtime.

Just as important, REFRESH P.M.® is preservative-free, to avoid the risk of preservative-induced irritation.

Active Ingredients: Mineral Oil 42.5% and White Petrolatum 57.3%

Purpose: Eye Lubricant

Uses: For the temporary relief of burning, irritation, and discomfort due to the dryness of the eye or exposure to wind or sun. May be used as a protectant against further irritation.

Warnings: For external use only. To avoid contamination, do not touch tip of container to any surface. Replace cap after using.

Stop use and ask a doctor if you experience eye pain, changes in vision, continued redness or irritation of the eye, or if the condition worsens or persists for more than 72 hrs.

Keep out of reach of children. If swallowed, get medical help, or contact a Poison Control Center right away.

Directions: Pull down the lower lid of the affected eye, and apply a small amount (one fourth inch) of ointment to the inside of the eyelid. Replace cap after using.

Other Information: Store away from heat. Protect from freezing. Use only if imprinted tape seals on top and bottom flaps are intact and clearly legible.
RETAIN CARTON FOR FUTURE REFERENCE

Inactive Ingredients: Lanolin alcohols

How Supplied: As a sterile eye lubricant in 3.5 g tube—NDC 0023-0240-04
® marks owned by Allergan, Inc.
©2007 Allergan, Inc.
Irvine, CA, U.S.A. 92612

Shown in Product Identification Guide, page 103

REFRESH TEARS®   OTC
(carboxymethylcellulose sodium) 0.5%
Lubricant Eye Drops

For mild-to-moderate dry eye, REFRESH TEARS® Lubricant Eye Drops restores the moisture your eyes crave, with a special formula, that has many of the same healthy qualities as your own natural tears.

Drug Facts

Active Ingredient: **Purpose:**
Carboxymethylcellulose .... Eye lubricant sodium 0.5%

Uses:
- For the temporary relief of burning, irritation, and discomfort due to the dryness of the eye, or exposure to wind or sun.
- May be used as a protectant against further irritation.

Warnings:
- **For external use only.**
- **To avoid contamination, do not touch tip of container to any surface. Replace cap after using.**
- **Do not use if solution changes color, or becomes cloudy.**

Stop use and ask a doctor if you experience eye pain, changes in vision, continued redness or irritation of the eye, or if the condition worsens or persists for more than 72 hours.

Keep out of reach of children. If swallowed, get medical help, or contact a Poison Control Center right away.

Directions: Instill 1 or 2 drops in the affected eye(s) as needed

Other Information:
- Use only if imprinted tape seals on top and bottom flaps are intact, and clearly legible.
- **RETAIN CARTON FOR FUTURE REFERENCE.**

Inactive Ingredients: Boric acid, calcium chloride, magnesium chloride, potassium chloride, purified water, PURITE® (stabilized oxychloro complex), sodium borate, and sodium chloride. May also contain hydrochloric acid and/or sodium hydroxide, to adjust pH

How Supplied: REFRESH TEARS® (carboxymethylcellulose sodium) 0.5% Lubricant Eye Drops are supplied in the following sizes:

3 mL bottle – NDC 0023-0798-03.
15 mL bottle – NDC 0023-0798-15.
30 mL bottle – NDC 0023-0798-30.
Two – 30 mL bottles – NDC 0023-0798-60
® marks owned by Allergan, Inc.
©2007 Allergan, Inc.
Irvine, CA 92612, U.S.A.
U.S. Patents 5,424,078; 5,736,165; 6,024,954; and 5,858,346

Shown in Product Identification Guide, page 103

RESTASIS®   ℞
[rĕ′stă-sĭs]
(cyclosporine ophthalmic emulsion) 0.05%
Sterile, Preservative-Free

Description: RESTASIS® (cyclosporine ophthalmic emulsion) 0.05% contains a topical immunomodulator with anti-inflammatory effects. Cyclosporine's chemical name is Cyclo [[(E)-(2S,3R,4R)-3-hydroxy-4-methyl-2-(methylamino)-6-octenoyl]-L-2-aminobutyryl-N-methylglycyl-N-methyl-L-leucyl-L-valyl-N-methyl-L-leucyl-L-alanyl-D-alanyl-N-methyl-L-leucyl-N-methyl-L-leucyl-N-methyl-L-valyl] and it has the following structure:
[See chemical structure at top of next column]
Cyclosporine is a fine white powder. RESTASIS® appears as a white opaque to slightly translucent homogeneous emulsion. It has an osmolality of 230 to 320 mOsmol/kg and a pH of 6.5-8.0.
Each mL of RESTASIS® ophthalmic emulsion contains: **Active:** cyclosporine 0.05%. **Inactives:**

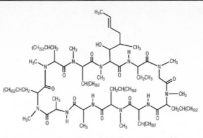

glycerin; castor oil; polysorbate 80; carbomer 1342; purified water and sodium hydroxide to adjust the pH.

Clinical Pharmacology:

Mechanism of action:
Cyclosporine is an immunosuppressive agent when administered systemically.
In patients whose tear production is presumed to be suppressed due to ocular inflammation associated with keratoconjunctivitis sicca, cyclosporine emulsion is thought to act as a partial immunomodulator. The exact mechanism of action is not known.

Pharmacokinetics:
Blood cyclosporin A concentrations were measured using a specific high pressure liquid chromatography-mass spectrometry assay. Blood concentrations of cyclosporine, in all the samples collected, after topical administration of RESTASIS® 0.05%, BID, in humans for up to 12 months, were below the quantitation limit of 0.1 ng/mL. There was no detectable drug accumulation in blood during 12 months of treatment with RESTASIS® ophthalmic emulsion.

Clinical Evaluations:
Four multicenter, randomized, adequate and well-controlled clinical studies were performed in approximately 1200 patients with moderate to severe keratoconjunctivitis sicca. RESTASIS® demonstrated statistically significant increases in Schirmer wetting of 10 mm versus vehicle at six months in patients whose tear production was presumed to be suppressed due to ocular inflammation. This effect was seen in approximately 15% of RESTASIS® ophthalmic emulsion treated patients versus approximately 5% of vehicle treated patients. Increased tear production was not seen in patients currently taking topical anti-inflammatory drugs or using punctal plugs. No increase in bacterial or fungal ocular infections was reported following administration of RESTASIS®.

Indications and Usage: RESTASIS® ophthalmic emulsion is indicated to increase tear production in patients whose tear production is presumed to be suppressed due to ocular inflammation associated with keratoconjunctivitis sicca. Increased tear production was not seen in patients currently taking topical anti-inflammatory drugs or using punctal plugs.

Contraindications: RESTASIS® is contraindicated in patients with active ocular infections and in patients with known or suspected hypersensitivity to any of the ingredients in the formulation.

Warning: RESTASIS® ophthalmic emulsion has not been studied in patients with a history of herpes keratitis.

Precautions:
General: For ophthalmic use only.

Information for Patients:
The emulsion from one individual single-use vial is to be used immediately after opening for administration to one or both eyes, and the remaining contents should be discarded immediately after administration.
Do not allow the tip of the vial to touch the eye or any surface, as this may contaminate the emulsion.
RESTASIS® should not be administered while wearing contact lenses. Patients with de-

creased tear production typically should not wear contact lenses. If contact lenses are worn, they should be removed prior to the administration of the emulsion. Lenses may be reinserted 15 minutes following administration of RESTASIS® ophthalmic emulsion.

Carcinogenesis, Mutagenesis, and Impairment of Fertility:
Systemic carcinogenicity studies were carried out in male and female mice and rats. In the 78-week oral (diet) mouse study, at doses of 1, 4, and 16 mg/kg/day, evidence of a statistically significant trend was found for lymphocytic lymphomas in females, and the incidence of hepatocellular carcinomas in mid-dose males significantly exceeded the control value.
In the 24-month oral (diet) rat study, conducted at 0.5, 2, and 8 mg/kg/day, pancreatic islet cell adenomas significantly exceeded the control rate in the low dose level. The hepatocellular carcinomas and pancreatic islet cell adenomas were not dose related. The low doses in mice and rats are approximately 1000 and 500 times greater, respectively, than the daily human dose of one drop (28 μL) of 0.05% RESTASIS® BID into each eye of a 60 kg person (0.001 mg/kg/day), assuming that the entire dose is absorbed.
Cyclosporine has not been found mutagenic/genotoxic in the Ames Test, the V79-HGPRT Test, the micronucleus test in mice and Chinese hamsters, the chromosome-aberration tests in Chinese hamster bone-marrow, the mouse dominant lethal assay, and the DNA-repair test in sperm from treated mice. A study analyzing sister chromatid exchange (SCE) induction by cyclosporine using human lymphocytes in vitro gave indication of a positive effect (i.e., induction of SCE). No impairment in fertility was demonstrated in studies in male and female rats receiving oral doses of cyclosporine up to 15 mg/kg/day (approximately 15,000 times the human daily dose of 0.001 mg/kg/day) for 9 weeks (male) and 2 weeks (female) prior to mating.

Pregnancy-Teratogenic effects:
Pregnancy category C.
Teratogenic effects: No evidence of teratogenicity was observed in rats or rabbits receiving oral doses of cyclosporine up to 300 mg/kg/day during organogenesis. These doses in rats and rabbits are approximately 300,000 times greater than the daily human dose of one drop (28 μL) 0.05% RESTASIS® BID into each eye of a 60 kg person (0.001mg/kg/day), assuming that the entire dose is absorbed.
Non-Teratogenic effects: Adverse effects were seen in reproduction studies in rats and rabbits only at dose levels toxic to dams. At toxic doses (rats at 30 mg/kg/day and rabbits at 100 mg/ kg/ day), cyclosporine oral solution, USP, was embryo- and fetotoxic as indicated by increased pre- and postnatal mortality and reduced fetal weight together with related skeletal retardations. These doses are 30,000 and 100,000 times greater, respectively than the daily human dose of one-drop (28 μL) of 0.05% RESTASIS® BID into each eye of a 60 kg person (0.001 mg/kg/day), assuming that the entire dose is absorbed. No evidence of embryofetal toxicity was observed in rats or rabbits receiving cyclosporine at oral doses up to 17 mg/kg/day or 30 mg/kg/day, respectively, during organogenesis. These doses in rats and rabbits are approximately 17,000 and 30,000 times greater, respectively, than the daily human dose.
Offspring of rats receiving a 45 mg/kg/day oral dose of cyclosporine from Day 15 of pregnancy until Day 21 post partum, a maternally toxic level, exhibited an increase in postnatal mor-

Continued on next page

Restasis—Cont.

tality; this dose is 45,000 times greater than the daily human topical dose, 0.001 mg/kg/day, assuming that the entire dose is absorbed. No adverse events were observed at oral doses up to 15 mg/kg/day (15,000 times greater than the daily human dose).

There are no adequate and well-controlled studies of RESTASIS® in pregnant women. RESTASIS® should be administered to a pregnant woman only if clearly needed.

Nursing Mothers:
Cyclosporine is known to be excreted in human milk following systemic administration but excretion in human milk after topical treatment has not been investigated. Although blood concentrations are undetectable after topical administration of RESTASIS® ophthalmic emulsion, caution should be exercised when RESTASIS® is administered to a nursing woman.

Pediatric Use:
The safety and efficacy of RESTASIS® ophthalmic emulsion have not been established in pediatric patients below the age of 16.

Geriatric Use:
No overall difference in safety or effectiveness has been observed between elderly and younger patients.

Adverse Reactions: The most common adverse event following the use of RESTASIS® was ocular burning (17%). Other events reported in 1% to 5% of patients included conjunctival hyperemia, discharge, epiphora, eye pain, foreign body sensation, pruritus, stinging, and visual disturbance (most often blurring).

Dosage and Administration: Invert the unit dose vial a few times to obtain a uniform, white, opaque emulsion before using. Instill one drop of RESTASIS® ophthalmic emulsion twice a day in each eye approximately 12 hours apart. RESTASIS® can be used concomitantly with artificial tears, allowing a 15 minute interval between products. Discard vial immediately after use.

How Supplied: RESTASIS® ophthalmic emulsion is packaged in single use vials. Each vial contains 0.4 mL fill in a 0.9 mL LDPE vial; 32 vials are packaged in a polypropylene tray with an aluminum peelable lid. The entire contents of this tray (32 vials) must be dispensed as one unit.

RESTASIS® 32 Vials 0.4 mL each - NDC 0023-9163-32

Storage: Store RESTASIS® ophthalmic emulsion at 15° to 25° C (59°-77° F).

KEEP OUT OF THE REACH OF CHILDREN.

Rx Only

Revised February 2004
©2004 Allergan, Inc., Irvine, CA 92612, U.S.A.
® marks owned by Allergan, Inc.
U.S. Patents 4,649,047; 4,839,342; and 5,474,979

INSPIRE

PHARMACEUTICALS, INC.

Inspire and the Inspire logo are registered trademarks of Inspire Pharmaceuticals, Inc. 71271US15P

Shown in Product Identification Guide, page 103

ZYMAR®　　　　　　　　　　　　　℞

[zi-mar]

(gatifloxacin ophthalmic solution) 0.3%
Sterile

Description: ZYMAR® (gatifloxacin ophthalmic solution) 0.3% is a sterile ophthalmic solution. It is an 8-methoxy fluoroquinolone anti-infective for topical ophthalmic use.

Structure and Empirical Formula:

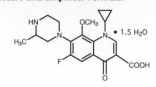

$C_{19}H_{22}FN_3O_4 \bullet 1.5\ H_2O$　　　Mol Wt 402.42

Chemical Name: (±)-1-cyclopropyl-6-fluoro-1, 4-dihydro-8-methoxy-7-(3-methyl-1-piperazinyl)-4-oxo-3-quinolinecarboxylic acid sesquihydrate

Contains: Active: gatifloxacin 0.3% (3 mg/mL).

Preservative: benzalkonium chloride 0.005%.

Inactives: edetate disodium; purified water and sodium chloride. May contain hydrochloric acid and/or sodium hydroxide to adjust pH to approximately 6.

ZYMAR® is a sterile, clear, pale yellow colored isotonic unbuffered solution. It has an osmolality of 260-330 mOsm/kg.

Clinical Pharmacology:

Pharmacokinetics: Gatifloxacin ophthalmic solution 0.3% or 0.5% was administered to one eye of 6 healthy male subjects each in an escalated dosing regimen starting with a single 2 drop dose, then 2 drops 4 times daily for 7 days and finally 2 drops 8 times daily for 3 days. At all time points, serum gatifloxacin levels were below the lower limit of quantification (5 ng/mL) in all subjects.

Microbiology: Gatifloxacin is an 8-methoxy fluoroquinolone with a 3-methylpiperazinyl substituent at C7. The antibacterial action of gatifloxacin results from inhibition of DNA gyrase and topoisomerase IV. DNA gyrase is an essential enzyme that is involved in the replication, transcription and repair of bacterial DNA. Topoisomerase IV is an enzyme known to play a key role in the partitioning of the chromosomal DNA during bacterial cell division.

The mechanism of action of fluoroquinolones including gatifloxacin is different from that of aminoglycoside, macrolide, and tetracycline antibiotics. Therefore, gatifloxacin may be active against pathogens that are resistant to these antibiotics and these antibiotics may be active against pathogens that are resistant to gatifloxacin. There is no cross-resistance between gatifloxacin and the aforementioned classes of antibiotics. Cross resistance has been observed between systemic gatifloxacin and some other fluoroquinolones.

Resistance to gatifloxacin *in vitro* develops via multiple step mutations. Resistance to gatifloxacin *in vitro* occurs at a general frequency of between 1×10^{-7} to 10^{-10}.

Gatifloxacin has been shown to be active against most strains of the following organisms both *in vitro* and clinically, in conjunctival infections as described in the INDICATIONS AND USAGE section.

Aerobes, Gram-Positive:
*Corynebacterium propinquum**
Staphylococcus aureus
Staphylococcus epidermidis
*Streptococcus mitis**
Streptococcus pneumoniae
Aerobes, Gram-Negative:
Haemophilus influenzae

---

* Efficacy for this organism was studied in fewer than 10 infections.

The following *in vitro* data are available, **but their clinical significance in ophthalmic infections is unknown.** The safety and effectiveness of ZYMAR® in treating ophthalmic infections due to the following organisms have not been established in adequate and well-controlled clinical trials.

The following organisms are considered susceptible when evaluated using systemic breakpoints. However, a correlation between the *in vitro* systemic breakpoint and ophthalmological efficacy has not been established. The following list of organisms is provided as guidance only in assessing the potential treatment of conjunctival infections.

Gatifloxacin exhibits *in vitro* minimal inhibitory concentrations (MICs) of 2µg/mL or less (systemic susceptible breakpoint) against most (≥90%) strains of the following ocular pathogens.

Aerobes, Gram-Positive:
Listeria monocytogenes
Staphylococcus saprophyticus
Streptococcus agalactiae
Streptococcus pyogenes
Streptococcus viridans Group
Streptococcus Groups C, F, G
Aerobes, Gram-Negative:
Acinetobacter lwoffii
Enterobacter aerogenes
Enterobacter cloacae
Escherichia coli
Citrobacter freundii
Citrobacter koseri
Haemophilus parainfluenzae
Klebsiella oxytoca
Klebsiella pneumoniae
Moraxella catarrhalis
Morganella morganii
Neisseria gonorrhoeae
Neisseria meningitidis
Proteus mirabilis
Proteus vulgaris
Serratia marcescens
Vibrio cholerae
Yersinia enterocolitica
Other Microorganisms:
Chlamydia pneumoniae
Legionella pneumophila
Mycobacterium marinum
Mycobacterium fortuitum
Mycoplasma pneumoniae
Anaerobic Microorganisms:
Bacteroides fragilis
Clostridium perfringens

Clinical Studies:
In a randomized, double-masked, multicenter clinical trial, where patients were dosed for 5 days, ZYMAR® solution was superior to its vehicle on day 5-7 in patients with conjunctivitis and positive conjunctival cultures. Clinical outcomes for the trial demonstrated clinical cure of 77% (40/52) for the gatifloxacin treated group versus 58% (28/48) for the placebo treated group. Microbiological outcomes for the same clinical trial demonstrated a statistically superior eradication rate for causative pathogens of 92% (48/52) for gatifloxacin vs. 72% (34/48) for placebo. Please note that microbiologic eradication does not always correlate with clinical outcome in anti-infective trials.

Indications and Usage: ZYMAR® solution is indicated for the treatment of bacterial conjunctivitis caused by susceptible strains of the following organisms:

Aerobic Gram-Positive Bacteria:
*Corynebacterium propinquum**
Staphylococcus aureus
Staphylococcus epidermidis
*Streptococcus mitis**
Streptococcus pneumoniae
Aerobic Gram-Negative Bacteria:
Haemophilus influenzae

---

* Efficacy for this organism was studied in fewer than 10 infections.

Contraindications: ZYMAR® solution is contraindicated in patients with a history of hypersensitivity to gatifloxacin, to other quinolones, or to any of the components in this medication.

Warnings: NOT FOR INJECTION.
ZYMAR® solution should not be injected sub-conjunctivally, nor should it be introduced directly into the anterior chamber of the eye.

In patients receiving systemic quinolones, including gatifloxacin, serious and occasionally fatal hypersensitivity (anaphylactic) reactions, some following the first dose, have been reported. Some reactions were accompanied by cardiovascular collapse, loss of consciousness, angioedema (including laryngeal, pharyngeal or facial edema), airway obstruction, dyspnea, urticaria, and itching. If an allergic reaction to gatifloxacin occurs, discontinue the drug. Serious acute hypersensitivity reactions may require immediate emergency treatment. Oxygen and airway management should be administered as clinically indicated.

Precautions:
General: As with other anti-infectives, prolonged use may result in overgrowth of non-susceptible organisms, including fungi. If superinfection occurs discontinue use and institute alternative therapy. Whenever clinical judgment dictates, the patient should be examined with the aid of magnification, such as slit lamp biomicroscopy and, where appropriate, fluorescein staining.

Patients should be advised not to wear contact lenses if they have signs and symptoms of bacterial conjunctivitis.

Information for Patients: Avoid contaminating the applicator tip with material from the eye, fingers or other source.

Systemic quinolones, including gatifloxacin, have been associated with hypersensitivity reactions, even following a single dose. Discontinue use immediately and contact your physician at the first sign of a rash or allergic reaction.

Drug Interactions: Specific drug interaction studies have not been conducted with ZYMAR® ophthalmic solution. However, the systemic administration of some quinolones has been shown to elevate plasma concentrations of theophylline, interfere with the metabolism of caffeine, and enhance the effects of the oral anticoagulant warfarin and its derivatives, and has been associated with transient elevations in serum creatinine in patients receiving systemic cyclosporine concomitantly.

Carcinogenesis, Mutagenesis, Impairment of Fertility
There was no increase in neoplasms among B6C3F1 mice given gatifloxacin in the diet for 18 months at doses averaging 81 mg/kg/day in males and 90 mg/kg/day in females. These doses are approximately 2000-fold higher than the maximum recommended ophthalmic dose of 0.04 mg/kg/day in a 50 kg human.

There was no increase in neoplasms among Fischer 344 rats given gatifloxacin in the diet for 2 years at doses averaging 47 mg/kg/day in males and 139 mg/kg/day in females (1000 and 3000-fold higher, respectively, than the maximum recommended ophthalmic dose). A statistically significant increase in the incidence of large granular lymphocyte (LGL) leukemia was seen in males treated with a high dose of approximately 2000-fold higher than the maximum recommended ophthalmic dose. Fischer 344 rats have a high spontaneous background rate of LGL leukemia and the incidence in high-dose males only slightly exceeded the historical control range established for this strain.

In genetic toxicity tests, gatifloxacin was positive in 1 of 5 strains used in bacterial reverse mutation assays; Salmonella strain TA102. Gatifloxacin was positive in *in vitro* mammalian cell mutation and chromosome aberration assays. Gatifloxacin was positive in *in vitro* unscheduled DNA synthesis in rat hepatocytes but not human leukocytes. Gatifloxacin was negative in *in vivo* micronucleus tests in mice, cytogenetics test in rats, and DNA repair test in rats. The findings may be due to the inhibitory effects of high concentrations on eukaryotic type II DNA topoisomerase.

There were no adverse effects on fertility or reproduction in rats given gatifloxacin orally at doses up to 200 mg/kg/day (approximately 4500-fold higher than the maximum recommended ophthalmic dose for ZYMAR®).

Pregnancy: Teratogenic Effects. Pregnancy Category C:
There were no teratogenic effects observed in rats or rabbits following oral gatifloxacin doses up to 50 mg/kg/day (approximately 1000-fold higher than the maximum recommended ophthalmic dose). However, skeletal/craniofacial malformations or delayed ossification, atrial enlargement, and reduced fetal weight were observed in fetuses from rats given ≥150 mg/kg/day (approximately 3000-fold higher than the maximum recommended ophthalmic dose). In a perinatal/postnatal study, increased late post-implantation loss and neonatal/perinatal mortalities were observed at 200 mg/kg/day (approximately 4500 times the maximum recommended ophthalmic dose).

Because there are no adequate and well-controlled studies in pregnant women, ZYMAR® solution should be used during pregnancy only if the potential benefit justifies the potential risk to the fetus.

Nursing Mothers: Gatifloxacin is excreted in the breast milk of rats. It is not known whether this drug is excreted in human milk. Because many drugs are excreted in human milk, caution should be exercised when gatifloxacin is administered to a nursing woman.

Pediatric Use: Safety and effectiveness in infants below the age of one year have not been established.

Geriatric use: No overall differences in safety or effectiveness have been observed between elderly and younger patients.

Adverse Reactions:
Ophthalmic Use: The most frequently reported adverse events in the overall study population were conjunctival irritation, increased lacrimation, keratitis, and papillary conjunctivitis. These events occurred in approximately 5-10% of patients. Other reported reactions occurring in 1-4% of patients were chemosis, conjunctival hemorrhage, dry eye, eye discharge, eye irritation, eye pain, eyelid edema, headache, red eye, reduced visual acuity and taste disturbance.

Dosage and Administration: The recommended dosage regimen for the treatment of bacterial conjunctivitis is:

Days 1 and 2: Instill one drop every two hours in the affected eye(s) while awake, up to 8 times daily.
Days 3 through 7: Instill one drop up to four times daily while awake.

How Supplied: ZYMAR® (gatifloxacin ophthalmic solution) 0.3% is supplied sterile in a white, low density polyethylene (LDPE) bottle with a controlled dropper tip and a tan, high impact polystyrene (HIPS) cap in the following size:

5 mL in 10 mL bottle- NDC 0023-9218-05
Note: Store at 15°–25°C (59°–77°F). Protect from freezing.

Animal Pharmacology: Quinolone antibacterials have been shown to cause bone or cartilage changes in immature animals. There was no evidence of bone cartilage changes following ocular administration of gatifloxacin in rabbits or dogs.

Rx only
Revised August 2004
©2004 Allergan, Inc., Irvine, CA 92612, U.S.A.
® marks owned by Allergan, Inc.

Licensed from: Kyorin Pharmaceuticals Co., Ltd.
U.S. PAT. 4,980,470; 5,880,283
71706US12P

Bausch & Lomb Incorporated
**ONE BAUSCH & LOMB PLACE
ROCHESTER NY 14604**

**8500 HIDDEN RIVER PARKWAY
TAMPA, FL 33637**

Direct Inquiries to:
Main Office
(585) 338-6000
Consumer Affairs
1-800-553-5340

Product List-Bauch & Lomb Pharma

NDC 24208	PRODUCT	
-601-10	ALAWAY™ Ketotifen Fumarate Ophthalmic Solution Antihistamine Eye Drops 10 mL	OTC
-353-	ALREX® loteprednol etabonate ophthalmic suspension, 0.2% 5 mL: -05 10 mL: -10	℞
-825-55	ATROPINE SULFATE OPHTHALMIC OINTMENT USP, 1% 3.5 gram tubes	℞
-750-	ATROPINE SULFATE OPHTHALMIC SOLUTION USP, 1% 5mL: -60 15mL: -06	℞
411-	BRIMONIDINE TARTRATE OPHTHALMIC SOLUTION, 0.2% 5mL: -05 10mL: -10 15mL: -15	℞
555-55	BACITRACIN ZINC & POLYMYXIN B SULFATE OPHTHALMIC OINTMENT USP 3.5 g tube	℞
367-	CARTEOLOL HYDROCHLORIDE OPHTHALMIC SOLUTION, USP, 1% 5 mL: -05 10 mL: -10 15 mL: -15	℞
300-10	CROLOM® cromolyn sodium ophthalmic solution USP, 4% 10 mL	℞
-735-	CYCLOPENTOLATE HYDROCHLORIDE OPHTHALMIC SOLUTION USP, 1% 2mL: -01 15mL: -06	℞
-720-02	DEXAMETHASONE SODIUM PHOSPHATE Ophthalmic Solution, USP, 0.1% 5 mL	℞

Continued on next page

Product List—Cont.

540 **DIPIVEFRIN HYDROCHLORIDE** ℞
Ophthalmic Solution USP, 0.1%
5 mL: -05
10 mL: -10
15 mL: -15

910- **ERYTHROMYCIN OPHTHALMIC** ℞
Ointment USP, 0.5%
50 × 1 g tube -19
3.5 g tube -55

732-05 **FLUORESCEIN SODIUM & BENOXINATE HCl OPHTHALMIC SOLUTION** ℞
USP, 0.25%/0.4%
5 ml

391-83 **FLUOR-I-STRIP® A.T.** ℞
1 mg Fluorescein Sodium
Ophthalmic Strips
Box of 300

391-82 **FLUORETS®** ℞
(fluorescein sodium
ophthalmic strips
USP 1 mg)
Box of 100

314-25 **FLURBIPROFEN** ℞
Sodium Ophthalmic
Solution USP,
0.03%
2.5 ml

-580- **GENTAMICIN SULFATE** ℞
Ophthalmic Solution
USP, 0.3%
5mL: -60
15mL: -64

-545- **LEVOBUNOLOL HYDROCHLORIDE OPHTHALMIC SOLUTION USP, 0.25%** ℞
5mL: -05
10mL: -10

-505- **LEVOBUNOLOL HYDROCHLORIDE OPHTHALMIC SOLUTION USP, 0.5%** ℞
5mL: -05
10mL: -10
15 mL: -15

-299- **LOTEMAX®** ℞
loteprednol etabonate
opthalmic suspension,
0.5%
5 mL -05
10 mL -10
15 mL -15

-402- **METIPRANOLOL OPHTHALMIC SOLUTION 0.3%** ℞
5 mL -05
10 mL -10

-280-15 **MUROCEL®** OTC
Methylcellulose Lubricant
Ophthalmic Solution USP,
1%
15 mL

-278-05 **MUROCOLL® 2** ℞
Phenylephrine
Hydrochloride 10% and
Scopolamine
Hydrobromide 0.3%
Ophthalmic Solution
5 mL

-385 **MURO™ 128® 5% OINTMENT** OTC
Sodium Chloride
Hypertonicity
Ophthalmic Ointment, 5%
3.5g: -55
TWIN PACK
2×3.5g: -56

-276-15 **MURO™ 128® 2%** OTC
Sodium Chloride
Hypertonicity
Ophthalmic Solution, 2%
15 mL

-277- **MURO™ 128® 5% SOLUTION** OTC
Sodium Chloride
Hypertonicity
Ophthalmic Solution, 5%
15 mL: -15
30 mL: -30

-785-55 **NEOMYCIN & POLYMYXIN B SULFATES, BACITRACIN ZINC AND HYDROCORTISONE OPHTHALMIC** ℞
Ointment USP
3.5 g tube

-780-55 **NEOMYCIN AND POLYMYXIN B SULFATES AND BACITRACIN ZINC OPHTHALMIC** ℞
Ointment USP
3.5 gram tubes

-795-35 **NEOMYCIN AND POLYMYXIN B SULFATES AND DEXAMETHASONE OPHTHALMIC OINTMENT USP** ℞
3.5 gram tubes

830-60 **NEOMYCIN AND POLYMYXIN B SULFATES AND DEXAMETHASONE Ophthalmic Suspension USP** ℞
5 mL

790-62 **NEOMYCIN AND POLYMYXIN B SULFATES AND GRAMICIDIN** ℞
Ophthalmic Solution USP
10 mL

OCUVITE® OTC
Antioxidant Vitamin and
Mineral Supplement
387-60 Bottle of 60 tablets
387-62 Bottle of 120 tablets

741-00 **OCUVITE® DF** OTC
Eye Vitamin Supplement
Bottle of 60 tablets

403-19 **OCUVITE® LUTEIN** OTC
Vitamin and Mineral
Supplement
403-73 Bottle of 36 capsules
Bottle of 72 capsules

432-62 **OCUVITE PRESERVISION** OTC
120s

432-72 **OCUVITE PRESERVISION** OTC
240s

632-10 **OCUVITE® PRESERVISION LUTEIN**
Vitamin and Mineral
Supplement
50 soft gels

532 **OCUVITE® PRESERVISION AREDS**
Vitamin and Mineral
Supplement
60 soft gels - 20
120 soft gels - 30
150 soft gels - 40

434-05 **OFLOXACIN OPHTHALMIC SOLUTION** ℞
5 mL

434-10 **OFLOXACIN OPHTHALMIC SOLUTION** ℞
10 mL

430 **OPCON-A®** OTC
Itching and Redness
reliever eyedrops
15 mL
TWIN PACK

2 × 15 mL
2 × 30 mL

-275- **OPTIPRANOLOL®** ℞
(metipranolol
ophthalmic solution) 0.3%
5 mL -07
10 mL -09

-740- **PHENYLEPHRINE HYDROCHLORIDE OPHTHALMIC SOLUTION USP, 2.5%** ℞
2mL: -59
5mL: -02
15mL: -06

-806-15 **PILOCARPINE HYDROCHLORIDE OPHTHALMIC SOLUTION USP, 0.5%** ℞
15mL

-676- **PILOCARPINE HYDROCHLORIDE OPHTHALMIC SOLUTION USP, 1%** ℞
15mL: -15

-681- **PILOCARPINE HYDROCHLORIDE OPHTHALMIC SOLUTION USP, 2%** ℞
15mL: -15

-811-15 **PILOCARPINE HYDROCHLORIDE OPHTHALMIC SOLUTION USP, 3%** ℞
15mL

-686- **PILOCARPINE HYDROCHLORIDE OPHTHALMIC SOLUTION USP, 4%** ℞
15mL: -15

-821-15 **PILOCARPINE HYDROCHLORIDE OPHTHALMIC SOLUTION USP, 6%** ℞
15mL

315-10 **POLYMYXIN B SULFATE AND TRIMETHOPRIM SULFATE OPHTHALMIC SOLUTION USP** ℞
10mL

715- **PREDNISOLONE SODIUM PHOSPHATE OPHTHALMIC SOLUTION USP, 1%** ℞
5 mL: -02
10 mL: -10
15 mL: -06

730-06 **PROPARACAINE HYDROCHLORIDE OPHTHALMIC SOLUTION USP, 0.5%** ℞
15 mL

317- **SULFACETAMIDE SODIUM AND PREDNISOLONE SODIUM PHOSPHATE** ℞
Ophthalmic Solution
10%/0.23%
(prednisolone phosphate)
5 mL: -05
10 mL: -10

-670-04 **SULFACETAMIDE SODIUM OPHTHALMIC SOLUTION USP, 10%** ℞
15mL

-920-64 **TETRACAINE HYDRO-CHLORIDE OPHTHALMIC SOLUTION USP, 0.5%** ℞
15mL

-330- **TIMOLOL MALEATE OPHTHALMIC SOLUTION USP, 0.25%** ℞
5 mL: -05
10 mL: -10
15 mL: -15

-324- **TIMOLOL MALEATE OPHTHALMIC SOLUTION USP, 0.5%** ℞

	5 mL: -05 10 mL: -10 15 mL: -15	
-290-05	**TOBRAMYCIN OPHTHALMIC SOLUTION USP, 0.3%** 5mL	℞
-590-64	**TROPICAMIDE OPHTHALMIC SOLUTION, USP 0.5%** 15 mL	℞
-585-	**TROPICAMIDE OPHTHALMIC SOLUTION, USP 1%** 2 mL: -59 15 mL: -64	
358	**ZYLET®** loteprednol etabonate 0.5% and tobramycin 0.3% ophthalmic suspension 2.5 mL 25 5 mL 05 10 mL 10	℞
416	**RETISERT®** fluocinolone acetonide intravitreal implant 0.59 mg 0.59 mg implant -01	℞

BAUSCH & LOMB ALAWAY™ OTC
Ketotifen Fumarate Ophthalmic Solution Antihistamine Eye Drops

Description: Alaway™ (ketotifen fumarate ophthalmic solution 0.025%) Antihistamine Eye Drops are indicated for temporary relief for itchy eyes due to ragweed, pollen, grass, animal hair and dander. The original prescription strength, now available over-the-counter, quickly stops the itch within minutes and provides up to 12 hours of symptom relief.

Drug Facts:
Active Ingredient: Ketotifen 0.025% (equivalent to ketotifen fumarate 0.035%)
Purpose: Antihistamine
Inactive ingredients: Benzalkonium chloride, 0.01%, glycerin, sodium hydroxide and/or hydrochloric acid and water for injection.
Uses: For the temporary relief of itchy eyes due to ragweed, pollen, grass, animal hair and dander.
Warnings: Do not use:
- if you are sensitive to any ingredient in this product
- if the solution changes color or becomes cloudy
- to treat contact lens related irritation
When using this product
- remove contact lenses before use
- wait at least 10 minutes before re-inserting contact lenses after use
- do not touch the tip of the container to any surface to avoid contamination
- replace cap after use
Stop use and ask a doctor if you experience any of the following:
- eye pain
- changes in vision
- redness of the eyes
- itching that worsens or lasts for more than 72 hours
Keep out of reach of children. If swallowed, get medical help or contact a Poison Control Center right away.
Directions: Adults and children 3 years and older: put 1 drop in the affected eye(s) twice daily, every 8-12 hours, no more than twice per day.
Children under 3 years of age: consult a doctor
Other information
STORE AT 4-25°C (39-77°F)
DO NOT USE IF TAPE SEAL ON CARTON OR IMPRINTED NECKBAND "SAFETY SEAL" ON BOTTLE IS NOT INTACT.

How Supplied: NDC 24208-601-10 Sterile 0.34 FL OZ (10mL) plastic dispenser bottle
Questions or Comments?
Toll Free Product Information
Call: 1-800-553-5340
Distributed by: Bausch & Lomb Incorporated. Rochester, NY 14609
Bausch & Lomb and Alaway are trademarks of Bausch & Lomb Incorporated
© Bausch & Lomb Incorporated
Rochester, NY 14609
Shown in Product Identification Guide, page 103

ALREX® ℞
[*ăl rĕx*]
loteprednol etabonate ophthalmic suspension 0.2%
STERILE OPHTHALMIC SUSPENSION
℞ only

Description: ALREX® (loteprednol etabonate ophthalmic suspension) contains a sterile, topical anti-inflammatory corticosteroid for ophthalmic use. Loteprednol etabonate is a white to off-white powder.
Loteprednol etabonate is represented by the following structural formula:

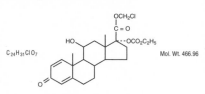

$C_{24}H_{31}ClO_7$ Mol. Wt. 466.96

Chemical Name:
chloromethyl 17α-[(ethoxycarbonyl)oxy]-11β-hydroxy-3-oxoandrosta-1,4-diene-17β-carboxylate.
Each mL contains:
ACTIVE: Loteprednol Etabonate 2 mg (0.2%); INACTIVES: Edetate Disodium, Glycerin, Povidone, Purified Water and Tyloxapol. Hydrochloric Acid and/or Sodium Hydroxide may be added to adjust the pH to 5.3-5.6. The suspension is essentially isotonic with a tonicity of 250 to 310 mOsmol/kg.
PRESERVATIVE ADDED: Benzalkonium Chloride 0.01%.
Clinical Pharmacology: Corticosteroids inhibit the inflammatory response to a variety of inciting agents and probably delay or slow healing. They inhibit the edema, fibrin deposition, capillary dilation, leukocyte migration, capillary proliferation, fibroblast proliferation, deposition of collagen, and scar formation associated with inflammation. There is no generally accepted explanation for the mechanism of action of ocular corticosteroids. However, corticosteroids are thought to act by the induction of phospholipase A₂ inhibitory proteins, collectively called lipocortins. It is postulated that these proteins control the biosynthesis of potent mediators of inflammation such as prostaglandins and leukotrienes by inhibiting the release of their common precursor arachidonic acid. Arachidonic acid is released from membrane phospholipids by phospholipase A₂. Corticosteroids are capable of producing a rise in intraocular pressure.
Loteprednol etabonate is structurally similar to other corticosteroids. However, the number 20 position ketone group is absent. It is highly lipid soluble which enhances its penetration into cells. Loteprednol etabonate is synthesized through structural modifications of prednisolone-related compounds so that it will undergo a predictable transformation to an inactive metabolite. Based upon *in vivo* and *in*

vitro preclinical metabolism studies, loteprednol etabonate undergoes extensive metabolism to inactive carboxylic acid metabolites.
Results from a bioavailability study in normal volunteers established that plasma levels of loteprednol etabonate and Δ¹ cortienic acid etabonate (PJ 91), its primary, inactive metabolite, were below the limit of quantitation (1 ng/mL) at all sampling times. The results were obtained following the ocular administration of one drop in each eye of 0.5% loteprednol etabonate 8 times daily for 2 days or 4 times daily for 42 days. This study suggests that limited (<1 ng/mL) systemic absorption occurs with ALREX.
Clinical Studies:
In two double-masked, placebo-controlled six-week environmental studies of 268 patients with seasonal allergic conjunctivitis, ALREX, when dosed four times per day was superior to placebo in the treatment of the signs and symptoms of seasonal allergic conjunctivitis. ALREX provided reduction in bulbar conjunctival injection and itching, beginning approximately 2 hours after instillation of the first dose and throughout the first 14 days of treatment.
Indications and Usage: ALREX Ophthalmic Suspension is indicated for the temporary relief of the signs and symptoms of seasonal allergic conjunctivitis.
Contraindications: ALREX, as with other ophthalmic corticosteroids, is contraindicated in most viral diseases of the cornea and conjunctiva including epithelial herpes simplex keratitis (dendritic keratitis), vaccinia, and varicella, and also in mycobacterial infection of the eye and fungal diseases of ocular structures. ALREX is also contraindicated in individuals with known or suspected hypersensitivity to any of the ingredients of this preparation and to other corticosteroids.
Warnings: Prolonged use of corticosteroids may result in glaucoma with damage to the optic nerve, defects in visual acuity and fields of vision, and in posterior subcapsular cataract formation. Steroids should be used with caution in the presence of glaucoma.
Prolonged use of corticosteroids may suppress the host response and thus increase the hazard of secondary ocular infections. In those diseases causing thinning of the cornea or sclera, perforations have been known to occur with the use of topical steroids. In acute purulent conditions of the eye, steroids may mask infection or enhance existing infection.
Use of ocular steroids may prolong the course and may exacerbate the severity of many viral infections of the eye (including herpes simplex). Employment of a corticosteroid medication in the treatment of patients with a history of herpes simplex requires great caution.
Precautions:
General: For ophthalmic use only. The initial prescription and renewal of the medication order beyond 14 days should be made by a physician only after examination of the patient with the aid of magnification, such as slit lamp biomicroscopy and, where appropriate, fluorescein staining.
If signs and symptoms fail to improve after two days, the patient should be re-evaluated.
If this product is used for 10 days or longer, intraocular pressure should be monitored.
Fungal infections of the cornea are particularly prone to develop coincidentally with long-term local steroid application. Fungus invasion must be considered in any persistent corneal ulceration where a steroid has been used or is in use. Fungal cultures should be taken when appropriate.
Information for Patients: This product is sterile when packaged. Patients should be advised

Continued on next page

Alrex—Cont.

not to allow the dropper tip to touch any surface, as this may contaminate the suspension. If redness or itching becomes aggravated, the patient should be advised to consult a physician.

Patients should be advised not to wear a contact lens if their eye is red. ALREX should not be used to treat contact lens related irritation. The preservative in ALREX, benzalkonium chloride, may be absorbed by soft contact lenses. Patients who wear soft contact lenses **and whose eyes are not red,** should be instructed to wait at least ten minutes after instilling ALREX before they insert their contact lenses.

Carcinogenesis, mutagenesis, impairment of fertility: Long-term animal studies have not been conducted to evaluate the carcinogenic potential of loteprednol etabonate. Loteprednol etabonate was not genotoxic *in vitro* in the Ames test, the mouse lymphoma tk assay, or in a chromosome aberration test in human lymphocytes, or *in vivo* in the single dose mouse micronucleus assay. Treatment of male and female rats with up to 50 mg/kg/day and 25 mg/kg/day of loteprednol etabonate, respectively, (1500 and 750 times the maximum clinical dose, respectively) prior to and during mating did not impair fertility in either gender.

Pregnancy: Teratogenic effects: Pregnancy Category C. Loteprednol etabonate has been shown to be embryotoxic (delayed ossification) and teratogenic (increased incidence of meningocele, abnormal left common carotid artery, and limb flexures) when administered orally to rabbits during organogenesis at a dose of 3 mg/kg/day (85 times the maximum daily clinical dose), a dose which caused no maternal toxicity. The no-observed-effect-level (NOEL) for these effects was 0.5 mg/kg/day (15 times the maximum daily clinical dose). Oral treatment of rats during organogenesis resulted in teratogenicity (absent innominate artery at ≥5 mg/kg/day doses, and cleft palate and umbilical hernia at ≥50 mg/kg/day) and embryotoxicity (increased post-implantation losses at 100 mg/kg/day and decreased fetal body weight and skeletal ossification with ≥50 mg/kg/day). Treatment of rats with 0.5 mg/kg/day (15 times the maximum clinical dose) during organogenesis did not result in any reproductive toxicity. Loteprednol etabonate was maternally toxic (significantly reduced body weight gain during treatment) when administered to pregnant rats during organogenesis at doses of ≥5 mg/kg/day.

Oral exposure of female rats to 50 mg/kg/day of loteprednol etabonate from the start of the fetal period through the end of lactation, a maternally toxic treatment regimen (significantly decreased body weight gain), gave rise to decreased growth and survival, and retarded development in the offspring during lactation; the NOEL for these effects was 5 mg/kg/day. Loteprednol etabonate had no effect on the duration of gestation or parturition when administered orally to pregnant rats at doses up to 50 mg/kg/day during the fetal period.

Nursing Mothers: It is not known whether topical ophthalmic administration of corticosteroids could result in sufficient systemic absorption to produce detectable quantities in human milk. Systemic steroids appear in human milk and could suppress growth, interfere with endogenous corticosteroid production, or cause other untoward effects. Caution should be exercised when ALREX is administered to a nursing woman.

Pediatric Use: Safety and effectiveness in pediatric patients have not been established.

Adverse Reactions: Reactions associated with ophthalmic steroids include elevated intra-ocular pressure, which may be associated with optic nerve damage, visual acuity and field defects, posterior subcapsular cataract formation, secondary ocular infection from pathogens including herpes simplex, and perforation of the globe where there is thinning of the cornea or sclera.

Ocular adverse reactions occurring in 5-15% of patients treated with loteprednol etabonate ophthalmic suspension (0.2%-0.5%) in clinical studies included abnormal vision/blurring, burning on instillation, chemosis, discharge, dry eyes, epiphora, foreign body sensation, itching, injection, and photophobia. Other ocular adverse reactions occurring in less than 5% of patients include conjunctivitis, corneal abnormalities, eyelid erythema, keratoconjunctivitis, ocular irritation/pain/discomfort, papillae, and uveitis. Some of these events were similar to the underlying ocular disease being studied.

Non-ocular adverse reactions occurred in less than 15% of patients. These include headache, rhinitis and pharyngitis.

In a summation of controlled, randomized studies of individuals treated for 28 days or longer with loteprednol etabonate, the incidence of significant elevation of intraocular pressure (≥10 mm Hg) was 2% (15/901) among patients receiving loteprednol etabonate, 7% (11/164) among patients receiving 1% prednisolone acetate and 0.5% (3/583) among patients receiving placebo. Among the smaller group of patients who were studied with ALREX, the incidence of clinically significant increases in IOP (≥10 mm Hg) was 1% (1/133) with ALREX and 1% (1/135) with placebo.

Dosage and Administration: SHAKE VIGOROUSLY BEFORE USING.

One drop instilled into the affected eye(s) four times daily.

How Supplied: ALREX® (loteprednol etabonate ophthalmic suspension, 0.2%) is supplied in a plastic bottle with a controlled drop tip in the following sizes:

5 mL (NDC 24208-353-05) - AB35307
10 mL (NDC 24208-353-10) - AB35309

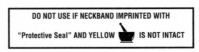

DO NOT USE IF NECKBAND IMPRINTED WITH
"Protective Seal" AND YELLOW ⚗ IS NOT INTACT

Storage: Store upright between 15°-25°C (59°-77°F). DO NOT FREEZE.
KEEP OUT OF REACH OF CHILDREN.
Revised April 2006.
Bausch & Lomb Incorporated, Tampa, Florida 33637
U.S. Patent No. 4,996,335
U.S. Patent No. 5,540,930
U.S. Patent No. 5,747,061
9007901 (Folded)
9005501 (Flat)
©Bausch & Lomb Incorporated
Alrex® is a registered trademark of Bausch & Lomb Incorporated

Shown in Product Identification Guide, page 103

BAUSCH & LOMB PRESERVISION® AREDS   OTC
Eye Vitamin and Mineral Supplement
AREDS: Soft Gel Formula.
Easy to swallow 2 per day Soft Gels Formula

Description: see Supplement Facts (table A) [See table A above]

Other Ingredients: Gelatin, Glycerin, Soybean Oil, Soy Lecithin, Yellow Beeswax, Silicon Dioxide, Titanium Dioxide, FD&C Yellow 6, FD&C Red #40, FD&C Blue #1, Contains Soy.

- Age-related macular degeneration (AMD) is the leading cause of vision loss and blindness in people over 55. The landmark National Institutes of Health AREDS trial proved that a high potency antioxidant vitamin and mineral supplement was effective in helping to preserve the sight of certain people most at risk.*
- The patented Bausch & Lomb PreserVision® Soft Gels are based on the AREDS Formula that is the ONLY eye vitamin and mineral supplement clinically proven effective in the 10 year National Institutes of Health (NIH) Age Related Eye Disease Study (AREDS). US Patent 6,660,297.
- Bausch & Lomb PreserVision® Soft Gels are a high potency antioxidant and mineral supplement with the antioxidant vitamins A, C, E, and selected minerals in amounts above those in ordinary multivitamins and generally cannot be obtained through diet alone.
- **Recommended Intake:** Instead of taking 4 tablets per day to get the high levels proven effective in the National Institutes of Health (NIH) Age Related Eye Disease Study (AREDS), you only need to take: 2 softgels per day – 1 in the morning. 1 in the evening taken with meals.

Bausch & Lomb PreserVision® is the #1 recommended eye vitamin and mineral supplement among vitreoretinal eye doctors.**

CURRENT AND FORMER SMOKERS:
Consult your eye doctor or eye care professional about the risks associated with smoking and Beta-Carotene.

> *** This statement has not been evaluated by the Food and Drug Administration. This product is not intended to diagnose, treat, cure or prevent any disease.**

** Data on file, Bausch & Lomb Incorporated.
How Supplied: NDC 24208-532-10 60 ct. NDC 24208-532-30 120 ct. NDC 24208-532-40 150 ct. Available in bottles of 60 count, 120 and 150 count soft gels.
Orange, oval shaped soft gelatin capsule.
DO NOT USE IF SEAL UNDER CLOSURE IS BROKEN
Keep this product out of the reach of children.
STORE AT ROOM TEMPERATURE
Made in the USA
Marketed by:
Bausch & Lomb Incorporated, Rochester NY 14609

Table A

Supplement Facts
Serving Size: 1 soft gel

Amount per serving	1 soft gel	% DV
Vitamin A (beta-carotene)	14,320 IU	286%
Vitamin C (ascorbic acid)	226 mg	377%
Vitamin E (dl-alpha tocopheryl acetate)	200 IU	667%
Zinc (zinc oxide)	34.8 mg	232%
Copper (cupric oxide)	0.8 mg	40%

Bausch & Lomb and Preservision are registered trademarks of Bausch & Lomb Incorporated.

© Bausch & Lomb Incorporated. All rights reserved.

Shown in Product Identification Guide, page 104

BAUSCH & LOMB
PRESERVISION® LUTEIN   OTC
Eye Vitamin and Mineral Supplement
Beta-carotene free formulation.
Easy to swallow 2 per day Soft Gels

Description: see Supplement Facts (table A) [See table above]

Other Ingredients: Gelatin, Glycerin, Soybean Oil, Soy Lecithin, Yellow Beeswax, Silicon Dioxide, Titanium Dioxide, FD&C Red #40, FD&C Blue #1. Contains Soy.

This product is Vitamin A (beta-carotene) Free.

- The Bausch & Lomb PreserVision® Lutein patented formula is based on the Bausch & Lomb PreserVision® AREDS formula*, with the beta-carotene substituted with 5 mg of FloraGlo® Lutein.
- Lutein is a carotenoid found in dark leafy green vegetables such as spinach. Carotenoids are concentrated in the macula, the part of the eye responsible for central vision. Studies suggest that lutein plays an essential role in maintaining healthy central vision by protecting against free radical damage and filtering blue light.**
- Lutein levels in your eye are related to the amount in your diet. Bausch & Lomb PreserVision® Lutein contains 5 mg of lutein per soft gel, which gives you 10 mg of lutein per day. The leading multivitamin contains only a fraction of the amount of lutein used in clinical studies.

*Bausch & Lomb Ocuvite® PreserVision® AREDS formula was the only antioxidant vitamin and mineral supplement proven effective in the 10-year National Institutes of Health (NIH) Age-Related Eye Disease Study (AREDS). AREDS was a 10-year, independent study conducted by the National Eye Institute (NEI) of the National Institutes of Health (NIH).

Recommended Intake: 2 soft gels per day — 1 in the morning, 1 in the evening taken with meals.

This statement has not been evaluated by the Food and Drug Administration. This product is not intended to diagnose, treat, cure or prevent any disease.

How Supplied: NDC 24208-632-10. Available in bottles of 50 count soft gels. Orange, oval shaped soft gelatin capsule.

DO NOT USE IF SEAL UNDER CLOSURE IS BROKEN.

Keep out of reach of children.

STORE AT ROOM TEMPERATURE

®FloraGLO is a registered trademark of Kemin Industries, Inc.

Made in the USA

Marketed by:

Bausch & Lomb Incorporated, Rochester NY 14609

© Bausch & Lomb Incorporated. All rights reserved.

Bausch & Lomb, Preservision and Ocuvite are registered trademarks of Bausch & Lomb Incorporated.

Shown in Product Identification Guide, page 104

Supplement Facts
Serving Size: 1 soft gel

Amount per serving	1 Soft Gel	% Daily Value
Vitamin C (ascorbic acid)	226 mg	377%
Vitamin E (dl-alpha tocopheryl acetate)	200 IU	667%
Zinc (zinc oxide)	34.8 mg	232%
Copper (cupric oxide)	0.8 mg	40%
Lutein	5 mg	†

† Daily value not established

CARTEOLOL HYDROCHLORIDE   ℞
Ophthalmic Solution USP, 1%
STERILE OPHTHALMIC SOLUTION

Rx only
FOR USE IN THE EYES ONLY

Description: Carteolol Hydrochloride Ophthalmic Solution, 1%, is a nonselective beta-adrenoceptor blocking agent for ophthalmic use. Carteolol hydrochloride is represented by the following structural formula:

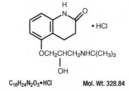

$C_{16}H_{24}N_2O_3 \cdot HCl$ Mol. Wt. 328.84

Chemical Name: (+)-5-[3-[(1, 1-dimethylethyl) amino]-2-hydroxypropoxy]-3, 4-dihydro-2(1 H)-quinolinone monohydrochloride.

Each mL of sterile solution contains:
ACTIVE: Carteolol Hydrochloride 10mg (1%), INACTIVES: Sodium Chloride, Monobasic and Dibasic Sodium Phosphate, Purified Water. PRESERVATIVE ADDED: Benzalkonium Chloride 0.005%. The product has a pH range of 6.2–7.2.

Clinical Pharmacology: Carteolol is a nonselective beta-adrenergic blocking agent with associated intrinsic sympathomimetic activity and without significant membrane- stabilizing activity.

Carteolol hydrochloride reduces normal and elevated intraocular pressure (IOP) whether or not accompanied by glaucoma. The exact mechanism of the ocular hypotensive effect of beta-blockers has not been definitely demonstrated.

In general, beta-adrenergic blockers reduce cardiac output in patients in good and poor cardiovascular health. In patients with severe impairment of myocardial function, beta-blockers may inhibit the sympathetic stimulation necessary to maintain adequate cardiac function. Beta-adrenergic blockers may also increase airway resistance in the bronchi and bronchioles due to unopposed parasympathetic activity.

Given topically twice daily in controlled domestic clinical trials ranging from 1.5 to 3 months, carteolol hydrochloride ophthalmic solution, 1% produced a median percent reduction of IOP 22% to 25%. No significant effects were noted on corneal sensitivity, tear secretion, or pupil size.

Indications and Usage: Carteolol hydrochloride ophthalmic solution, 1%, has been shown to be effective in lowering intraocular pressure and may be used in patients with chronic open-angle glaucoma and intraocular hypertension. It may be used alone or in combination with other intraocular pressure lowering medications.

Contraindications: Carteolol is contraindicated in those individuals with bronchial asthma or with a history of bronchial asthma, or severe chronic obstructive pulmonary disease

(see Warnings); sinus bradycardia; second- and third-degree atrioventricular block; overt cardiac failure (see Warnings); cardiogenic shock; or hypersensitivity to any component of this product.

Warnings: Carteolol has not been detected in plasma following ocular instillation. However, as with other topically applied ophthalmic preparations, carteolol may be absorbed systemically. The same adverse reactions found with systemic administration of beta- adrenergic blocking agents may occur with topical administration. For example, severe respiratory reactions and cardiac reactions, including death due to bronchospasm in patients with asthma and rarely death in association with cardiac failure, have been reported with topical application of beta-adrenergic blocking agents (see Contraindications).

Cardiac Failure: Sympathetic stimulation may be essential for support of the circulation in individuals with diminished myocardial contractility, and its inhibition by beta-adrenergic receptor blockade may precipitate more severe failure.

In Patients Without a History of Cardiac Failure: Continued depression of the myocardium with beta-blocking agents over a period of time can, in some cases, lead to cardiac failure. At the first sign or symptom of cardiac failure, carteolol hydrochloride should be discontinued.

Non-allergic Bronchospasm: In patients with non-allergic bronchospasm or with a history of non-allergic bronchospasm (e.g., chronic bronchitis, emphysema), carteolol should be administered with caution since it may block bronchodilation produced by endogenous and exogenous catecholamine stimulation of beta$_2$ receptors.

Major Surgery: The necessity or desirability of withdrawal of beta-adrenergic blocking agents prior to major surgery is controversial. Beta-adrenergic receptor blockade impairs the ability of the heart to respond to beta-adrenergically mediated reflex stimuli. This may augment the risk of general anesthesia in surgical procedures. Some patients receiving beta-adrenergic receptor blocking agents have been subject to protracted severe hypotension during anesthesia. For these reasons, in patients undergoing elective surgery, gradual withdrawal of beta-adrenergic receptor blocking agents may be appropriate.

If necessary during surgery, the effects of beta-adrenergic blocking agents may be reversed by sufficient doses of such agonists as isoproterenol, dopamine, dobutamine or levarterenol (see Overdosage).

Diabetes Mellitus: Beta-adrenergic blocking agents should be administered with caution in patients subject to spontaneous hypoglycemia or to diabetic patients (especially those with labile diabetes) who are receiving insulin or oral hypoglycemic agents. Beta-adrenergic receptor blocking agents may mask the signs and symptoms of acute hypoglycemia.

Thyrotoxicosis: Beta-adrenergic blocking agents may mask certain clinical signs (e.g., tachycardia) of hyperthyroidism. Patients sus-

Continued on next page

Carteolol HCl—Cont.

pected of developing thyrotoxicosis should be managed carefully to avoid abrupt withdrawal of beta-adrenergic blocking agents which might precipitate a thyroid storm.

Precautions: General: Carteolol hydrochloride ophthalmic solution should be used with caution in patients with known hypersensitivity to other beta-adrenoceptor blocking agents.

Use with caution in patients with known diminished pulmonary function.

In patients with angle-closure glaucoma, the immediate objective of treatment is to reopen the angle. This requires constricting the pupil with a miotic. Carteolol has little or no effect on the pupil. When carteolol is used to reduce elevated intraocular pressure in angle-closure glaucoma, it should be used with a miotic and not alone.

Information to the Patient: For topical use only. To prevent contaminating the dropper tip and solution, care should be taken not to touch the eyelids or surrounding areas with the dropper tip of the bottle. Keep bottle tightly closed when not in use. Protect from light.

Risk from Anaphylactic Reaction: While taking beta-blockers, patients with a history of atopy or a history of severe anaphylactic reaction to a variety of allergens may be more reactive to repeated accidental, diagnostic or therapeutic challenge with such allergens. Such patients may be unresponsive to the usual doses of epinephrine used to treat anaphylactic reactions.

Muscle Weakness: Beta-adrenergic blockade has been reported to potentiate muscle weakness consistent with certain myasthenic symptoms (e.g., diplopia, ptosis and generalized weakness).

Drug Interactions: Carteolol should be used with caution in patients who are receiving a beta-adrenergic blocking agent orally, because of the potential for additive effects on systemic beta-blockade.

Close observation of the patient is recommended when a beta-blocker is administered to patients receiving catecholamine-depleting drugs such as reserpine, because of possible additive effects and the production of hypotension and/or marked bradycardia, which may produce vertigo, syncope, or postural hypotension.

Carcinogenesis, Mutagenesis, Impairment of Fertility: Carteolol hydrochloride did not produce carcinogenic effects at doses up to 40 mg/kg/day in two-year oral rat and mouse studies. Tests of mutagenicity, including the Ames Test, recombinant (rec)-assay, *in vivo* cytogenetics and dominant lethal assay demonstrated no evidence for mutagenic potential. Fertility of male and female rats and male and female mice was unaffected by administration of carteolol hydrochloride dosages up to 150 mg/kg/day.

Pregnancy: Teratogenic Effects: Pregnancy Category C: Carteolol hydrochloride increased resorptions and decreased fetal weights in rabbits and rats at maternally toxic doses approximately 1052 and 5264 times the maximum recommended human oral dose (10 mg/70 kg/day), respectively. A dose-related increase in wavy ribs was noted in the developing rat fetus when pregnant females received daily doses of approximately 212 times the maximum recommended human oral dose. No such effects were noted in pregnant mice subjected to up to 1052 times the maximum recommended human oral dose. There are no adequate and well-controlled studies in pregnant women. Carteolol hydrochloride ophthalmic solution should be used during pregnancy only if the potential benefit justifies the potential risk to the fetus.

Nursing Mothers: It is not known whether this drug is excreted in human milk, although in animal studies carteolol has been shown to be excreted in breast milk. Caution should be exercised when carteolol hydrochloride ophthalmic solution is administered to nursing mothers.

Pediatric Use: Safety and effectiveness in pediatric patients have not been established.

Adverse Reactions: The following adverse reactions have been reported in clinical trials with carteolol hydrochloride ophthalmic solution:

Ocular: Transient eye irritation, burning, tearing, conjunctival hyperemia and edema occurred in about 1 of 4 patients. Ocular symptoms including blurred and cloudy vision, photophobia, decreased night vision, and ptosis and ocular signs including blepharoconjunctivitis, abnormal corneal staining, and corneal sensitivity occurred occasionally.

Systemic: As is characteristic of nonselective adrenergic blocking agents, carteolol may cause bradycardia and decreased blood pressure (see Warnings). The following systemic events have occasionally been reported with the use of carteolol hydrochloride: cardiac arrhythmia, heart palpitation, dyspnea, asthenia, headache, dizziness, insomnia, sinusitis, and taste perversion.

The following additional adverse reactions have been reported with ophthalmic use of beta$_1$ and beta$_2$(nonselective) adrenergic receptor blocking agents:

Body As a Whole: Headache

Cardiovascular: Arrhythmia, syncope, heart block, cerebral vascular accident, cerebral ischemia, congestive heart failure, palpitation (see Warnings).

Digestive: Nausea

Psychiatric: Depression

Skin: Hypersensitivity, including localized and generalized rash

Respiratory: Bronchospasm (predominantly in patients with pre-existing bronchospastic disease), respiratory failure (see Warnings)

Endocrine: Masked symptoms of hypoglycemia in insulin-dependent diabetics (see Warnings)

Special Senses: Signs and symptoms of keratitis, blepharoptosis, visual disturbances including refractive changes (due to withdrawal of miotic therapy in some cases), diplopia, ptosis.

Other reactions associated with the oral use of nonselective adrenergic receptor blocking agents should be considered potential effects with ophthalmic use of these agents.

Overdosage: No specific information on emergency treatment of overdosage in humans is available. Should accidental ocular overdosage occur, flush eye(s) with water or normal saline. The most common effects expected with overdosage of a beta-adrenergic blocking agent are bradycardia, bronchospasm, congestive heart failure and hypotension.

In case of ingestion, treatment with carteolol hydrochloride ophthalmic solution should be discontinued and gastric lavage considered. The patient should be closely observed and vital signs carefully monitored. The prolonged effects of carteolol must be considered when determining the duration of corrective therapy. On the basis of the pharmacologic profile, the following additional measures should be considered as appropriate:

Symptomatic Sinus Bradycardia or Heart Block: Administer atropine. If there is no response to vagal blockade, administer isoproterenol cautiously.

Bronchospasm: Administer a beta$_2$-stimulating agent such as isoproterenol and/or a theophylline derivative.

Congestive Heart Failure: Administer diuretics and digitalis glycosides as necessary.

Hypotension: Administer vasopressors such as intravenous dopamine, epinephrine or norepinephrine bitartrate.

Dosage and Administration: The usual dose is one drop of carteolol hydrochloride ophthalmic solution, 1%, in the affected eye(s) twice a day.

If the patient's IOP is not at a satisfactory level on this regimen, concomitant therapy with pilocarpine and other miotics, and/or epinephrine or dipivefrin, and/or systemically administered carbonic anhydrase inhibitors, such as acetazolamide, can be instituted.

How Supplied: Carteolol Hydrochloride Ophthalmic Solution, 1% is supplied as a sterile ophthalmic solution in a plastic bottle with a controlled drop tip in the following sizes:

5 mL bottles - Prod. No. 36707
10 mL bottles - Prod. No. 36709
15 mL bottles - Prod. No. 36711

Storage: Store between 15°–30°C (59°–86°F). Protect from light.

DO NOT USE IF IMPRINTED NECKBAND IS NOT INTACT

KEEP OUT OF REACH OF CHILDREN
Bausch & Lomb
Incorporated
Tampa, Florida 33637   REV. 2/04-92

FLUOR–I–STRIP® -A.T.   ℞

[floo-or 'a 'strip]

(Fluorescein Sodium Ophthalmic Strips)
For Applanation Tonometry

Composition   (Per Strip):
Diagnostic dye: Fluorescein Sodium 1 mg
Preservative: Chlorobutanol (chloral derivative) 0.5%
Surface active agent: Polysorbate 80
Buffering agents: Potassium Chloride, Boric Acid, Sodium Carbonate

Description: FLUOR-I-STRIP-A.T. consists of sterile ophthalmic strips, specially prepared for diagnostic use in applanation tonometry.

Indications: For staining the anterior segment of the eye when:
a) delineating a corneal injury, herpetic lesion or foreign body,
b) determining the site of an intraocular injury,
c) fitting contact lenses,
d) making the fluorescein test to ascertain postoperative closure of the sclerocorneal (also referred to as corneoscleral) wound in delayed anterior chamber reformation,
e) making the lacrimal drainage test.

Directions for Use: To open envelope, grasp pull-tabs firmly and separate slowly. Separate the two strips by tearing off white tab end. Anesthetize the eyes. Retract upper lid and touch tip of strip to the bulbar conjunctiva on the temporal side until an adequate amount of stain is available for a clearly defined end-point reading.

Warning: Never use fluorescein while the patient is wearing *soft contact lenses* because the lenses may become stained. Whenever fluorescein is used, flush the eyes with sterile, normal saline solution, and wait at least one hour before replacing the lenses.

Storage: Store at room temperature (approximately 25°C).

How Supplied: Boxes of 300 strips, 2 in each envelope NDC 24208-391-83
Manufactured by
Wyeth-Ayerst Laboratories
Rouses Point, NY 12979
Marketed by
Bausch & Lomb Incorporated
Tampa, FL 33637

LOTEMAX®   ℞

[lō tĕ max]
loteprednol etabonate
ophthalmic suspension 0.5%
STERILE OPHTHALMIC SUSPENSION
Rx only

Description: LOTEMAX® (loteprednol etabonate ophthalmic suspension) contains a sterile, topical anti-inflammatory corticosteroid for ophthalmic use. Loteprednol etabonate is a white to off-white powder.

Loteprednol etabonate is represented by the following structural formula:

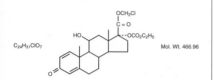

$C_{24}H_{31}ClO_7$ Mol. Wt. 466.96

Chemical Name:
chloromethyl 17α-[(ethoxycarbonyl)oxy]-11β-hydroxy-3-oxoandrosta-1,4-diene-17β-carboxylate

Each mL contains:
ACTIVE: Loteprednol Etabonate 5 mg (0.5%); INACTIVES: Edetate Disodium, Glycerin, Povidone, Purified Water and Tyloxapol. Hydrochloric Acid and/or Sodium Hydroxide may be added to adjust the pH to 5.5-5.6. The suspension is essentially isotonic with a tonicity of 250 to 310 mOsmol/kg.
PRESERVATIVE ADDED: Benzalkonium Chloride 0.01%.

Clinical Pharmacology: Corticosteroids inhibit the inflammatory response to a variety of inciting agents and probably delay or slow healing. They inhibit the edema, fibrin deposition, capillary dilation, leukocyte migration, capillary proliferation, fibroblast proliferation, deposition of collagen, and scar formation associated with inflammation. There is no generally accepted explanation for the mechanism of action of ocular corticosteroids. However, corticosteroids are thought to act by the induction of phospholipase A_2 inhibitory proteins, collectively called lipocortins. It is postulated that these proteins control the biosynthesis of potent mediators of inflammation such as prostaglandins and leukotrienes by inhibiting the release of their common precursor arachidonic acid. Arachidonic acid is released from membrane phospholipids by phospholipase A_2. Corticosteroids are capable of producing a rise in intraocular pressure.

Loteprednol etabonate is structurally similar to other corticosteroids. However, the number 20 position ketone group is absent. It is highly lipid soluble which enhances its penetration into cells. Loteprednol etabonate is synthesized through structural modifications of prednisolone-related compounds so that it will undergo a predictable transformation to an inactive metabolite. Based upon *in vivo* and *in vitro* preclinical metabolism studies, loteprednol etabonate undergoes extensive metabolism to inactive carboxylic acid metabolites.

Results from a bioavailability study in normal volunteers established that plasma levels of loteprednol etabonate and Δ^1 cortienic acid etabonate (PJ 91), its primary, inactive metabolite, were below the limit of quantitation (1 ng/mL) at all sampling times. The results were obtained following the ocular administration of one drop in each eye of 0.5% loteprednol etabonate 8 times daily for 2 days or 4 times daily for 42 days. This study suggests that limited (<1 ng/ml) systemic absorption occurs with LOTEMAX.

Clinical Studies:
Post-Operative Inflammation: Placebo-controlled clinical studies demonstrated that

LOTEMAX is effective for the treatment of anterior chamber inflammation as measured by cell and flare.

Giant Papillary Conjunctivitis: Placebo-controlled clinical studies demonstrated that LOTEMAX was effective in reducing the signs and symptoms of giant papillary conjunctivitis after 1 week of treatment and continuing for up to 6 weeks while on treatment.

Seasonal Allergic Conjunctivitis: A placebo-controlled clinical study demonstrated that LOTEMAX was effective in reducing the signs and symptoms of allergic conjunctivitis during peak periods of pollen exposure.

Uveitis: Controlled clinical studies of patients with uveitis demonstrated that LOTEMAX was less effective than prednisolone acetate 1%. Overall, 72% of patients treated with LOTEMAX experienced resolution of anterior chamber cell by day 28, compared to 87% of patients treated with 1% prednisolone acetate. The incidence of patients with clinically significant increases in IOP (≥10 mmHg) was 1% with LOTEMAX and 6% with prednisolone acetate 1%.

Indications and Usage: LOTEMAX is indicated for the treatment of steroid responsive inflammatory conditions of the palpebral and bulbar conjunctiva, cornea and anterior segment of the globe such as allergic conjunctivitis, acne rosacea, superficial punctate keratitis, herpes zoster keratitis, iritis, cyclitis, selected infective conjunctivitides, when the inherent hazard of steroid use is accepted to obtain an advisable diminution in edema and inflammation.

LOTEMAX is less effective than prednisolone acetate 1% in two 28-day controlled clinical studies in acute anterior uveitis, where 72% of patients treated with LOTEMAX experienced resolution of anterior chamber cells, compared to 87% of patients treated with prednisolone acetate 1%. The incidence of patients with clinically significant increases in IOP (≥10 mmHg) was 1% with LOTEMAX and 6% with prednisolone acetate 1%. LOTEMAX should not be used in patients who require a more potent corticosteroid for this indication. LOTEMAX is also indicated for the treatment of post-operative inflammation following ocular surgery.

Contraindications: LOTEMAX, as with other ophthalmic corticosteroids, is contraindicated in most viral diseases of the cornea and conjunctiva including epithelial herpes simplex keratitis (dendritic keratitis), vaccinia, and varicella, and also in mycobacterial infection of the eye and fungal diseases of ocular structures. LOTEMAX is also contraindicated in individuals with known or suspected hypersensitivity to any of the ingredients of this preparation and to other corticosteroids.

Warnings: Prolonged use of corticosteroids may result in glaucoma with damage to the optic nerve, defects in visual acuity and fields of vision, and in posterior subcapsular cataract formation. Steroids should be used with caution in the presence of glaucoma.

Prolonged use of corticosteroids may suppress the host response and thus increase the hazard of secondary ocular infections. In those diseases causing thinning of the cornea or sclera, perforations have been known to occur with the use of topical steroids. In acute purulent conditions of the eye, steroids may mask infection or enhance existing infection.

Use of ocular steroids may prolong the course and may exacerbate the severity of many viral infections of the eye (including herpes simplex). Employment of a corticosteroid medication in the treatment of patients with a history of herpes simplex requires great caution.

The use of steroids after cataract surgery may delay healing and increase the incidence of bleb formation.

Precautions: **General:** For ophthalmic use only. The initial prescription and renewal of

the medication order beyond 14 days should be made by a physician only after examination of the patient with the aid of magnification, such as slit lamp biomicroscopy and, where appropriate, fluorescein staining.

If signs and symptoms fail to improve after two days, the patient should be re-evaluated.

If this product is used for 10 days or longer, intraocular pressure should be monitored even though it may be difficult in children and uncooperative patients (see WARNINGS).

Fungal infections of the cornea are particularly prone to develop coincidentally with long-term local steroid application. Fungus invasion must be considered in any persistent corneal ulceration where a steroid has been used or is in use. Fungal cultures should be taken when appropriate.

Information for Patients: This product is sterile when packaged. Patients should be advised not to allow the dropper tip to touch any surface, as this may contaminate the suspension. If pain develops, redness, itching or inflammation becomes aggravated, the patient should be advised to consult a physician. As with all ophthalmic preparations containing benzalkonium chloride, patients should be advised not to wear soft contact lenses when using LOTEMAX®.

Carcinogenesis, mutagenesis, impairment of fertility: Long-term animal studies have not been conducted to evaluate the carcinogenic potential of loteprednol etabonate. Loteprednol etabonate was not genotoxic *in vitro* in the Ames test, the mouse lymphoma tk assay, or in a chromosome aberration test in human lymphocytes, or *in vivo* in the single dose mouse micronucleus assay. Treatment of male and female rats with up to 50 mg/kg/day and 25 mg/kg/day of loteprednol etabonate, respectively, (600 and 300 times the maximum clinical dose, respectively) prior to and during mating did not impair fertility in either gender.

Pregnancy: Teratogenic effects: Pregnancy Category C. Loteprednol etabonate has been shown to be embryotoxic (delayed ossification) and teratogenic (increased incidence of meningocele, abnormal left common carotid artery, and limb flexures) when administered orally to rabbits during organogenesis at a dose of 3 mg/kg/day (35 times the maximum daily clinical dose), a dose which caused no maternal toxicity. The no-observed-effect-level (NOEL) for these effects was 0.5 mg/kg/day (6 times the maximum daily clinical dose). Oral treatment of rats during organogenesis resulted in teratogenicity (absent innominate artery at ≥5 mg/kg/day doses, and cleft palate and umbilical hernia at ≥50 mg/kg/day) and embryotoxicity (increased post-implantation losses at 100 mg/kg/day and decreased fetal body weight and skeletal ossification with ≥50 mg/kg/day). Treatment of rats with 0.5 mg/kg/day (6 times the maximum clinical dose) during organogenesis did not result in any reproductive toxicity. Loteprednol etabonate was maternally toxic (significantly reduced body weight gain during treatment) when administered to pregnant rats during organogenesis at doses of ≥5 mg/kg/day.

Oral exposure of female rats to 50 mg/kg/day of loteprednol etabonate from the start of the fetal period through the end of lactation, a maternally toxic treatment regimen (significantly decreased body weight gain), gave rise to decreased growth and survival, and retarded development in the offspring during lactation; the NOEL for these effects was 5 mg/kg/day. Loteprednol etabonate had no effect on the duration of gestation or parturition when administered orally to pregnant rats at doses up to 50 mg/kg/day during the fetal period.

Continued on next page

Lotemax—Cont.

Nursing Mothers: It is not known whether topical ophthalmic administration of corticosteroids could result in sufficient systemic absorption to produce detectable quantities in human milk. Systemic steroids appear in human milk and could suppress growth, interfere with endogenous corticosteroid production, or cause other untoward effects. Caution should be exercised when LOTEMAX is administered to a nursing woman.

Pediatric Use: Safety and effectiveness in pediatric patients have not been established.

Adverse Reactions: Reactions associated with ophthalmic steroids include elevated intraocular pressure, which may be associated with optic nerve damage, visual acuity and field defects, posterior subcapsular cataract formation, secondary ocular infection from pathogens including herpes simplex, and perforation of the globe where there is thinning of the cornea or sclera.

Ocular adverse reactions occurring in 5-15% of patients treated with loteprednol etabonate ophthalmic suspension (0.2%-0.5%) in clinical studies included abnormal vision/blurring, burning on instillation, chemosis, discharge, dry eyes, epiphora, foreign body sensation, itching, injection, and photophobia. Other ocular adverse reactions occurring in less than 5% of patients include conjunctivitis, corneal abnormalities, eyelid erythema, keratoconjunctivitis, ocular irritation/pain/discomfort, papillae, and uveitis. Some of these events were similar to the underlying ocular disease being studied.

Non-ocular adverse reactions occurred in less than 15% of patients. These include headache, rhinitis and pharyngitis.

In a summation of controlled, randomized studies of individuals treated for 28 days or longer with loteprednol etabonate, the incidence of significant elevation of intraocular pressure ($\geq$10 mmHg) was 2% (15/901) among patients receiving loteprednol etabonate, 7% (11/164) among patients receiving 1% prednisolone acetate and 0.5% (3/583) among patients receiving placebo.

Dosage and Administration: SHAKE VIGOROUSLY BEFORE USING.

Steroid Responsive Disease Treatment: Apply one to two drops of LOTEMAX into the conjunctival sac of the affected eye(s) four times daily. During the initial treatment within the first week, the dosing may be increased, up to 1 drop every hour, if necessary. Care should be taken not to discontinue therapy prematurely. If signs and symptoms fail to improve after two days, the patient should be re-evaluated (See PRECAUTIONS).

Post-Operative Inflammation: Apply one to two drops of LOTEMAX into the conjunctival sac of the operated eye(s) four times daily beginning 24 hours after surgery and continuing throughout the first 2 weeks of the postoperative period.

How Supplied: LOTEMAX® (loteprednol etabonate ophthalmic suspension) is supplied in a plastic bottle with a controlled drop tip in the following sizes:

2.5 mL (NDC 24208-299-25) - AB29904
  5 mL (NDC 24208-299-05) - AB29907
10 mL (NDC 24208-299-10) - AB29909
15 mL (NDC 24208-299-15) - AB29911

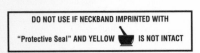

DO NOT USE IF NECKBAND IMPRINTED WITH "Protective Seal" AND YELLOW IS NOT INTACT

Storage: Store upright between 15°–25°C (59°–77°F). DO NOT FREEZE.
KEEP OUT OF REACH OF CHILDREN.
Revised April 2006

Bausch & Lomb Incorporated, Tampa, Florida 33637
U.S. Patent No. 4,996,335
U.S. Patent No. 5,540,930
U.S. Patent No. 5,747,061
©Bausch & Lomb Incorporated
Lotemax is a registered trademark of Bausch & Lomb Incorporated.

9007802 (Folded)
9005902 (Flat)
Shown in Product Identification Guide, page 104

MURO® 128® 2%   **OTC**
[mŭ 'rō 128]
Sodium Chloride Hypertonicity Ophthalmic Solution, 2%

MURO™ 128® 5%   **OTC**
Sodium Chloride Hypertonicity Ophthalmic Solution, 5%
STERILE OPHTHALMIC SOLUTION

Description: Muro™ 128® 2% Solution is a sterile ophthalmic solution used to draw water out of the cornea of the eye.

Each mL Contains: ACTIVE: Sodium Chloride 2%; INACTIVES: Boric Acid, Hypromellose, Propylene Glycol, Purified Water, Sodium Borate. Sodium Hydroxide and/ or Hydrochloric Acid may be added to adjust pH. PRESERVATIVES: Methylparaben 0.028%, Propylparaben 0.012%

Description: Muro™ 128® 5% Solution is a sterile ophthalmic solution used to draw water out of the cornea of the eye.

Each mL Contains: ACTIVE: Sodium Chloride 5%; INACTIVES: Boric Acid, Hypromellose, Propylene Glycol, Purified Water, Sodium Borate. Sodium Hydroxide and/ or Hydrochloric Acid may be added to adjust pH. PRESERVATIVES: Methylparaben 0.023%, Propylparaben 0.01%

Uses: For the temporary relief of corneal edema.

Warnings: Do not use this product except under the advice and supervision of a doctor.

If you experience eye pain, changes in vision, continued redness or irritation of the eye, or if the condition worsens or persists, consult a doctor.

To avoid contamination of the product, do not touch the tip of the container to any surface. Replace cap after using.

This product may cause temporary burning and irritation on being instilled into the eye.

If the solution changes color or becomes cloudy, do not use.

In case of accidental ingestion, seek professional assistance or contact a Poison Control Center immediately.

Directions: Instill 1 or 2 drops in the affected eye(s) every 3 or 4 hours, or as directed by a doctor.

FOR OPHTHALMIC USE ONLY

How Supplied: Muro™ 128® 2% Solution is supplied in a plastic controlled drop tip bottle in the following size:

½ Fl. Oz. (15 mL) (NDC 24208-276-15)—Prod. No. AB15511

How Supplied: Muro™ 128® 5% Solution is supplied in ½ Fl. Oz. (15 mL) or 1 Fl. Oz. (30 mL) plastic controlled dropper tip bottles.
15 mL [NDC 24208-277-15]—Prod. No. AB15611
30 mL [NDC 24208-277-30]—Prod. No. AB15616

DO NOT USE IF IMPRINTED NECKBAND IS NOT INTACT

Storage: Store between 15°–30°C [59°–86°F].

KEEP TIGHTLY CLOSED. **STORE UPRIGHT AND IMMEDIATELY REPLACE CAP AFTER USE.**
KEEP OUT OF REACH OF CHILDREN.
Bausch & Lomb Incorporated
Tampa, FL 33637
MURO is a trademark of MURO Pharmaceutical, Inc.
128 is a registered trademark of Bausch & Lomb Incorporated
2/04-03
Shown in Product Identification Guide, page 104

MURO® 128® 5% OINTMENT   **OTC**
[mŭ 'rō 128]
Sodium Chloride Hypertonicity Ophthalmic Ointment, 5%
FOR TEMPORARY RELIEF OF CORNEAL EDEMA
STERILE OPHTHALMIC OINTMENT

Description: Muro™ 128® 5% Ointment is a sterile ophthalmic ointment used to draw water out of the cornea of the eye.

Each Gram Contains: ACTIVE: Sodium Chloride 5% INACTIVES: Lanolin, Mineral Oil, Purified Water, White Petrolatum.

Uses: For the temporary relief of corneal edema.

Warnings: Do not use this product except under the advice and supervision of a doctor.

If you experience eye pain, changes in vision, continued redness or irritation of the eye, or if the condition worsens or persists, consult a doctor.

To avoid contamination of the product, do not touch the tip of the container to any surface. Replace cap after using.

This product may cause temporary burning and irritation on being instilled into the eye.

In case of accidental ingestion, seek professional assistance or contact a Poison Control Center immediately.

Directions: Pull down lower lid of the affected eye(s) and apply a small amount (approximately ¼ inch) of the ointment to the inside of the eyelid every 3 or 4 hours, or as directed by a doctor.

FOR OPHTHALMIC USE ONLY

How Supplied: Muro™ 128® 5% Ointment is supplied in ⅛ oz (3.5 g) tube.
[NDC 24208-385-55]—Prod. No. AB15834
TWIN PACK: 2 x ⅛ oz (2 x 3.5 g)
[NDC 24208-385-56]—Prod. No. AB15899

NOTE: Tubes are filled by weight (⅛ oz/3.5g) not volume.

See Crimp of tube for Lot Number and Expiration Date.

DO NOT USE IF BOTTOM RIDGE OF TUBE CAP IS EXPOSED AND IMPRINTED SEAL ON BOX IS BROKEN OR MISSING.

KEEP OUT OF REACH OF CHILDREN.
Storage: Store between 15°–30°C (59°–86°F). DO NOT FREEZE.
KEEP TIGHTLY CLOSED.
Bausch & Lomb Incorporated
Tampa, FL 33637
™/® denotes trademark of Bausch & Lomb Incorporated
11/03-72
Shown in Product Identification Guide, page 104

BAUSCH & LOMB OCUVITE®   **OTC**
Adult Formula
Eye Vitamin and Mineral Supplement

The #1 recommended supplement brand among eye-care professionals is now available in an Adult Formula!

Easy to swallow soft gels.
• Essential Eye Nutrition
• Contains 2 mg of Lutein and 100 mg of Omega-3

Description: see Supplement Facts (table A) [See first table A above]

Other Ingredients: Soybean Oil, Gelatin, Glycerin, Fish Oil (anchovy, sardine), Yellow Beeswax, Silicon Dioxide, Soy Lecithin (Contains peanut oil), Titanium Dioxide, Blue #2, Yellow #6, Green #3

• Ocuvite® Adult formula is an antioxidant supplement with 2 mg of Lutein and 100 mg of Omega-3
• Lutein is clinically proven to help you maintain optimal retinal health.*
• Omega-3 essential fatty acids are structural components of retinal tissues. The retina is particularly rich in long-chain polyunsaturated fatty acids (PUFA) like Omega-3.[1] DHA is a major component of Omega-3. The brain and retina show the highest content of DHA in any tissues. DHA is used continuously for the biogenesis and maintenance of photoreceptor membranes.[2]

> ***This statement has not been evaluated by the Food and Drug Administration. This product is not intended to diagnose, treat, cure or prevent any disease.**

References:
1. Uauy R, Lipids, 2001; Vertuani S, Current Pharmac Des, 2004.
2. San Giovanni JP, Progr Ret Eye Res, 2005.

Directions for use: Take 1 Soft Gel daily, in the morning taken with food. Do not exceed the dose indicated without seeking medical advice.

DO NOT USE IF SEAL UNDER CLOSURE IS BROKEN

Keep out of reach of children

STORE AT ROOM TEMPERATURE

How supplied: NDC 24208-466-30. Available in bottles of 50 count soft gels

FOR MORE INFORMATION, CALL 1-800-553-5340

Bausch & Lomb – Committed to research and leadership in ocular nutritionals

Bausch & Lomb and Ocuvite are registered trademarks of Bausch & Lomb Incorporated.

©Bausch & Lomb Incorporated.

All Rights Reserved

Marketed by:

Bausch & Lomb Incorporated, Rochester, NY 14609

Shown in Product Identification Guide, page 104

BAUSCH & LOMB OCUVITE®   OTC Adult 50+ Formula

Eye Vitamin and Mineral Supplement

The #1 recommended supplement brand among eye-care professionals now in an Adult 50+ Formula!

Easy to swallow soft gels.
• Advanced Eye Nutrition
• Contains 6 mg Lutein and 150 mg of Omega-3

Description: see Supplement Facts (table A) [See second table A above]

Other Ingredients: Gelatin, Fish Oil (anchovy, sardine), Glycerin, Yellow Beeswax, Silicon Dioxide, Soy Lecithin (Contains peanut oil), Caramel color, Titanium Dioxide, Blue 2 Lake, Yellow #6, Yellow 6 Lake, Red #40, Red 40 Lake.

• Ocuvite® Adult 50+ formula is an antioxidant supplement with 6 mg of Lutein and 150 mg of Omega-3
• As we age, free radicals pose a greater threat to eye health. Our bodies don't neutralize them as effectively as before. The right amount of natural antioxidants, such as

6 mg of Lutein found in Ocuvite® Adult 50+ can help maintain eye health as you age.*
• Omega-3 essential fatty acids are structural components of retinal tissues. The retina is particularly rich in long-chain polyunsaturated fatty acids (PUFA) like Omega-3.[1] DHA is a major component of Omega-3. The brain and retina show the highest content of DHA in any tissues. DHA is used continuously for the biogenesis and maintenance of photoreceptor membranes.[2]

> ***This statement has not been evaluated by the Food and Drug Administration. This product is not intended to diagnose, treat, cure or prevent any disease.**

References:
1. Uauy R, Lipids, 2001; Vertuani S, Current Pharmac Des, 2004.
2. San Giovanni JP, Progr Ret Eye Res, 2005.

Directions for use: Take 1 Soft Gel daily, in the morning taken with food. Do not exceed the dose indicated without seeking medical advice.

How Supplied: NDC 24208-465-30. – Available in bottles of 50 count soft gels

DO NOT USE IF SEAL UNDER CLOSURE IS BROKEN

Keep out of reach of children

STORE AT ROOM TEMPERATURE

FOR MORE INFORMATION, CALL 1-800-553-5340

Bausch & Lomb – Committed to research and leadership in ocular nutritionals

Bausch & Lomb and Ocuvite are registered trademarks of Bausch & Lomb Incorporated.

©Bausch & Lomb Incorporated.

All Rights Reserved

Marketed by:

Bausch & Lomb Incorporated, Rochester, NY 14609

Shown in Product Identification Guide, page 104

BAUSCH & LOMB OCUVITE® DF   OTC

Eye Vitamin Supplement

Nutritional support for people with Diabetes Specially Formulated to SUPPORT EYE HEALTH*

Description: see Supplement Facts (See table A below) [See first table A at top of next page]

Other Ingredients: Dibasic calcium phosphate, microcrystalline cellulose, polyvinyl alcohol, hydroxypropylcellulose, croscarmellose sodium, silicon dioxide, hydrogenated vegetable oil (soybean oil, castor oil), stearic acid, magnesium stearate, caramel color, carmine, titanium dioxide.

People with diabetes are at an increased risk of vision loss. Oxidative stress is one of the major contributing factors for this vision loss. A combination of nutrients, like alpha lipoic acid and the antioxidant genistein, have been shown to combat the effects of oxidative stress.*

Recommended Intake: Take two tablets daily; 1 in the morning, 1 in the evening taken with meals.

> *** These statements have not been evaluated by the Food and Drug Administration. This product is not intended to diagnose, treat, cure or prevent any disease.**

How Supplied:

NDC 24208 741-00

Available in bottles of 60 count tablets.

DO NOT USE IF SEAL UNDER CLOSURE IS BROKEN

Keep out of reach of children

STORE AT up to 25° C (77° F) IN A DRY PLACE

Marketed by:

Bausch & Lomb Incorporated, Rochester, NY 14609

FOR MORE INFORMATION, CALL 1-800-553-5340

Continued on next page

Table A

Supplement Facts

Serving Size: 1 Soft Gel
Servings per container: 50

Amount per Serving	1 Soft Gel	% of Daily Value
Vitamin C (ascorbic acid)	100 mg	166.5%
Vitamin E (d-alpha tocopherol)	15 IU	50%
Zinc (as zinc oxide)	9 mg	60%
Copper (as cupric oxide)	1 mg	50%
Lutein	2 mg	+
Omega-3	100mg	+

+ Daily Value not established

Table A

Supplement Facts

Serving Size: 1 Soft Gel
Servings per container: 50

Amount per Serving	1 Soft Gel	% of Daily Value
Vitamin C (ascorbic acid)	150 mg	250%
Vitamin E (d-alpha tocopherol)	30 IU	100%
Zinc (as zinc oxide)	9 mg	60%
Copper (as cupric oxide)	1 mg	50%
Lutein	6 mg	+
Omega-3	150mg	+

+ Daily Value not established

Ocuvite DF—Cont.

Bausch & Lomb and Ocuvite are registered trademarks of Bausch & Lomb Incorporated.
Shown in Product Identification Guide, page 104

BAUSCH & LOMB OCUVITE® LUTEIN   OTC

[lu 'teen]
Vitamin and Mineral Supplement

Description: see Supplement Facts (table A) [See second table A above]

Other Ingredients: Lactose monohydrate, Gelatin, Crospovidone, Magnesium Stearate, Titanium dioxide, Silicon dioxide Yellow #6, Blue #2. Contains lactose and casein (milk).

- Lutein is a carotenoid. Carotenoids are the yellow pigments found in fruits and vegetables, particularly dark, leafy green vegetables such as spinach. Carotenoids are concentrated in the macula, the part of the eye responsible for central vision. Clinical studies suggest that Lutein plays an essential role in maintaining healthy central vision by protecting against free radical damage and filtering blue light.*
- Lutein levels in your eye are related to the amount in your diet. Ocuvite® Lutein contains 6 mg of Lutein per capsule. The leading multi-vitamin contains only a fraction of the amount of lutein used in clinical studies.
- Ocuvite® Lutein helps supplement your diet with 100% of the US Daily Values for the antioxidant vitamins C, E, and essential minerals, zinc and copper that can play an important role in your ocular health.*
- Ocuvite® Lutein is an advanced antioxidant supplement formulated to provide nutritional support for the eye.* The Ocuvite® Lutein formulation contains essential antioxidant vitamins, minerals and 6 mg of Lutein.

Recommended Intake: Adults: One capsule, one or two times daily or as directed by their physician.

> ***These statements have not been evaluated by the Food and Drug Administration. This product is not intended to diagnose, treat, cure or prevent any disease.**

How Supplied: Yellow capsule with Ocuvite Lutein printed in black.
NDC 24208-403-19—Bottle of 36
NDC 24208-403-73—Bottle of 72
DO NOT USE IF SEAL UNDER CLOSURE IS BROKEN.
Keep this product out of the reach of children.
STORE AT ROOM TEMPERATURE
Made in U.S.A.
Marketed by
Bausch & Lomb
Rochester, NY 14609
Bausch & Lomb, Ocuvite are registered trademarks of Bausch & Lomb Incorporated.
Shown in Product Identification Guide, page 104

BAUSCH & LOMB PRESERVISION® AREDS   OTC

High Potency Eye Vitamin and Mineral Supplement Original, 4 per day tablets

Description: see Supplement Facts (table A) [See third table A above]

Table A

Supplement Facts
Serving Size: 1 tablet

	Amount	% of Daily Value
Vitamin C (ascorbic acid)	100 mg	167%
Vitamin E (d-alpha tocopheryl succinate)	100 IU	333%
Vitamin B-1 (thiamine mononitrate)	0.75 mg	50%
Niacin (niacinamide)	10 mg	50%
Vitamin B-6 (pyridoxine hydrochloride)	1 mg	50%
Alpha Lipoic Acid	140 mg	+
Genistein	25 mg	+

+ (DV) Daily value not establihsed

Table A

Supplement Facts
Serving Size: 1 capsule

	Amount	% Daily Value
Vitamin C (ascorbic acid)	60 mg	100%
Vitamin E (dl-alpha tocopheryl acetate)	30 IU	100%
Zinc (zinc oxide)	15 mg	100%
Copper (cupric oxide)	2 mg	100%
Lutein	6 mg	†

† Daily value not established

Table A

Supplement Facts
Serving Size: 4 tablets daily; 2 in the morning, 2 in the evening taken with meals.

Contents	Two tablets Amount	% of Daily Value	Daily Dosage (4 tablets) Amount	% of Daily Value
Vitamin A (100% as beta-carotene)	14,320 IU	286%	28,640 IU	573%
Vitamin C (ascorbic acid)	226 mg	376%	452 mg	753%
Vitamin E (dl-alpha tocopheryl acetate)	200 IU	666%	400 IU	1333%
Zinc (zinc oxide)	34.8 mg	232%	69.6 mg	464%
Cooper (cupric oxide)	0.8 mg	40%	1.6 mg	80%

Other Ingredients: Lactose Monohydrate, Microcrystalline Cellulose, Crospovidone, Stearic Acid, Magnesium Stearate, Silicon Dioxide, Polysorbate 80, Triethyl Citrate, Yellow 6, Yellow 6 Lake, Red 40, Red 40 Lake. Contains Soy.

- Age-related macular degeneration is the leading cause of vision loss and blindness in people over 55. The National Institutes of Health (NIH) Age Related Eye Disease Study (AREDS) proved that a unique high-potency vitamin and mineral supplement was effective in helping to preserve the sight of certain people most at risk.*
- Bausch & Lomb **Ocuvite® PreserVision®** was the only eye vitamin and mineral supplement clinically proven effective in the NIH AREDS Study.
- Bausch & Lomb **Ocuvite® PreserVision®** is a high-potency antioxidant supplement with the antioxidant vitamins A, C, E and select minerals at levels that are well above those in ordinary multivitamins and generally cannot be attained through diet alone.

For a FREE 16-page brochure on Age-Related Macular Degeneration call toll-free 1-866-467-3263 (1-866-HOPE-AMD)

Recommended Intake: To get the same levels proven in the NIH AREDS Study it is important to take 4 tablets per day – 2 in the morning, 2 in the evening taken with meals.
Current and Former Smokers: Consult your eye care professional about the risks associated with smoking and using Beta-Carotene. Bausch & Lomb Ocuvite PreserVision is the #1 recommended eye vitamin and mineral supplement brand among Retinal Specialists.[1]

> ***This statement has not been evaluated by the Food and Drug Administration. This product is not intended to diagnose, treat, cure or prevent any disease.**

How Supplied: NDC 24208-432-62 120 ct. bottle NDC 24208-432-72 240 ct. bottle Orange, eye shaped film coated tablet, engraved BL 01 on one side, scored on the other side. Available in bottles of 120 or 240 count tablets
DO NOT USE IF SEAL UNDER CLOSURE IS BROKEN.
Keep this product out of the reach of children.
STORE AT ROOM TEMPERATURE.
Made in USA

Marketed by
Bausch & Lomb
Rochester, NY 14609
References: 1. Data on file, Bausch & Lomb, Inc.
© Bausch & Lomb Incorporated. All Rights Reserved.
Bausch & Lomb, Ocuvite and PreserVision are registered trademarks of Bausch & Lomb Incorporated.

Shown in Product Identification Guide, page 104

OFLOXACIN ℞

[ō-flŏks-ă-sĭn]
Ophthalmic Solution 0.3%
STERILE
Rx only

Description: Ofloxacin Ophthalmic Solution 0.3% is a sterile ophthalmic solution. It is a fluorinated carboxyquinolone anti-infective for topical ophthalmic use.

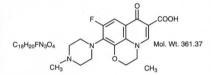

$C_{18}H_{20}FN_3O_4$ Mol. Wt. 361.37

Chemical Name:
(±)-9-Fluoro-2,3-dihydro-3-methyl-10-(4-methyl-1-piperazinyl)-7-oxo-7H-pyrido[1,2,3-de]-1,4 benzoxazine-6-carboxylic acid.
Each mL Contains: Active:
ofloxacin 0.3% (3 mg/mL)
Preservative Added:
benzalkonium chloride (0.005%)
Inactives: sodium chloride and purified water. Hydrochloric Acid and/or Sodium Hydroxide may be added to adjust pH. Ofloxacin ophthalmic solution is unbuffered and formulated with a pH of 6.4 (range - 6.0 to 6.8). It has an osmolality of 300 mOsm/kg. Ofloxacin is a fluorinated 4-quinolone which differs from other fluorinated 4-quinolones in that there is a six member (pyridobenzoxazine) ring from positions 1 to 8 of the basic ring structure.
Clinical Pharmacology:
Pharmacokinetics: Serum, urine and tear concentrations of ofloxacin were measured in 30 healthy women at various time points during a ten-day course of treatment with ofloxacin ophthalmic solution. The mean serum ofloxacin concentration ranged from 0.4 ng/mL to 1.9 ng/mL. Maximum ofloxacin concentration increased from 1.1 ng/mL on day one to 1.9 ng/mL on day 11 after QID dosing for 10 1/2 days. Maximum serum ofloxacin concentrations after ten days of topical ophthalmic dosing were more than 1000 times lower than those reported after standard oral doses of ofloxacin.
Tear ofloxacin concentrations ranged from 5.7 to 31 µg/g during the 40 minute period following the last dose on day 11. Mean tear concentration measured four hours after topical ophthalmic dosing was 9.2 µg/g.
Corneal tissue concentrations of 4.4 µg/mL were observed four hours after beginning topical ocular application of two drops of ofloxacin ophthalmic solution every 30 minutes. Ofloxacin was excreted in the urine primarily unmodified.
Microbiology: Ofloxacin has *in vitro* activity against a broad range of gram-positive and gram-negative aerobic and anaerobic bacteria. Ofloxacin is bactericidal at concentrations equal to or slightly greater than inhibitory concentrations. Ofloxacin is thought to exert a bactericidal effect on susceptible bacterial cells by inhibiting DNA gyrase, an essential

bacterial enzyme which is a critical catalyst in the duplication, transcription, and repair of bacterial DNA.
Cross-resistance has been observed between ofloxacin and other fluoroquinolones. There is generally no cross-resistance between ofloxacin and other classes of antibacterial agents such as beta-lactams or aminoglycosides. Ofloxacin has been shown to be active against most strains of the following organisms both *in vitro* and clinically, in conjunctival and/or corneal ulcer infections as described in the **INDICATIONS AND USAGE** section.
AEROBES, GRAM-POSITIVE:
Staphylococcus aureus
Staphylococcus epidermidis
Streptococcus pneumoniae
AEROBES, GRAM-NEGATIVE:
Enterobacter cloacae
Haemophilus influenzae
Proteus mirabilis
Pseudomonas aeruginosa
*Serratia marcescens**
ANAEROBIC SPECIES:
Propionibacterium acnes
*Efficacy for this organism was studied in fewer than 10 infections
The safety and effectiveness of ofloxacin ophthalmic solution in treating ophthalmologic infections due to the following organisms have not been established in adequate and well-controlled clinical trials. Ofloxacin ophthalmic solution has been shown to be active *in vitro* against most strains of these organisms but the clinical significance in ophthalmologic infections is unknown.
AEROBES, GRAM-POSITIVE:
Enterococcus faecalis
Listeria monocytogenes
Staphylococcus capitis
Staphylococcus hominus
Staphylococcus simulans
Streptococcus pyogenes
AEROBES, GRAM-NEGATIVE:
Acinetobacter calcoaceticus var. anitratus
Acinetobacter calcoaceticus var. lwoffi
Citrobacter diversus
Citrobacter freundii
Enterobacter aerogenes
Enterobacter agglomerans
Escherichia coli
Haemophilus parainfluenzae
Klebsiella oxytoca
Klebsiella pneumoniae
Moraxella (Branhamella) catarrhalis
Moraxella lacunata
Morganella morganii
Neisseria gonorrhoeae
Pseudomonas acidovorans
Pseudomonas fluorescens
Shigella sonnei
OTHER:
Chlamydia trachomatis
Clinical Studies:
Conjunctivitis: In a randomized, double-masked, multicenter clinical trial, ofloxacin ophthalmic solution was superior to its vehicle after 2 days of treatment in patients with conjunctivitis and positive conjunctival cultures. Clinical outcomes for the trial demonstrated a clinical improvement rate of 86% (54/63) for the ofloxacin treated group versus 72% (48/67) for the placebo treated group after 2 days of therapy. Microbiological outcomes for the same clinical trial demonstrated an eradication rate for causative pathogens of 65% (41/63) for the ofloxacin treated group versus 25% (17/67) for the vehicle treated group after 2 days of therapy. Please note that microbiologic eradication does not always correlate with clinical outcome in anti-infective trials.
Corneal Ulcers: In a randomized, double-masked, multi-center clinical trial of 140 subjects with positive cultures, ofloxacin ophthalmic solution treated subjects had an overall clinical success rate (complete re-

epithelialization and no progression of the infiltrate for two consecutive visits) of 82% (61/74) compared to 80% (53/66) for the fortified antibiotic group, consisting of 1.5% tobramycin and 10% cefazolin solutions. The median time to clinical success was 11 days for the ofloxacin treated group and 10 days for the fortified treatment group.
Indications and Usage: Ofloxacin ophthalmic solution is indicated for the treatment of infections caused by susceptible strains of the following bacteria in the conditions listed below:
CONJUNCTIVITIS:
Gram-positive bacteria:
Staphylococcus aureus
Staphylococcus epidermidis
Streptococcus pneumoniae
Gram-negative bacteria:
Enterobacter cloacae
Haemophilus influenzae
Proteus mirabilis
Pseudomonas aeruginosa
CORNEAL ULCERS:
Gram-positive bacteria:
Staphylococcus aureus
Staphylococcus epidermidis
Streptococcus pneumoniae
Gram-negative bacteria:
Pseudomonas aeruginosa
*Serratia marcescens**
Anaerobic species:
Propionibacterium acnes

---

*Efficacy for this organism was studied in fewer than 10 infections
Contraindications: Ofloxacin ophthalmic solution is contraindicated in patients with a history of hypersensitivity to ofloxacin, to other quinolones, or to any of the components in this medication.
Warnings:
NOT FOR INJECTION.
Ofloxacin ophthalmic solution should not be injected subconjunctivally, nor should it be introduced directly into the anterior chamber of the eye.
Serious and occasionally fatal hypersensitivity (anaphylactic) reactions, some following the first dose, have been reported in patients receiving systemic quinolones, including ofloxacin. Some reactions were accompanied by cardiovascular collapse, loss of consciousness, angioedema (including laryngeal, pharyngeal or facial edema), airway obstruction, dyspnea, urticaria, and itching. A rare occurrence of Stevens-Johnson syndrome, which progressed to toxic epidermal necrolysis, has been reported in a patient who was receiving topical ophthalmic ofloxacin. If an allergic reaction to ofloxacin occurs, discontinue the drug. Serious acute hypersensitivity reactions may require immediate emergency treatment. Oxygen and airway management, including intubation should be administered as clinically indicated.
Precautions:
General: As with other anti-infectives, prolonged use may result in overgrowth of non-susceptible organisms, including fungi. If superinfection occurs discontinue use and institute alternative therapy. Whenever clinical judgment dictates, the patient should be examined with the aid of magnification, such as slit lamp biomicroscopy and, where appropriate, fluorescein staining. Ofloxacin should be discontinued at the first appearance of a skin rash or any other sign of hypersensitivity reaction.
The systemic administration of quinolones, including ofloxacin, has led to lesions or erosions of the cartilage in weight-bearing joints and other signs of arthropathy in immature animals of various species. Ofloxacin, administered systemically at 10 mg/kg/day in young

Continued on next page

Ofloxacin—Cont.

dogs (equivalent to 110 times the maximum recommended daily adult ophthalmic dose) has been associated with these types of effects.

Information for Patients: Avoid contaminating the applicator tip with material from the eye, fingers or other source.

Systemic quinolones, including ofloxacin, have been associated with hypersensitivity reactions, even following a single dose. Discontinue use immediately and contact your physician at the first sign of a rash or allergic reaction.

Drug Interactions: Specific drug interaction studies have not been conducted with ofloxacin ophthalmic solution. However, the systemic administration of some quinolones has been shown to elevate plasma concentrations of theophylline, interfere with the metabolism of caffeine, and enhance the effects of the oral anticoagulant warfarin and its derivatives, and has been associated with transient elevations in serum creatinine in patients receiving cyclosporine concomitantly.

Carcinogenesis, Mutagenesis, Impairment of Fertility: Long term studies to determine the carcinogenic potential of ofloxacin have not been conducted.

Ofloxacin was not mutagenic in the Ames test, *in vitro* and *in vivo* cytogenic assay, sister chromatid exchange assay (Chinese hamster and human cell lines), unscheduled DNA synthesis (UDS) assay using human fibroblasts, the dominant lethal assay, or mouse micronucleus assay. Ofloxacin was positive in the UDS test using rat hepatocyte, and in the mouse lymphoma assay.

In fertility studies in rats, ofloxacin did not affect male or female fertility or morphological or reproductive performance at oral dosing up to 360 mg/kg/day (equivalent to 4000 times the maximum recommended daily ophthalmic dose).

Pregnancy: Teratogenic Effects. Pregnancy Category C: Ofloxacin has been shown to have an embryocidal effect in rats and in rabbits when given in doses of 810 mg/kg/day (equivalent to 9000 times the maximum recommended daily ophthalmic dose) and 160 mg/kg/day (equivalent to 1800 times the maximum recommended daily ophthalmic dose). These dosages resulted in decreased fetal body weight and increased fetal mortality in rats and rabbits, respectively. Minor fetal skeletal variations were reported in rats receiving doses of 810 mg/kg/day. Ofloxacin has not been shown to be teratogenic at doses as high as 810 mg/kg/day and 160 mg/kg/day when administered to pregnant rats and rabbits, respectively.

Nonteratogenic Effects: Additional studies in rats with doses up to 360 mg/kg/day during late gestation showed no adverse effect on late fetal development, labor, delivery, lactation, neonatal viability, or growth of the newborn. There are, however, no adequate and well-controlled studies in pregnant women. Ofloxacin ophthalmic solution should be used during pregnancy only if the potential benefit justifies the potential risk to the fetus.

Nursing Mothers: In nursing women a single 200 mg oral dose resulted in concentrations of ofloxacin in milk which were similar to those found in plasma. It is not known whether ofloxacin is excreted in human milk following topical ophthalmic administration. Because of the potential for serious adverse reactions from ofloxacin in nursing infants, a decision should be made whether to discontinue nursing or to discontinue the drug, taking into account the importance of the drug to the mother.

Pediatric Use: Safety and effectiveness in infants below the age of one year have not been established.

Quinolones, including ofloxacin, have been shown to cause arthropathy in immature animals after oral administration; however, topical ocular administration of ofloxacin to immature animals has not shown any arthropathy. There is no evidence that the ophthalmic dosage form of ofloxacin has any effect on weight bearing joints.

Geriatric Use: No overall differences in safety or effectiveness have been observed between elderly and younger patients.

Adverse Reactions:

Ophthalmic Use: The most frequently reported drug-related adverse reaction was transient ocular burning or discomfort. Other reported reactions include stinging, redness, itching, chemical conjunctivitis/keratitis, ocular/periocular/facial edema, foreign body sensation, photophobia, blurred vision, tearing, dryness, and eye pain. Rare reports of dizziness and nausea have been received.

Dosage and Administration: The recommended dosage regimen for the treatment of **bacterial conjunctivitis** is:

Days 1 and 2	Instill one to two drops every two to four hours in the affected eye(s).
Days 3 through 7	Instill one to two drops four times daily.

The recommended dosage regimen for the treatment of **bacterial corneal ulcer** is:

Days 1 and 2	Instill one to two drops into the affected eye every 30 minutes, while awake. Awaken at approximately four and six hours after retiring and instill one to two drops.
Days 3 through 7 to 9	Instill one to two drops hourly, while awake.
Days 7 to 9 through treatment completion	Instill one to two drops, four times daily.

DO NOT USE IF IMPRINTED "Protective Seal" WITH YELLOW ☞ IS NOT INTACT.

How Supplied: Ofloxacin Ophthalmic Solution 0.3% is supplied sterile in plastic dropper bottles in the following sizes:

5 mL	NDC 24208-434-05	AB43407
10 mL	NDC 24208-434-10	AB43409

Storage: Store at 15°–25°C (59°–77°F)
KEEP OUT OF REACH OF CHILDREN.
FOR OPHTHALMIC USE ONLY.
Bausch & Lomb Incorporated
Tampa, FL 33637
©Bausch & Lomb Incorporated

XO51054 (**FOLDED**)
XM10124 (**FLAT**)
R.2/04-01

Shown in Product Identification Guide, page 104

OPTIPRANOLOL® ℞
(metipranolol ophthalmic solution) 0.3%
Rx only

Description: OPTIPRANOLOL® (metipranolol ophthalmic solution) 0.3% contains metipranolol, a non-selective beta-adrenergic receptor blocking agent. Metipranolol is a white, odorless, crystalline powder.

The chemical name of metipranolol is (±)-1-(4-Hydroxy-2,3,5-trimethylphenoxy)-3-(isopropylamino)-2-propanol-4-acetate.

The chemical structure of metipranolol is:

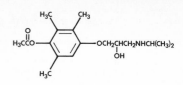

$C_{17}H_{27}NO_4$ Mol. Wt. 309.40

Each mL of OPTIPRANOLOL® contains 3 mg metipranolol. INACTIVES: Povidone, Glycerin, Hydrochloric Acid, Sodium Chloride, Edetate Disodium, and Purified Water. Sodium Hydroxide and/or Hydrochloric Acid may be added to adjust pH. PRESERVATIVE: Benzalkonium Chloride 0.004%.

Clinical Pharmacology: Metipranolol blocks beta$_1$ and beta$_2$(non-selective) adrenergic receptors. It does not have significant intrinsic sympathomimetic activity, and has only weak local anesthetic (membrane-stabilizing) and myocardial depressant activity.

Orally administered beta-adrenergic blocking agents reduce cardiac output in both healthy subjects and patients with heart disease. In patients with severe impairment of myocardial function, beta-adrenergic receptor antagonists may inhibit the sympathetic stimulatory effect necessary to maintain adequate cardiac output.

Beta-adrenergic receptor blockade in the bronchi and bronchioles may result in significantly increased airway resistance from unopposed para-sympathetic activity. Such an effect is potentially dangerous in patients with asthma or other bronchospastic conditions (see CONTRAINDICATIONS and WARNINGS).

OPTIPRANOLOL® Ophthalmic Solution, when applied topically in the eye, has the action of reducing elevated as well as normal intraocular pressure (IOP), whether or not accompanied by glaucoma. Elevated intraocular pressure is a major risk factor in the pathogenesis of glaucomatous visual field loss. The higher the level of intraocular pressure, the greater the likelihood of glaucomatous visual field loss and optic nerve damage.

The primary mechanism of the ocular hypotensive action of metipranolol is most likely due to a reduction in aqueous humor production. A slight increase in outflow may be an additional mechanism. OPTIPRANOLOL Ophthalmic Solution reduces IOP with little or no effect on pupil size or accommodation.

In controlled studies of patients with intraocular pressure greater than 24 mmHg at baseline, OPTIPRANOLOL Ophthalmic Solution reduced the average intraocular pressure approximately 20–26%.

The onset of action of OPTIPRANOLOL Ophthalmic Solution, as measured by a reduction in intraocular pressure, occurs within 30 minutes after a single administration. The maximum effect occurs at about 2 hours. A reduction in intraocular pressure can be demonstrated 24 hours after a single dose. Clinical studies in patients with glaucoma treated for up to two years indicate that an intraocular pressure lowering effect is maintained.

Animal Pharmacology: In rabbits administered metipranolol in one eye at 2 to 4 fold increased concentrations, multi-focal interstitial nephritis was observed in male animals, and lympho-hystiocytic and heterophilic interstitial pneumonia was observed in female animals. The clinical relevance of these findings in unknown.

Indications and Usage: OPTIPRANOLOL Ophthalmic Solution is indicated in the treatment of elevated intraocular pressure in patients with ocular hypertension or open angle glucoma.

Contraindications: Hypersensitivity to any component of this product. OPTIPRANOLOL Ophthalmic Solution is contraindicated in patients with bronchial asthma or a history of bronchial asthma, or severe chronic obstructive pulmonary disease; symptomatic sinus bradycardia; greater than a first degree atrioventricular block; cardiogenic shock; or overt cardiac failure.

Warnings: As with other topically applied ophthalmic drugs, this drug may be absorbed systemically. Thus, the same adverse reactions found with systemic administration of beta-adrenergic blocking agents may occur with topical administration. For example, severe respiratory reactions and cardiac reactions, including death due to bronchospasm in patients with asthma, and rarely, death in association with cardiac failure, have been reported following topical application of beta-adrenergic blocking agents (see CONTRAINDICATIONS). Since OPTIPRANOLOL Ophthalmic Solution had a minor effect on heart rate and blood pressure in clinical studies, caution should be observed in treating patients with a history of cardiac failure. Treatment with OPTIPRANOLOL Ophthalmic Solution should be discontinued at the first evidence of cardiac failure.

OPTIPRANOLOL Ophthalmic Solution, or other beta-blockers, should not, in general, be administered to patients with chronic obstructive pulmonary disease (e.g., chronic bronchitis, emphysema) of mild or moderate severity (see CONTRAINDICATIONS). However, if the drug is necessary in such patients, then it should be administered with caution since it may block bronchodilation produced by endogenous and exogenous catecholamine stimulation of beta₂ receptors.

Precautions: General: Because of potential effects of beta-adrenergic receptor blocking agents relative to blood pressure and pulse, these should be used with caution in patients with cerebrovascular insufficiency. If signs or symptoms suggesting reduced cerebral blood flow develop following initiation of therapy with OPTIPRANOLOL Ophthalmic Solution, alternative therapy should be considered.

Some authorities recommend gradual withdrawal of beta-adrenergic receptor blocking agents in patients undergoing elective surgery. If necessary during surgery, the effects of beta-adrenergic receptor blocking agents may be reversed by sufficient doses of such agonists as isoproterenol, dopamine, dobutamine or levarterenol.

While OPTIPRANOLOL Ophthalmic Solution has demonstrated a low potential for systemic effect, it should be used with caution in patients with diabetes (especially labile diabetes,) because of possible masking of signs and symptoms of acute hypoglycemia.

Beta-adrenergic receptor blocking agents may mask certain signs and symptoms of hyperthyroidism, and their abrupt withdrawal might precipitate a thyroid storm.

Beta-adrenergic blockade has been reported to potentiate muscle weakness consistent with certain myasthenic symptoms (e.g., diplopia, ptosis, and generalized weakness).

Risk of anaphylactic reaction: While taking beta-blockers, patients with a history of severe anaphylactic reaction to a variety of allergens may be more reactive to repeated challenge, either accidental, diagnostic, or therapeutic. Such patients may be unresponsive to the usual doses of epinephrine used to treat allergic reaction.

Information for Patients: Patients should be instructed to avoid allowing the tip of the dispensing container to contact the eye or surrounding structures. Patients should be advised that OPTIPRANOLOL contains benzalkonium chloride which may be absorbed by soft contact lenses. Contact lenses should be removed prior to administration of the solution. Lenses may be reinserted 15 minutes following OPTIPRANOLOL administration.

Drug Interactions: OPTIPRANOLOL Ophthalmic Solution should be used with caution in patients who are receiving a beta-adrenergic blocking agent orally, because of the potential for additive effects on systemic beta-blockade.

Close observation of the patient is recommended when a beta-blocker is administered to patients receiving catecholamine-depleting drugs such as reserpine, because of possible additive effects and the production of hypotension and/or bradycardia.

Caution should be used in the coadministration of beta-adrenergic receptor blocking agents, such as metipranolol, and oral or intravenous calcium channel antagonists, because of possible precipitation of left ventricular failure, and hypotension. In patients with impaired cardiac function, who are receiving calcium channel antagonists, coadministration should be avoided.

The concomitant use of beta-adrenergic receptor blocking agents with digitalis and calcium channel antagonists may have additive effects, prolonging atrioventricular conduction time.

Caution should be used in patients using concomitant adrenergic psychotropic drugs.

Ocular: In patients with angle-closure glaucoma, the immediate treatment objective is to re-open the angle by constriction of the pupil with a miotic agent. OPTIPRANOLOL Ophthalmic Solution has little or no effect on the pupil, therefore, when it is used to reduce intraocular pressure in angle-closure glaucoma, it should be used only with concomitant administration of a miotic agent.

Carcinogenesis, Mutagensis, Impairment of Fertility: Lifetime studies with metipranolol have been conducted in mice at oral doses of 5, 50, and 100 mg/kg/day and in rats at oral doses of up to 70 mg/kg/day. Metipranolol demonstrated no carcinogenic effect. In the mouse study, female animals receiving the low, but not the intermediate or high dose, had an increased number of pulmonary adenomas. The significance of this observation is unknown. In a variety of in vitro and in vivo bacterial and mammalian cell assays, metipranolol was nonmutagenic.

Reproduction and fertility studies of metipranolol in rats and mice showed no adverse effect on male fertility at oral doses of up to 50 mg/kg/ day, and female fertility at oral doses of up to 25 mg/kg/day.

Pregnancy: Teratogenic effects: Pregnancy Category C: No drug related effects were reported for the segment II teratology study in fetal rats after administration, during organogenesis, to dams of up to 50 mg/kg/day. OPTIPRANOLOL Ophthalmic Solution has been shown to increase fetal resorption, fetal death, and delayed development when administered orally to rabbits at 50 mg/kg/day during organogenesis.

There are no adequate and well-controlled studies in pregnant women. OPTIPRANOLOL Ophthalmic Solution should be used during pregnancy only if the potential benefit justifies the potential risk to the fetus.

Nursing Mothers: It is not known whether OPTIPRANOLOL Ophthalmic Solution is excreted in human milk. Because many drugs are excreted in human milk, caution should be exercised when OPTIPRANOLOL Ophthalmic Solution is administered to nursing women.

Pediatric Use: Safety and effectiveness in children have not been established.

Geriatric Use: No overall differences in safety or effectiveness have been observed between elderly and younger patients.

Adverse Reactions: In clinical trials, the use of OPTIPRANOLOL Ophthalmic Solution has been associated with transient local discomfort.

Other ocular adverse reactions, such as abnormal vision, blepharitis, blurred vision, browache, conjunctivitis, edema, eyelid dermatitis, photophobia, tearing, and uveitis have been reported in small numbers of patients.

Other systemic adverse reactions, such as allergic reaction, angina, anxiety, arthritis, asthenia, atrial fibrillation, bradycardia, bronchitis, coughing, depression, dizziness, dyspnea, epistaxis, headache, hypertension, myalgia, myocardial infarct, nausea nervousness, palpitation, rash, rhinitis and somnolence have also been reported in small numbers of patients.

Overdosage: No information is available on overdosage of OPTIPRANOLOL Ophthalmic Solution in humans. The symptoms which might be expected with an overdose of a systemically administered beta-adrenergic receptor blocking agent are bradycardia, hypotension and accute cardiac failure.

Dosage and Administration: The recommended dose is one drop of OPTIPRANOLOL Ophthalmic Solution in the affected eye(s) twice a day.

If the patients's IOP is not at a satisfactory level on this regimen, use of more frequent administration or a larger dose of OPTIPRANOLOL Ophthalmic Solution is not known to be of benefit. Concomitant therapy to lower intraocular pressure can be instituted. In clinical trials, OPTIPRANOLOL Ophthalmic Solution was safely used during concomitant therapy with pilocarpine, epinephrine or acetazolamide.

How Supplied: OPTIPRANOLOL® (metipranolol ophthalmic solution) 0.3% is supplied in a plastic with a controlled drop tip and a yellow plastic screw-top cap as follows:
5 mL: NDC 24208-275-07-AB40207
10 mL NDC 24208-275-09-AB40209
Storage: Store between, 15°–30°C (59°–86°F). Replace cap immediately after use.

DO NOT USE IF IMPRINTED NECKBAND IS NOT INTACT.

FOR OPHTHALMIC USE ONLY
Bausch & Lomb
Incorporated, Inc.
Tampa, FL 33637   Rev. 11/03-91
©Bausch & Lomb Incorporated, Inc.
Shown in Product Identification Guide, page 104

RETISERT®   ℞
[rĕ-tĭ-sərt]
(fluocinolone acetonide intravitreal implant)
0.59 mg STERILE
Rx only

Description: RETISERT® (fluocinolone acetonide intravitreal implant) 0.59 mg is a sterile implant designed to release fluocinolone acetonide locally to the posterior segment of the eye at a nominal initial rate of 0.6 µg/day, decreasing over the first month to a steady state

Continued on next page

Retisert—Cont.

between 0.3-0.4 µg/day over approximately 30 months. The drug substance is the synthetic corticosteroid fluocinolone acetonide, represented by the following structural formula:

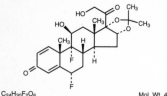

$C_{24}H_{30}F_2O_6$

Mol. Wt. 452.50

Chemical Name: Pregna-1,4-diene-3,20-dione,6,9-difluoro-11,21-dihydroxy-16,17-[(1-methyl-ethylidene)bis(oxy)]-, (6α ,11β,16α)-.
Fluocinolone acetonide is a white crystalline powder, insoluble in water, and soluble in methanol. It has a melting point of 265-266°C. Each RETISERT consists of a tablet containing 0.59 mg of the active ingredient, Fluocinolone Acetonide, USP, and the following inactives: microcrystalline cellulose, polyvinyl alcohol, and magnesium stearate.
Clinical Pharmacology: Corticosteroids inhibit the inflammatory response to a variety of inciting agents and probably delay or slow healing. They inhibit the edema, fibrin deposition, capillary dilation, leukocyte migration, capillary proliferation, fibroblast proliferation, deposition of collagen, and scar formation associated with inflammation. There is no generally accepted explanation for the mechanism of action of ocular corticosteroids. However, corticosteroids are thought to act by the induction of phospholipase A_2 inhibitory proteins, collectively called lipocortins. It is postulated that these proteins control the biosynthesis of potent mediators of inflammation such as prostaglandins and leukotrienes by inhibiting the release of their common precursor arachidonic acid. Arachidonic acid is released from membrane phospholipids by phospholipase A_2. Corticosteroids are capable of producing a rise in intraocular pressure.

Pharmacokinetics: In a subset of patients who received the intravitreal implant, and had blood samples taken at various times (weeks 1, 4 and 34) after implantation, plasma levels of fluocinolone acetonide were below the limit of detection (0.2 ng/mL) at all times. Aqueous and vitreous humor samples were assayed for fluocinolone acetonide in a further subset of patients. While detectable concentrations of fluocinolone acetonide were seen throughout the observation interval (up to 34 months), the concentrations were highly variable, ranging from below the limit of detection (0.2 ng/mL) to 589 ng/mL.

Clinical Studies: In two randomized, double-masked, multicenter controlled clinical trials, 227 patients with chronic (a one year or greater history) non-infectious uveitis affecting the posterior segment of one or both eyes who received a 0.59 mg RETISERT were studied. The primary efficacy endpoint in both trials was the rate of recurrence of uveitis affecting the posterior segment of the study eye in the 34 week period post-implantation compared to the rate of recurrence in the 34 week period pre-implantation. The rates of recurrence ranged from approximately 7% (7/108) to 14% (16/116) for the 34 week period post-implantation as compared to approximately 40% (46/116) to 54% (58/108) for the 34 week period pre-implantation.
Indications and Usage: RETISERT is indicated for the treatment of chronic non-infectious uveitis affecting the posterior segment of the eye.
Contraindications: RETISERT is contraindicated in most viral diseases of the cornea and

conjunctiva including epithelial herpes simplex keratitis (dendritic keratitis), vaccinia, and varicella, and also in mycobacterial infections of the eye and fungal diseases of ocular structures. RETISERT is also contraindicated in individuals with known or suspected hypersensitivity to any of the ingredients of this preparation and to other corticosteroids.
Warnings: As with any surgical procedure there is risk involved. Potential complications accompanying intraocular surgery to place RETISERT into the vitreous cavity may include, but are not limited to, the following: cataract formation, choroidal detachment, temporary decreased visual acuity, endophthalmitis, hypotony, increased intraocular pressure, exacerbation of intraocular inflammation, retinal detachment, vitreous hemorrhage, vitreous loss, and wound dehiscence.
Following implantation of RETISERT, nearly all patients will experience an immediate and temporary decrease in visual acuity in the implanted eye which lasts for approximately one to four weeks post-operatively. This decrease in visual acuity is likely a result of the surgical procedure.
Prolonged use of corticosteroids may result in glaucoma with damage to the optic nerve, defects in visual acuity and fields of vision, and in posterior subcapsular cataract formation. Steroids should be used with caution in the presence of glaucoma. Patients must be monitored for elevated IOP.
Based on clinical trials with RETISERT, within 34 weeks post-implantation, approximately 60% of patients will require IOP lowering medications to control intraocular pressure. Within an average post-implantation period of approximately 2 years, approximately 32% of patients are expected to require filtering procedures to control intraocular pressure.
Within an average post-implantation period of approximately 2 years, nearly all phakic eyes are expected to develop cataracts and require cataract surgery.
Use of ocular steroids may prolong the course and may exacerbate the severity of many viral infections of the eye (including herpes simplex). Employment of a corticosteroid medication in the treatment of patients with a history of herpes simplex requires great caution.
Prolonged use of corticosteroids may suppress the host response and thus increase the hazard of secondary ocular infections. In acute purulent conditions of the eye, steroids may mask infection or enhance existing infection.
The use of steroids after cataract surgery may delay healing and increase the incidence of bleb formation.
Precautions:
General
As with all intraocular surgery, sterility of the surgical field and RETISERT should be rigorously maintained. RETISERT should be handled only by the suture tab in order to avoid damaging the implant since this could affect the release rate of fluocinolone acetonide inside the eye. Care should be taken during implantation and explantation to avoid sheer forces on the implant that could disengage the silicone cup reservoir (which contains a fluocinolone acetonide tablet) from the suture tab. RETISERT should not be resterilized by any method.
In vitro stability studies show that the strength of the adhesive bond between the silicone cup reservoir and the suture tab is reduced with prolonged hydration, indicating a potential for the separation of these components. Physicians should monitor the integrity of the implant during ophthalmologic examinations.
RETISERT should be used with caution in most viral diseases of the cornea and con-

junctiva including epithelial herpes simplex keratitis (dendritic keratitis), vaccinia, and varicella.
Since resistance to infections is known to be reduced by corticosteroids, simultaneous bilateral implantation should not be carried out, in order to limit the potential for bilateral post-operative infection.
Information for Patients: RETISERT is designed to locally treat inflammation in the eye, but it is not known to treat the underlying disease. Medication to treat the underlying disease may be prescribed concurrently as deemed appropriate by a physician. Patients should be advised to have ophthalmologic follow-up examinations of both eyes at appropriate intervals following implantation of RETISERT.
As with any surgical procedure, there is risk involved. Potential complications accompanying intraocular surgery to place RETISERT into the vitreous cavity may include, but are not limited to, the following: cataract formation, choroidal detachment, temporary decreased visual acuity, endophthalmitis, hypotony, increased intraocular pressure, exacerbation of intraocular inflammation, retinal detachment, vitreous hemorrhage, vitreous loss, and wound dehiscence.
Following implantation of RETISERT, nearly all patients will experience an immediate and temporary decrease in visual acuity in the implanted eye which lasts for approximately one to four weeks post-operatively. This decrease in visual acuity is likely a result of the surgical implant procedure.
Based on clinical trials with RETISERT, within 34 weeks post-implantation, approximately 60% of patients will require IOP lowering medications to control intraocular pressure. Within an average post-implantation period of approximately 2 years, approximately 32% of patients are expected to require filtering procedures to control intraocular pressure.
Within an average post-implantation period of approximately 2 years, nearly all phakic eyes are expected to develop cataracts and require cataract surgery.
Carcinogenesis, mutagenesis, impairment of fertility: Long-term animal studies have not been performed on RETISERT to evaluate the carcinogenic potential or the effect on fertility of fluocinolone acetonide.
Fluocinolone acetonide was not genotoxic *in vitro* in the Ames test, the mouse lymphoma TK assay, or *in vivo* in the mouse bone marrow micronucleus assay.
Pregnancy: Teratogenic effects: Pregnancy Category C. No adequate animal reproduction studies have been conducted with fluocinolone acetonide.
Corticosteroids are generally teratogenic in laboratory animals when administered systemically at relatively low dosage levels. Fluocinolone acetonide when administered subcutaneously at a dose of 0.13 mg/kg/day (approximately 10,000 times the daily clinical dose of RETISERT), during Days 6 to 18 of pregnancy in the rabbit, induced abortion at the end of the third and at the beginning of the fourth gestational week. When administered subcutaneously to rats and rabbits during gestation at a maternal toxic dose of 50 µg/kg/day (approximately 4,000 times the clinical dose of RETISERT), fluocinolone acetonide caused abortions and malformations in a few surviving fetuses.
There are no adequate and well-controlled studies in pregnant women. RETISERT should be used during pregnancy only if the potential benefit justifies the potential risk to the fetus.
Nursing Mothers: It is not known whether ocular administration of corticosteroids could result in sufficient systemic absorption to pro-

duce detectable quantities in human milk. Systemic steroids appear in human milk and could suppress growth, interfere with endogenous corticosteroid production, or cause other untoward effects. Caution should be exercised when RETISERT is implanted in a nursing woman.

Pediatric Use: Safety and effectiveness in pediatric patients below the age of 12 years have not been established.

Geriatric Use: No overall differences in safety and effectiveness have been observed between elderly and younger patients.

Adverse Reactions: Adverse reactions associated with ocular administration of corticosteroids include elevated intraocular pressure with possible development of glaucoma, optic nerve damage, and visual acuity and field defects, posterior subcapsular cataract formation, delayed wound healing, and perforation of the globe where there is thinning of the sclera.

The development of secondary ocular infection (bacterial, fungal, and viral) has occurred after use of ophthalmic steroids. Fungal and viral infections of the cornea are particularly prone to develop coincidentally with long-term applications of steroids. The possibility of fungal invasion should be considered in any persistent corneal ulceration where steroid treatment has been used (see **Warnings**).

The most frequently reported ocular adverse events in the overall study population were cataract, increased intraocular pressure, procedural complication, and eye pain. These events occurred in approximately 50-90% of patients. Procedural complication includes cataract fragments in the eye post-op, implant expulsion, injury, mechanical complication of implant, migration of implant, post-op complications, post-op wound complications, and wound dehiscence.

Based on clinical trials with RETISERT, within an average post-implantation period of approximately 2 years, nearly all phakic eyes are expected to develop cataracts and require cataract surgery.

Within 34 weeks post-implantation, approximately 60% of patients will require IOP lowering medications to control intraocular pressure. Within an average post-implantation period of approximately 2 years, approximately 32% of patients are expected to require filtering procedures to control intraocular pressure.

Ocular adverse events occurring in approximately 10-35% of patients include reduced visual acuity, conjunctival hemorrhage, conjunctival hyperemia, glaucoma, blurred vision, abnormal sensation in the eye, eye irritation, hypotony, pruritus, vitreous floaters, maculopathy, vitreous hemorrhage, ptosis, eye inflammation, eyelid edema, increased tearing, and dry eye.

Ocular adverse events occurring in approximately 5-9% of patients included macular edema, visual disturbance, eye discharge, conjunctival edema/chemosis, photophobia, blepharitis, corneal edema, photopsia, retinal hemorrhage, choroidal detachment, vitreous opacities, and eye swelling.

The most frequently reported non-ocular adverse event was headache (31%).

Other non-ocular adverse events occurring in approximately 5-15% of patients were nasopharyngitis, arthralgia, sinusitis, dizziness, pyrexia, nausea, cough, influenza, upper respiratory tract infection, vomiting, limb pain, back pain, rash, and pain.

Dosage and Administration: RETISERT is surgically implanted into the posterior segment of the affected eye through a pars plana incision. The implant contains one tablet of 0.59 mg of fluocinolone acetonide. RETISERT is designed to release fluocinolone acetonide at a nominal initial rate of 0.6 µg/day, decreasing over the first month to a steady state between 0.3-0.4 µg/

day over approximately 30 months. Following depletion of fluocinolone acetonide from RETISERT as evidenced by recurrence of uveitis, RETISERT may be replaced.

Handling and Disposal: Caution should be exercised in handling RETISERT in order to avoid damage to the implant, which may result in an increased rate of drug release from the implant. Thus, RETISERT should be handled only by the suture tab. Care should be taken during implantation and explantation to avoid sheer forces on the implant that could disengage the silicone cup reservoir (which contains a fluocinolone acetonide tablet) from the suture tab. Aseptic technique should be maintained at all times prior to and during the surgical implantation procedure. RETISERT should not be resterilized by any method.

How Supplied: The implant consists of a tablet encased in a silicone elastomer cup containing a release orifice and a polyvinyl alcohol membrane positioned between the tablet and the orifice. The silicone elastomer cup assembly is attached to a polyvinyl alcohol suture tab with silicone adhesive. Each RETISERT is approximately 3 mm × 2 mm × 5 mm.

Each implant is stored in a clear polycarbonate case within a foil pouch within a Tyvek peel-able overwrap. Each packaged implant is provided in a carton which includes the package insert.

0.59 mg RETISERT – NDC 24208-416-01

Storage: Store in the original container at 15° - 25°C (59° - 77°F).

Protect from freezing.

Revised April 2007

U.S. Patent # 6,217,895,

U.S. Patent # 6,548,078

™/® denote trademarks of

Bausch & Lomb Incorporated.

© Bausch & Lomb Incorporated

Marketed by:

Bausch & Lomb Incorporated, Rochester, NY 14609

Manufactured by:

Bausch & Lomb Incorporated, Waterford, Ireland

Shown in Product Identification Guide, page 104

ZYLET® ℞

[zī-lĕt]

loteprednol etabonate 0.5% and tobramycin 0.3% ophthalmic suspension

STERILE

Description: Zylet (loteprednol etabonate and tobramycin ophthalmic suspension), is a sterile, multiple dose topical anti-inflammatory corticosteroid and antibiotic combination for ophthalmic use. Both loteprednol etabonate and tobramycin are white to off-white powders. The chemical structures of loteprednol etabonate and tobramycin are shown below.

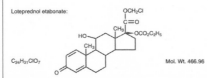

Loteprednol etabonate:

$C_{24}H_{31}ClO_7$ Mol. Wt. 466.96

Chemical name: chloromethyl 17α-[(ethoxycarbonyl)oxy]-11 β-hydroxy-3-oxoandrosta-1, 4-diene-17 β-carboxylate

[See chemical structure at top of next column]

Chemical Name:

O-3-Amino-3-deoxy-α-D-glucopyranosyl-(1→4)-*O*-[2,6-diamino-2,3,6-trideoxy-α-D-*ribo*-hexopyranosyl-(1→6)]-2-deoxystreptamine

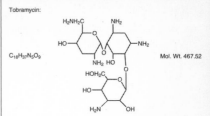

Tobramycin:

$C_{18}H_{37}N_5O_9$ Mol. Wt. 467.52

Each mL contains:

Actives: Loteprednol Etabonate 5 mg (0.5%) and Tobramycin 3 mg (0.3%). Inactives: Edetate Disodium, Glycerin, Povidone, Purified Water, Tyloxapol, and Benzalkonium Chloride 0.01% (preservative). Sulfuric Acid and/or Sodium Hydroxide may be added to adjust the pH to 5.7-5.9. The suspension is essentially isotonic with a tonicity of 260 to 320 mOsmol/kg.

Clinical Pharmacology: Corticosteroids inhibit the inflammatory response to a variety of inciting agents and probably delay or slow healing. They inhibit the edema, fibrin deposition, capillary dilation, leukocyte migration, capillary proliferation, fibroblast proliferation, deposition of collagen, and scar formation associated with inflammation. There is no generally accepted explanation for the mechanism of action of ocular corticosteroids. However, corticosteroids are thought to act by the induction of phospholipase A_2 inhibitory proteins, collectively called lipocortins. It is postulated that these proteins control the biosynthesis of potent mediators of inflammation such as prostaglandins and leukotrienes by inhibiting the release of their common precursor arachidonic acid. Arachidonic acid is released from membrane phospholipids by phospholipase A_2. Corticosteroids are capable of producing a rise in intraocular pressure.

Loteprednol etabonate is structurally similar to other corticosteroids. However, the number 20 position ketone group is absent. It is highly lipid soluble which enhances its penetration into cells. Loteprednol etabonate is synthesized through structural modifications of prednisolone-related compounds so that it will undergo a predictable transformation to an inactive metabolite. Based upon *in vivo* and *in vitro* preclinical metabolism studies, loteprednol etabonate undergoes extensive metabolism to inactive carboxylic acid metabolites.

The antibiotic component in the combination (tobramycin) is included to provide action against susceptible organisms. *In vitro* studies have demonstrated that tobramycin is active against susceptible strains of the following microorganisms:

Staphylococci, including *S. aureus* and *S. epidermidis* (coagulase-positive and coagulase-negative), including penicillin-resistant strains. Streptococci, including some of the Group A-beta-hemolytic species, some non-hemolytic species, and some *Streptococcus pneumoniae*. *Pseudomonas aeruginosa, Escherichia coli, Klebsiella pneumoniae, Enterobacter aerogenes, Proteus mirabilis, Morganella morganii*, most *Proteus vulgaris* strains, *Haemophilus influenzae* and *H. aegyptius, Moraxella lacunata, Acinetobacter calcoaceticus* and some *Neisseria* species.

Pharmacokinetics:

In a controlled clinical study of ocular penetration, the levels of loteprednol etabonate in the aqueous humor were found to be comparable between Lotemax and Zylet treatment groups. Results from a bioavailability study in normal volunteers established that plasma levels of loteprednol etabonate and Δ^1 cortienic acid etabonate (PJ 91), its primary, inactive metab-

Continued on next page

Zylet—Cont.

olite, were below the limit of quantitation (1 ng/mL) at all sampling times. The results were obtained following the ocular administration of one drop in each eye of 0.5% loteprednol etabonate ophthalmic suspension 8 times daily for 2 days or 4 times daily for 42 days. This study suggests that limited (<1 ng/mL) systemic absorption occurs with 0.5% loteprednol etabonate.

Indications and Usage: Zylet is indicated for steroid-responsive inflammatory ocular conditions for which a corticosteroid is indicated and where superficial bacterial ocular infection or a risk of bacterial ocular infection exists.

Ocular steroids are indicated in inflammatory conditions of the palpebral and bulbar conjunctiva, cornea and anterior segment of the globe such as allergic conjunctivitis, acne rosacea, superficial punctate keratitis, herpes zoster keratitis, iritis, cyclitis, and where the inherent risk of steroid use in certain infective conjunctivitides is accepted to obtain a diminution in edema and inflammation. They are also indicated in chronic anterior uveitis and corneal injury from chemical, radiation or thermal burns, or penetration of foreign bodies.

The use of a combination drug with an anti-infective component is indicated where the risk of superficial ocular infection is high or where there is an expectation that potentially dangerous numbers of bacteria will be present in the eye.

The particular anti-infective drug in this product (tobramycin) is active against the following common bacterial eye pathogens: Staphylococci, including *S. aureus* and *S. epidermidis* (coagulase-positive and coagulase-negative), including penicillin-resistant strains. Streptococci, including some of the Group A-beta-hemolytic species, some nonhemolytic species, and some *Streptococcus pneumoniae*. *Pseudomonas aeruginosa*, *Escherichia coli*, *Klebsiella pneumoniae*, *Enterobacter aerogenes*, *Proteus mirabilis*, *Morganella morganii*, most *Proteus vulgaris* strains, *Haemophilus influenzae*, and *H. aegyptius*, *Moraxella lacunata*, *Acinetobacter calcoaceticus* and some *Neisseria* species.

Contraindications: Zylet, as with other steroid anti-infective ophthalmic combination drugs, is contraindicated in most viral diseases of the cornea and conjunctiva including epithelial herpes simplex keratitis (dendritic keratitis), vaccinia, and varicella, and also in mycobacterial infection of the eye and fungal diseases of ocular structures. Zylet is also contraindicated in individuals with known or suspected hypersensitivity to any of the ingredients of this preparation and to other corticosteroids.

Warnings: NOT FOR INJECTION INTO THE EYE.

Prolonged use of corticosteroids may result in glaucoma with damage to the optic nerve, defects in visual acuity and fields of vision, and in posterior subcapsular cataract formation. Steroids should be used with caution in the presence of glaucoma. Sensitivity to topically applied aminoglycosides may occur in some patients. If sensitivity reaction does occur, discontinue use.

Prolonged use of corticosteroids may suppress the host response and thus increase the hazard of secondary ocular infections. In those diseases causing thinning of the cornea or sclera, perforations have been known to occur with the use of topical steroids.

In acute purulent conditions of the eye, steroids may mask infection or enhance existing infection.

Use of ocular steroids may prolong the course and may exacerbate the severity of many viral infections of the eye (including herpes sim-

plex). Employment of a corticosteroid medication in the treatment of patients with a history of herpes simplex requires great caution.

The use of steroids after cataract surgery may delay healing and increase the incidence of bleb formation.

Precautions: General: For ophthalmic use only. The initial prescription and renewal of the medication order beyond 14 days should be made by a physician only after examination of the patient with the aid of magnification, such as slit lamp biomicroscopy and, where appropriate, fluorescein staining.

If signs and symptoms fail to improve after 2 days, the patient should be re-evaluated.

If this product is used for 10 days or longer, intraocular pressure should be monitored even though it may be difficult in children and uncooperative patients (See WARNINGS).

Fungal infections of the cornea are particularly prone to develop coincidentally with long-term local steroid application. Fungus invasion must be considered in any persistent corneal ulceration where a steroid has been used or is in use. Fungal cultures should be taken when appropriate.

As with other antibiotic preparations, prolonged use may result in overgrowth of non-susceptible organisms, including fungi. If superinfection occurs, appropriate therapy should be initiated.

Cross-sensitivity to other aminoglycoside antibiotics may occur; if hypersensitivity develops with this product, discontinue use and institute appropriate therapy.

Information for Patients: This product is sterile when packaged. Patients should be advised not to allow the dropper tip to touch any surface, as this may contaminate the suspension. If pain develops, redness, itching or inflammation becomes aggravated, the patient should be advised to consult a physician. As with all ophthalmic preparations containing benzalkonium chloride, patients should be advised not to wear soft contact lenses when using Zylet.

Carcinogenesis, mutagenesis, impairment of fertility: Long-term animal studies have not been conducted to evaluate the carcinogenic potential of loteprednol etabonate or tobramycin.

Loteprednol etabonate was not genotoxic *in vitro* in the Ames test, the mouse lymphoma TK assay, a chromosome aberration test in human lymphocytes, or in an *in vivo* mouse micronucleus assay.

Oral treatment of male and female rats at 50 mg/kg/day and 25 mg/kg/day of loteprednol etabonate, respectively, (500 and 250 times the maximum clinical dose, respectively) prior to and during mating did not impair fertility in either gender. No impairment of fertility was noted in studies of subcutaneous tobramycin in rats at 100 mg/kg/day (1700 times the maximum daily clinical dose).

Pregnancy: Teratogenic effects: Pregnancy Category C.

Loteprednol etabonate was shown to be teratogenic when administered orally to rats and rabbits during organogenesis at 5 and 3 mg/kg/day, respectively (50 and 30 times the maximum daily clinical dose in rats and rabbits, respectively). An oral dose of loteprednol etabonate in rats at 50 mg/kg/day (500 times the maximum daily clinical dose) during late pregnancy through the weaning period showed a decrease in the growth and survival of pups without dystocia. However, no adverse effect in the pups was observed at 5 mg/kg/day (50 times the maximum daily clinical dose).

Parenteral doses of tobramycin did not show any harm to fetuses up to 100 mg/kg/day (1700 times the maximum daily clinical dose) in rats and rabbits.

There are no adequate and well controlled studies in pregnant women. Zylet should be

used during pregnancy only if the potential benefit justifies the potential risk to the fetus.

Nursing Mothers: It is not known whether topical ophthalmic administration of corticosteroids could result in sufficient systemic absorption to produce detectable quantities in human milk. Systemic steroids appear in human milk and could suppress growth, interfere with endogenous corticosteroid production, or cause other untoward effects. Caution should be exercised when Zylet is administered to a nursing woman.

Pediatric Use: Safety and effectiveness in pediatric patients have not been established.

Geriatric Use: No overall differences in safety and effectiveness have been observed between elderly and younger patients.

Adverse Reactions Adverse reactions have occurred with steroid/anti-infective combination drugs which can be attributed to the steroid component, the anti-infective component, or the combination.

Zylet:

In a 42 day safety study comparing Zylet to placebo, the incidence of ocular adverse events reported in greater than 10% of subjects included injection (approximately 20%) and superficial punctate keratitis (approximately 15%). Increased intraocular pressure was reported in 10% (Zylet) and 4% (placebo) of subjects. Nine percent (9%) of Zylet subjects reported burning and stinging upon instillation. Ocular reactions reported with an incidence less than 4% include vision disorders, discharge, itching, lacrimation disorder, photophobia, corneal deposits, ocular discomfort, eyelid disorder, and other unspecified eye disorders.

The incidence of non-ocular adverse events reported in approximately 14% of subjects was headache; all other non-ocular events had an incidence of less than 5%.

Loteprednol etabonate ophthalmic suspension 0.2% - 0.5%:

Reactions associated with ophthalmic steroids include elevated intraocular pressure, which may be associated with infrequent optic nerve damage, visual acuity and field defects, posterior subcapsular cataract formation, delayed wound healing and secondary ocular infection from pathogens including herpes simplex, and perforation of the globe where there is thinning of the cornea or sclera.

In a summation of controlled, randomized studies of individuals treated for 28 days or longer with loteprednol etabonate, the incidence of significant elevation of intraocular pressure (≥ 10 mm Hg) was 2% (15/901) among patients receiving loteprednol etabonate, 7% (11/164) among patients receiving 1% prednisolone acetate and 0.5% (3/583) among patients receiving placebo.

Tobramycin ophthalmic solution 0.3%:

The most frequent adverse reactions to topical tobramycin are hypersensitivity and localized ocular toxicity, including lid itching and swelling and conjunctival erythema. These reactions occur in less than 4% of patients. Similar reactions may occur with the topical use of other aminoglycoside antibiotics. Other adverse reactions have not been reported; however, if topical ocular tobramycin is administered concomitantly with systemic aminoglycoside antibiotics, care should be taken to monitor the total serum concentration.

Secondary Infection: The development of secondary infection has occurred after use of combinations containing steroids and antimicrobials. Fungal infections of the cornea are particularly prone to develop coincidentally with long-term applications of steroids. The possibility of fungal invasion must be considered in any persistent corneal ulceration where steroid treatment has been used.

Secondary bacterial ocular infection following suppression of host responses also occurs.

Dosage and Administration: SHAKE VIGOROUSLY BEFORE USING.

Apply one or two drops of Zylet into the conjunctival sac of the affected eye(s) every four to six hours. During the initial 24 to 48 hours, the dosing may be increased, to every one to two hours. Frequency should be decreased gradually as warranted by improvement in clinical signs. Care should be taken not to discontinue therapy prematurely. Not more than 20 mL should be prescribed initially and the prescription should not be refilled without further evaluation as outlined in PRECAUTIONS above.

How Supplied: Zylet (loteprednol etabonate and tobramycin ophthalmic suspension) is supplied in a white low density polyethylene plastic bottle with a white controlled drop tip and a white polypropylene cap in the following sizes:
2.5 mL (NDC 24208-358-25) in a 7.5 mL bottle
5 mL (NDC 24208-358-05) in a 7.5 mL bottle
10 mL (NDC 24208-358-10) in a 10 mL bottle

USE ONLY IF IMPRINTED NECKBAND IS INTACT.

Storage: Store upright at 15°-25°C (59°-77°F). PROTECT FROM FREEZING. KEEP OUT OF REACH OF CHILDREN.

Rx only

Revised January 2006

Manufactured by:
Bausch & Lomb Incorporated
Tampa, Florida 33637

©Bausch & Lomb Incorporated

U.S. Patent Numbers: 4,996,335; 5,540,930; 5,747,061

Zylet is a registered trademark of Bausch & Lomb Incorporated

Shown in Product Identification Guide, page 104

Corneal Science Corporation

3209-129 GRESHAM LAKE ROAD RALEIGH, NC 27615

Direct Inquries To:
800-325-6789
919-876-4444
Fax 919-878-5040
www.cornealscience.com

VIVA® Lubricating Eye Drops   OTC
[vē´vä]

Active Ingredient: **Purpose:**
Polysorbate 80 1%   Eye Lubricant and Demulcent

Inactive Ingredients: Citric acid, edetate disodium, purified water, sodium chloride and the antioxidants: mannitol, pyruvate, retinyl palmitate, and sodium citrate.

Description of VIVA® Lubricating Eye Drops:
VIVA® Lubricating Eye Drops are preservative-free in a multi-dose bottle. It is a patented, non-oily/glycerin free (no blurring of vision) sterile isotonic buffered "micro-gel" ophthalmic lubricant that is designed to provide instant moisturizing Dry Eye relief and protect the eyes from further damage and prevent further irritation. It is a tear-balanced, anti-oxidant based low viscosity solution that also contains iron chelating agents. It is designed to promote healing, restore electrolyte

balance and to scavenge for the free-radical by-products of inflammation. Though a low viscosity solution, the ingredients create a complex with the lipocalin in the tears which increases the lipid integrity and therefore, the "dwell time" of the solution on the eye. Clinical studies show that TBUT is increased by an average of 132% over baseline while the product is in regular use. It is labeled to be discarded after 30 days of use by the consumer.

VIVA Lubricating Eye Drops available in 10mL and 15mL for dosing flexibility

Uses: Temporary relief of discomfort, burning and irritation due to dryness of the eye or from exposure to wind, sun, computer use, environmental conditions, prescription medication, post surgical Dry Eye, or systemically induced Dry Eye.

FDA Approved Indication: **FOR USE AS A LUBRICANT AND FOR PROTECTION AGAINST FURTHER IRRITATION OR TO RELIEVE DRYNESS OF THE EYE.**

Directions: Instill 1 or 2 drops in the affected eye(s) as needed.

Discard bottle and contents 30 days after opening. Store at room temperature.

Warnings: For external use only. To avoid contamination replace cap after use. Do not use if solution changes color or becomes cloudy.

Stop use and ask a doctor:

If you experience eye pain, changes in vision, continued redness or irritation, or if condition persists for more than 72 hours. Keep this and all other drugs out of reach of children.

How Supplied: In 10mL NDC 54891 00102, and 15mL NDC 54891 00101 bottles.

Shown in Product Identification Guide, page 104

VIVA LUBRICATING REDNESS RELIEF EYE DROPS   OTC

Active Ingredients: **Purpose**
Polysorbate 80   1%   Eye Lubricant
Naphazoline HCl   0.025%   Redness Reliever

Inactive Ingredients: Citric Acid, Edetate Disodium, Purified Water, Sodium Chloride, and the antioxidants: mannitol, pyruvate, retinyl palmitate and sodium citrate

Description of VIVA Lubricating Redness Relief Eye Drops
VIVA Lubricating Redness Relief Eye Drops is a unique sterile, isotonic, buffered ophthalmic solution that builds on the lubricant/antioxidant based characteristics of VIVA Lubricating Eye Drops (See Description of VIVA Lubricating Eye Drops under Section: Pharmaceutical Product Information). VIVA Lubricating Redness Relief Eye Drops provides a formula with antioxidants, iron-chelating agents, lubricant/demulcent (polysorbate 80) and redness reliever (naphazoline HCl). The naphazoline HCl in this formula is in a concentration indicated by studies that provides the maximum dosage that is effective for the indication of redness relief for the patient with dry red eyes due to minor eye irritations. Higher doses of naphazoline HCl are not any more effective than the dose contained in this formula. VIVA Lubricating Redness Relief Eye Drops is a low-viscosity, no-blur, no-sting, rapid dispersement redness relief formula. Studies in the literature indicate that 0.025% naphazoline HCl (the redness reliever in VIVA Lubricating Redness Relief Eye Drops) is more effective than 0.05% tetrahydrozoline in whitening and duration of effectiveness and blocking the recurring erythema (redness) that results from a histaminic reaction. Longer

duration effectiveness can be used to suggest less dosing to patients. Less dosing may reduce the potential for a "rebound effect". VIVA Lubricating Redness Relief can be used by contact lens wearers for the indicated uses if the patient removes lenses for 10 to 15 minutes.

Uses:
Relieves redness of the eye due to minor eye irritations. Temporary relief of discomfort, burning, and irritation due to dryness of the eye. Lubricant and protectant against further irritation or to relieve dryness of the eye.

Directions:
Put 1 or 2 drops in the affected eye(s) up to 4 times daily

Warnings:
For external use only

Ask a doctor before use if you have narrow angle glaucoma

Do not use if solution changes color or becomes cloudy

Do not touch the tip of container to any surface to avoid contamination

To avoid contamination replace cap after use

Overuse may cause more redness of the eye.

Pupils may become enlarged temporarily

Remove contact lenses before using

Do not put contact lenses for at least 15 minutes.

Stop use and ask a doctor if:
Redness or irritation of the eyes continues
You feel eye pain
Changes in vision occur
Condition persists for more than 72 hours
Condition worsens

Keep out of the reach of children
If swallowed, get medical help or contact a Poison Control Center right away.

How Supplied: In 10 mL (0.33 fl. Oz) NDC 54891 00107

VIVA UltraTears™
Lubricating Eye Drops + MR   OTC

Therapy for Severe Dry Eyes

Active Ingredients: **Purpose**
Polysorbate 80   1%   Lubricant
Hypromellose   0.3%   Lubricant
Glycerin   0.125%   Lubricant
Zinc Sulfate   0.25%   Astringent

Inactive Ingredients:
citric acid, edetate disodium, purified water, sodium chloride and the antioxidants: mannitol, pyruvate, retinyl palmitate, and sodium citrate.

Description of VIVA UltraTears Lubricating Eye Drops + MR™:
VIVA UltraTears Lubricating Eye Drops + MR™ is a sterile, isotonic, buffered "micro-gel" ophthalmic solution for Severe Dry Eye that builds on the lubricant/antioxidant based characteristics of VIVA Lubricating Eye Drops (See Description of VIVA Lubricating Eye Drops under Section: Pharmaceutical Product Information). This product provides an expanded VIVA formula offering "triple layer protection" with antioxidants, iron-chelating agents and active ingredients including Polysorbate 80, Hypromellose and Glycerin as lubricants/demulcents as well as Zinc Sulfate as an astringent. Patients that present with severe dry eye can experience pain, redness, blurred vision, severe itching and frequent mucus discharge. The by-products of inflammation called free-radicals and the cytokines that lead to inflammation and desensitization of the cornea are abundant in the severe dry eye patient causing the dry eye. VIVA UltraTears Lubricating Eye Drops + MR for Severe Dry Eye is for the patient with severe dry eyes that needs long-lasting multi-layered

Continued on next page

VIVA UltraTears—Cont.

protection for all three layers of the tears and the very dry cornea while providing astringent relief from itching, burning, watery eyes and mucous discharge. It is the only formula for severe dry eyes that is antioxidant based and balanced to restore tears to their natural state while protecting the cornea that frequently feels "bone-dry". It is designed to be less blurry for a shorter period of time than very high viscosity, "gel-like" thicker formulas yet provide relief and protection for long periods of time and relief from the frequent mucus discharge that accompanies most severe dry eye.

Uses: Temporary relief of discomfort, burning, and irritation due to dryness of the eye. Lubricant and protectant against further irritation or to relieve dryness of the eye.

Directions: Put 1 or 2 drops in the affected eye(s) up to 4 times daily

Warnings: For external use only

Do not use if solution changes color or becomes cloudy

Do not touch the tip of container to any surface to avoid contamination

To avoid contamination replace cap after use

Stop use and ask a doctor if:

You feel eye pain

Changes in vision occur

Condition of redness or irritation persist for more than 72 hours

Keep out of the reach of children

If swallowed, get medical help or contact a Poison Control Center right away.

How Supplied: In 15 mL (0.5 fl. Oz) NDC 54891 00106.

(OSI) Eyetech
140 E. HANOVER AVENUE
CEDAR KNOLLS, NJ 07927

(OSI) Eyetech, Inc.
Direct inquiries to:
Phone: 973 775 4500
Fax 1: 973 539 9661
Fax 2: 973 539 2665

MACUGEN®   ℞
(pegaptanib sodium injection)

Description: MACUGEN® (pegaptanib sodium injection) is a sterile, aqueous solution containing pegaptanib sodium for intravitreous injection. Macugen is supplied in a single-dose, pre-filled syringe and is formulated as a 3.47 mg/mL solution, measured as the free acid form of the oligonucleotide. The active ingredient is 0.3 mg of the free acid form of the oligonucleotide without polyethylene glycol, in a nominal volume of 90 μL. This dose is equivalent to 1.6 mg of pegaptanib sodium (pegylated oligonucleotide) or 0.32 mg when expressed as the sodium salt form of the oligonucleotide moiety. The product is a sterile, clear, preservative-free solution containing sodium chloride, monobasic sodium phosphate monohydrate, dibasic sodium phosphate heptahydrate, hydrochloric acid, and/or sodium hydroxide to adjust the pH and water for injection.

Pegaptanib sodium is a covalent conjugate of an oligonucleotide of twenty-eight nucleotides in length that terminates in a pentylamino linker, to which two 20-kilodalton monomethoxy polyethylene glycol (PEG) units are covalently attached via the two amino groups on a lysine residue.

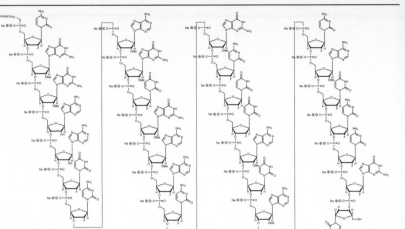

Pegaptanib sodium is represented by the following structural formula:
[See figure above]
Where R is

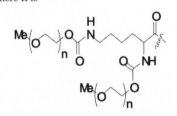

and n is approximately 450.

The chemical name for pegaptanib sodium is as follows: RNA, ((2'-deoxy-2'-fluoro)C-G_m-G_m-A-A-(2'-deoxy-2'-fluoro)U-(2'-deoxy-2'-fluoro)C-A_m-G_m-(2'-deoxy-2'-fluoro)U-G_m-A_m-A_m-(2'-deoxy-2'-fluoro)U-G_m-(2'-deoxy-2'-fluoro)C-(2'-deoxy-2'-fluoro)U-(2'-deoxy-2'-fluoro)U-A_m-(2'-deoxy-2'-fluoro)U-A_m-(2'-deoxy-2'-fluoro)C-A_m-(2''-deoxy-2'fluoro)U-(2'-deoxy-2'-fluoro)C-(2'-deoxy-2'-fluoro)C-G_m-(3'→3')-dT), 5'-ester with α,α'-[4,12-dioxo-6-[[[5-(phosphoonoxy)pentyl]amino]carbonyl]-3,13-dioxa-5,11-diaza-1,15-pentadecanediyl]-bis[ω -methoxypoly(oxy-1,2-ethanediyl)], sodium salt.

The molecular formula for pegaptanib sodium is $C_{294}H_{342}F_{13}N_{107}Na_{28}O_{188}P_{28}[C_2H_4O]_n$ (where n is approximately 900) and the molecular weight is approximately 50 kilodaltons. Macugen is formulated to have an osmolality of 280-360 mOsm/Kg, and a pH of 6–7.

Clinical Pharmacology:
Mechanism of Action

Pegaptanib is a selective vascular endothelial growth factor (VEGF) antagonist. VEGF is a secreted protein that selectively binds and activates its receptors located primarily on the surface of vascular endothelial cells. VEGF induces angiogenesis, and increases vascular permeability and inflammation, all of which are thought to contribute to the progression of the neovascular (wet) form of age-related macular degeneration (AMD), a leading cause of blindness. VEGF has been implicated in blood retinal barrier breakdown and pathological ocular neovascularization.

Pegaptanib is an aptamer, a pegylated modified oligonucleotide, which adopts a three-dimensional conformation that enables it to bind to extracellular VEGF. Under in vitro testing conditions, pegaptanib binds to the major pathological VEGF isoform, extracellular $VEGF_{165}$, thereby inhibiting $VEGF_{165}$ binding to its VEGF receptors. The inhibition of $VEGF_{164}$, the rodent counterpart of human $VEGF_{165}$, was effective at suppressing pathological neovascularization.

Pharmacokinetics
Absorption

In animals, pegaptanib is slowly absorbed into the systemic circulation from the eye after intravitreous administration. The rate of absorption from the eye is the rate limiting step in the disposition of pegaptanib in animals and is likely to be the rate limiting step in humans. In humans, a mean maximum plasma concentration of about 80 ng/mL occurs within 1 to 4 days after a 3 mg monocular dose (10 times the recommended dose). The mean area under the plasma concentration-time curve (AUC) is about 25 μg·hr/mL at this dose.

Distribution/Metabolism/Excretion

Twenty-four hours after intravitreous administration of a radiolabeled dose of pegaptanib to both eyes of rabbits, radioactivity was mainly distributed in vitreous fluid, retina, and aqueous fluid. After intravitreous and intravenous administrations of radiolabeled pegaptanib to rabbits, the highest concentrations of radioactivity (excluding the eye for the intravitreous dose) were obtained in the kidney. In rabbits, the component nucleotide, 2'-fluorouridine is found in plasma and urine after single radiolabeled pegaptanib intravenous and intravitreous doses. In rabbits, pegaptanib is eliminated as parent drug and metabolites primarily in the urine.

Based on preclinical data, pegaptanib is metabolized by endo- and exonucleases.

In humans, after a 3 mg monocular dose (10 times the recommended dose), the average (± standard deviation) apparent plasma half-life of pegaptanib is 10 (±4) days.

Special Populations

Plasma concentrations do not appear to be affected by age or gender, but have not been studied in patients under the age of 50.

Renal Insufficiency

Dose adjustment for patients with renal impairment is not needed when administering the 0.3 mg dose.

Following a single 3 mg dose (10 times the recommended dose), in patients with severe (N = 7), moderate (N = 18), and mild (N = 10) renal impairment, the mean (CV%) pegaptanib AUC values were 37.8 (17%), 26.7 (31%), and 23.6 (21%) μg.hr/mL, respectively. The corresponding Cmax values were 96.8 (23%), 81.6 (29.2%), and 66.5 (47%) ng/mL, respectively.

In patients with renal impairment, following administration of 3 mg pegaptanib doses every 6 weeks, the last detectable pegaptanib concentrations in plasma after the fourth dose were highly variable (ranging from 8 ng/mL to 66 ng/ mL) and the variability was more pronounced in patients with severe renal impairment.

Hemodialysis
Macugen has not been studied in patients requiring hemodialysis.

Hepatic Impairment
Macugen has not been studied in patients with hepatic impairment.

Clinical Studies
Macugen was studied in two controlled, double-masked, and identically designed randomized studies in patients with neovascular AMD. Patients were randomized to receive control (sham treatment) or 0.3 mg, 1 mg or 3 mg Macugen administered as intravitreous injections every 6 weeks for 48 weeks. A total of approximately 1200 patients were enrolled with 892 patients receiving Macugen and 298 receiving a sham injection. The median age of the patients was 77 years. Patients received a mean 8.5 treatments out of a possible 9 total treatments across all treatment arms. Patients were re-randomized between treatment and no treatment during the second year. Patients who continued treatment in year 2 received a mean of 16 treatments out of a possible total 17 overall.

The two trials enrolled patients with neovascular AMD characteristics including classic, occult, and mixed lesions of up to 12 disc areas and baseline visual acuity in the study eye between 20/40 and 20/320. The primary efficacy endpoint was the proportion of patients losing less than 15 letters of visual acuity, from baseline up to 54 week assessment. Verteporfin photodynamic therapy (PDT) usage was permitted at the discretion of the investigators in patients with predominantly classic lesions.

The groups treated with Macugen 0.3 mg exhibited a statistically significant result in both trials for the primary efficacy endpoint at 1 year: Study EOP1003, Macugen 73% vs. Sham 60%; Study EOP1004, Macugen 67% vs. Sham 53%. Concomitant use of PDT overall was low. More sham treated patients (75/296) received PDT than Macugen 0.3 mg treated patients (58/294).

On average, Macugen 0.3 mg treated patients and sham treated patients continued to experience vision loss. However, the rate of vision decline in the Macugen treated group was slower than the rate in the patients who received sham treatment. See Figure 1.

[See figure 1 above]

At the end of the first year (week 54), approximately 1050 of the original 1200 patients were re-randomized to either continue the same treatment or to discontinue treatment through week 102. See Figure 2.

Macugen was less effective during the second year than during the first year. The percentage of patients losing less than 15 letters from baseline to week 102 was: Study EOP1003, Macugen 38/67 (57%); Sham 30/54 (56%); Study EOP1004, Macugen 40/66 (61%); Sham 18/53 (34%).

[See figure 2 above]

Dose levels above 0.3 mg did not demonstrate any additional benefit.

The safety or efficacy of Macugen beyond 2 years has not been demonstrated.

Indications and Usage: Macugen is indicated for the treatment of neovascular (wet) age-related macular degeneration.

Contraindications: Macugen is contraindicated in patients with ocular or periocular infections.

Macugen is contraindicated in patients with known hypersensitivity to pegaptanib sodium or any other excipient in this product.

Warnings: Intravitreous injections including those with Macugen have been associated with endophthalmitis. Proper aseptic injection technique should always be utilized when administering Macugen. In addition, patients should be monitored during the week following the injec-

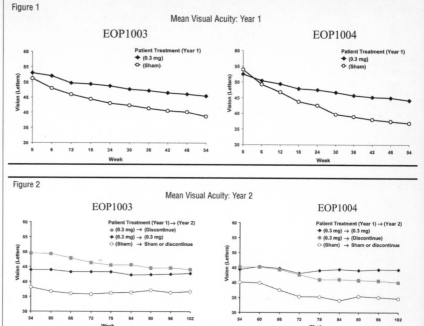

Figure 1

Mean Visual Acuity: Year 1

EOP1003

EOP1004

Figure 2

Mean Visual Acuity: Year 2

EOP1003

EOP1004

tion to permit early treatment, should an infection occur (see **DOSAGE AND ADMINISTRATION**).

Increases in intraocular pressure have been seen within 30 minutes of injection with Macugen. Therefore, intraocular pressure as well as the perfusion of the optic nerve head should be monitored and managed appropriately.

Precautions:
General
FOR OPHTHALMIC INTRAVITREAL INJECTION ONLY.

Rare cases of anaphylaxis/anaphylactoid reactions, including angioedema, have been reported in the post-marketing experience following the Macugen intravitreal administration procedure (see ADVERSE EVENTS and DOSAGE AND ADMINISTRATION).

Information for Patients
In the days following Macugen administration, patients are at risk for the development of endophthalmitis. If the eye becomes red, sensitive to light, painful or develops a change in vision, the patient should seek the immediate care with their ophthalmologist.

Drug Interactions
Drug interaction studies have not been conducted with Macugen. Pegaptanib is metabolized by nucleases and is generally not affected by the cytochrome P450 system.

Two early clinical studies conducted in patients who received Macugen alone and in combination with PDT revealed no apparent difference in the plasma pharmacokinetics of pegaptanib.

Carcinogenesis, Mutagenesis, Impairment of Fertility
Carcinogenicity studies with pegaptanib have not been conducted.

Pegaptanib and its monomer component nucleotides (2'-MA, 2'-MG, 2'-FU, 2'-FC) were evaluated for genotoxicity in a battery of *in vitro* and *in vivo* assay systems. Pegaptanib, 2'-O-methyladenosine (2'-MA), and 2'-O-methylguanosine (2'-MG) were negative in all assay systems evaluated. 2'-fluorouridine (2'-FU) and 2'-fluorocytidine (2'-FC) were non-clastogenic and were negative in all *S. typhimurium* tester strains, but produced a non-dose related increase in revertant frequency in

a single *E. coli* tester strain. Pegaptanib, 2'-FU, and 2'-FC tested negative in cell transformation assays.

No data are available to evaluate male or female mating or fertility indices.

Pregnancy
Teratogenic Effects: Pregnancy Category B. Pegaptanib produced no maternal toxicity and no evidence of teratogenicity or fetal mortality in mice at intravenous doses of up to 40 mg/kg/day (about 7,000 times the recommended human monocular ophthalmic dose of 0.3 mg/eye). Pegaptanib crosses the placenta in mice. There are no studies in pregnant women. The potential risk to humans is unknown. Macugen should be used during pregnancy only if the potential benefit to the mother justifies the potential risk to the fetus.

Nursing Mothers
It is not known whether pegaptanib is excreted in human milk. Because many drugs are excreted in human milk, caution should be exercised when Macugen is administered to a nursing woman.

Pediatric Use
Safety and effectiveness of Macugen in pediatric patients have not been studied.

Geriatric Use
Approximately 94% (834/892) of the patients treated with Macugen were ≥ 65 years of age and approximately 62% (553/892) were ≥ 75 years of age. No difference in treatment effect or systemic exposure was seen with increasing age.

Adverse Events: Serious adverse events related to the injection procedure occurring in < 1% of intravitreous injections included endophthalmitis (see **WARNINGS**), retinal detachment, and iatrogenic traumatic cataract. The most frequently reported adverse events in patients treated with Macugen 0.3 mg for up to two years were anterior chamber inflammation, blurred vision, cataract, conjunctival hemorrhage, corneal edema, eye discharge, eye irritation, eye pain, hypertension, increased intraocular pressure (IOP), ocular discomfort, punctate keratitis, reduced visual

Continued on next page

Macugen—Cont.

acuity, visual disturbance, vitreous floaters, and vitreous opacities. These events occurred in approximately 10-40% of patients.

The following events were reported in 6-10% of patients receiving Macugen 0.3 mg therapy:

Ocular: blepharitis, conjunctivitis, photopsia, vitreous disorder.

Non-Ocular: bronchitis, diarrhea, dizziness, headache, nausea, urinary tract infection.

The following events were reported in 1-5% of patients receiving Macugen 0.3 mg therapy:

Ocular: allergic conjunctivitis, conjunctival edema, corneal abrasion, corneal deposits, corneal epithelium disorder, endophthalmitis, eye inflammation, eye swelling, eyelid irritation, meibomianitis, mydriasis, periorbital hematoma, retinal edema, vitreous hemorrhage.

Non-Ocular: arthritis, bone spur, carotid artery occlusion, cerebrovascular accident, chest pain, contact dermatitis, contusion, diabetes mellitus, dyspepsia, hearing loss, pleural effusion, transient ischemic attack, urinary retention, vertigo, vomiting.

Post Marketing Experience: Anaphylaxis/anaphylactoid reactions, including angioedema, have been identified during postapproval use of Macugen. Because these reactions are reported voluntarily from a population of uncertain size, it is not always possible to reliably estimate their frequency or establish a causal relationship to drug exposure (see PRECAUTIONS and DOSAGE AND ADMINSTRATION).

Overdosage: Doses of Macugen up to 10 times the recommended dosage of 0.3 mg have been studied. No additional adverse events have been noted but there is decreased efficacy with doses above 1 mg.

Dosage and Administration: Macugen 0.3 mg should be administered once every six weeks by intravitreous injection into the eye to be treated.

Macugen should be inspected visually for particulate matter and discoloration prior to administration. Administration of the syringe contents involves attaching the threaded plastic plunger rod to the rubber stopper inside the barrel of the syringe. Do not pull back on the plunger. Remove the syringe needle cap. Holding the syringe with the needle pointing up, check the syringe for bubbles. If there are bubbles, gently tap the syringe with your finger until the bubbles rise to the top of the syringe. Slowly push the plunger up to force all the bubbles out of the syringe.

The injection procedure should be carried out under controlled aseptic conditions, which includes the use of sterile gloves, a sterile drape, and a sterile eyelid speculum (or equivalent). The patient's medical history for hypersensitivity reactions should be evaluated prior to performing the intravitreal procedure (see PRECAUTIONS and ADVERSE EVENTS). Adequate anesthesia and a broad-spectrum microbicide should be given prior to the injection.

Following the injection, patients should be monitored for elevation in intraocular pressure and for endophthalmitis. Monitoring may consist of a check for perfusion of the optic nerve head immediately after the injection, tonometry within 30 minutes following the injection, and biomicroscopy between two and seven days following the injection. Patients should be instructed to report any symptoms suggestive of endophthalmitis without delay.

No special dosage modification is required for any of the populations that have been studied (i.e. gender, elderly).

The safety and efficacy of Macugen therapy administered to both eyes concurrently have not been studied.

How Supplied: Macugen (pegaptanib sodium injection) is supplied in a single use 1 mL glass syringe with a gray rubber plunger containing 0.3 mg in a 90 µL deliverable volume. Each syringe is fitted with a fixed 27 gauge needle covered with a gray rubber needle shield and a rigid plastic outside sheath. All are contained in a foil pouch. The accompanying polystyrene plunger rod and white flange are in a separate foil pouch. The two foil pouches are packaged in a carton.

Storage

Store in the refrigerator at 2° to 8°C (36° to 46°F). Do not freeze or shake vigorously.

Rx only.

NDC 68782-001-01

Manufactured by:

Gilead Sciences, Inc
650 Cliffside Drive
San Dimas, CA 91773

(OSI) Eyetech
140 E. Hanover Avenue
Cedar Knolls, NJ 07927
Phone 973-775-9661
Fax 973-539-9661

Inspire Pharmaceuticals, Inc.

**4222 EMPEROR BOULEVARD
SUITE 200
DURHAM, NC 27703**

Direct Inquiries to:
Telephone: 919-941-9777
Fax: 919-941-9797
E-mail: info@inspirepharm.com

ELESTAT® ℞
[ĕl-ĕ-stăt]
**(epinastine HCl ophthalmic solution) 0.05%
Sterile**

Description: ELESTAT® (epinastine HCl ophthalmic solution) 0.05% is a clear, colorless, sterile isotonic solution containing epinastine HCl, an antihistamine and an inhibitor of histamine release from the mast cell for topical administration to the eyes.

Epinastine HCl is represented by the following structural formula:

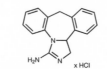

$C_{16}H_{15}N_3$ • HCl Mol. Wt. 285.78

Chemical Name: 3-Amino-9, 13b-dihydro-1H-dibenz[c,f]imidazo[1,5-a]azepine hydrochloride

Each mL contains: Active: Epinastine HCl 0.05% (0.5mg/mL) equivalent to epinastine 0.044% (0.44mg/mL); **Preservative:** Benzalkonium chloride 0.01%; **Inactives:** Edetate disodium; purified water; sodium chloride; sodium phosphate, monobasic; and sodium hydroxide and/or hydrochloric acid (to adjust the pH). ELESTAT® has a pH of approximately 7 and an osmolality range of 250 to 310 mOsm/kg.

Clinical Pharmacology: Epinastine is a topically active, direct H_1-receptor antagonist and an inhibitor of the release of histamine from the mast cell. Epinastine is selective for the histamine H_1-receptor and has affinity for the histamine H_2-receptor. Epinastine also possesses affinity for the $α_1$-, $α_2$-, and 5-HT_2- receptors. Epinastine does not penetrate the blood/brain

barrier and, therefore, is not expected to induce side effects of the central nervous system.

Fourteen subjects, with allergic conjunctivitis, received one drop of ELESTAT® ophthalmic solution in each eye twice daily for seven days. On day seven average maximum epinastine plasma concentrations of 0.04 ± 0.014 ng/ml were reached after about two hours indicating low systemic exposure. While these concentrations represented an increase over those seen following a single dose, the day 1 and day 7 Area Under the Curve (AUC) values were unchanged indicating that there is no increase in systemic absorption with multiple dosing. Epinastine is 64% bound to plasma proteins. The total systemic clearance is approximately 56 L/hr and the terminal plasma elimination half-life is about 12 hours. Epinastine is mainly excreted unchanged. About 55% of an intravenous dose is recovered unchanged in the urine with about 30% in feces. Less than 10% is metabolized. The renal elimination is mainly via active tubular secretion.

Clinical studies: Epinastine HCl 0.05% has been shown to be significantly superior to vehicle for improving ocular itching in patients with allergic conjunctivitis in clinical studies using two different models: (1) conjunctival antigen challenge (CAC) where patients were dosed and then received antigen instilled into the inferior conjunctival fornix; and (2) environmental field studies where patients were dosed and evaluated during allergy season in their natural habitat. Results demonstrated a rapid onset of action for epinastine HCl 0.05% within 3 to 5 minutes after conjunctival antigen challenge. Duration of effect was shown to be 8 hours, making a twice daily regimen suitable. This dosing regimen was shown to be safe and effective for up to 8 weeks, without evidence of tachyphylaxis.

Indications and Usage: ELESTAT® ophthalmic solution is indicated for the prevention of itching associated with allergic conjunctivitis.

Contraindications: ELESTAT® ophthalmic solution is contraindicated in those patients who have shown hypersensitivity to epinastine or to any of the other ingredients.

Warnings: ELESTAT® is for topical ophthalmic use only and not for injection or oral use.

Precautions:

Information for Patients: Patients should be advised not to wear a contact lens if their eye is red. ELESTAT® ophthalmic solution should not be used to treat contact lens related irritation. The preservative in ELESTAT®, benzalkonium chloride, may be absorbed by soft contact lenses. Contact lenses should be removed prior to instillation of ELESTAT® ophthalmic solution and may be reinserted after 10 minutes following its administration.

Patients should be instructed to avoid allowing the tip of the dispensing container to contact the eye, surrounding structures, fingers, or any other surface in order to avoid contamination of the solution by common bacteria known to cause ocular infections. Serious damage to the eye and subsequent loss of vision may result from using contaminated solutions. Bottle should be kept tightly closed when not in use.

Carcinogenesis, Mutagenesis, Impairment of Fertility: In 18-month or 2-year dietary carcinogenicity studies in mice or rats, respectively, epinastine was not carcinogenic at doses up to 40 mg/kg [approximately 30,000 times higher than the maximum recommended ocular human dose of 0.0014 mg/kg/day (MROHD) on a mg/kg basis, assuming 100% absorption in humans and animals].

Epinastine in newly synthesized batches was negative for mutagenicity in the Ames/ Salmo-

nella assay and *in vitro* chromosome aberration assay using human lymphocytes. Positive results were seen with early batches of epinastine in two *in vitro* chromosomal aberration studies conducted in 1980s with human peripheral lymphocytes and with V79 cells, respectively. Epinastine was negative in the *in vivo* clastogenicity studies, including the mouse micronucleus assay and chromosome aberration assay in Chinese hamsters. Epinastine was also negative in the cell transformation assay using Syrian hamster embryo cells, V79/HGPRT mammalian cell point mutation assay, and *in vivo/in vitro* unscheduled DNA synthesis assay using rat primary hepatocytes.

Epinastine had no effect on fertility of male rats. Decreased fertility in female rats was observed at an oral dose up to approximately 90,000 times the MROHD.

Pregnancy: Teratogenic Effects: Pregnancy Category C In an embryofetal developmental study in pregnant rats, maternal toxicity with no embryofetal effects was observed at an oral dose that was approximately 150,000 times the MROHD. Total resorptions and abortion were observed in an embryofetal study in pregnant rabbits at an oral dose that was approximately 55,000 times the MROHD. In both studies, no drug-induced teratogenic effects were noted.

Epinastine reduced pup body weight gain following an oral dose to pregnant rats that was approximately 90,000 times the MROHD.

There are, however, no adequate and well-controlled studies in pregnant women. Because animal reproduction studies are not always predictive of human response, ELESTAT® ophthalmic solution should be used during pregnancy only if the potential benefit justifies the potential risk to the fetus.

Nursing Mothers: A study in lactating rats revealed excretion of epinastine in the breast milk. It is not known whether this drug is excreted in human milk. Because many drugs are excreted in human milk, caution should be exercised when ELESTAT® ophthalmic solution is administered to a nursing woman.

Pediatric Use: Safety and effectiveness in pediatric patients below the age of 3 years have not been established.

Geriatric Use: No overall differences in safety or effectiveness have been observed between elderly and younger patients.

Adverse Reactions: The most frequently reported ocular adverse events occurring in approximately 1-10% of patients were burning sensation in the eye, folliculosis, hyperemia, and pruritus.

The most frequently reported non-ocular adverse events were infection (cold symptoms and upper respiratory infections) seen in approximately 10% of patients, and headache, rhinitis, sinusitis, increased cough, and pharyngitis seen in approximately 1-3% of patients. Some of these events were similar to the underlying disease being studied.

Dosage and Administration: The recommended dosage is one drop in each eye twice a day.

Treatment should be continued throughout the period of exposure (i.e., until the pollen season is over or until exposure to the offending allergen is terminated), even when symptoms are absent.

How Supplied: ELESTAT® (epinastine HCl ophthalmic solution) 0.05% is supplied sterile in opaque white LDPE plastic bottles with dropper tips and white high impact polystyrene (HIPS) caps as follows:

5 mL in 10 mL bottle   NDC 0023-9201-05
Storage: Store at 15-25°C (59-77°F). Keep bottle tightly closed and out of the reach of children.

Rx Only   August 2004
© 2007 Allergan, Inc.
Irvine, CA 92612, U.S.A.
® marks owned by Allergan, Inc.
Licensed from Boehringer Ingelheim Int. GmbH
Inspire and the Inspire logo are registered trademarks of Inspire Pharmaceuticals Inc.
71634US11P

Johnson & Johnson Healthcare Product Division of McNeil PPC, Inc.
**199 GRANDVIEW ROAD
SKILLMAN, NJ 08558**

Direct Inquiries to:
Consumer Affairs
1 888 734 7648

VISINE TEARS®   OTC
Lubricant Eye Drops
Dry Eye Relief

Description: Visine Tears® Lubricant Eye Drops cools and comforts your dry, scratchy, irritated eyes, and helps them feel their best. It relieves the dryness caused by computer use, reading, wind, heat and air conditioning, while it protects your eyes from further irritation. This "natural tears formula" contains 10 important ingredients found in your own natural tears. Visine Tears is safe to use as often as needed.

Active Ingredients:	Purpose:
Glycerin 0.2%	Lubricant
Hypromellose 0.2%	Lubricant
Polyethylene glycol 400 1%	Lubricant

Uses:
• for the temporary relief of burning and irritation due to dryness of the eye
• for protection against further irritation
Warnings:
When using this product
• remove contact lenses before using
• do not use if this solution changes color or becomes cloudy
• do not touch tip of container to any surface to avoid contamination
• replace cap after each use
Stop use and ask a doctor if
• you feel eye pain
• changes in vision occur
• redness or irritation of the eye lasts
• condition worsens or lasts more than 72 hours
If pregnant or breast-feeding, ask a health professional before use.
Keep out of reach of children. If swallowed, get medical help or contact a Poison Control Center right away.
Directions:
• put 1 or 2 drops in the affected eye(s) as needed
• children under 6 years of age: ask a doctor
Other Information:
• store at 15° to 25°C (59° to 77°F)
Inactive Ingredients: ascorbic acid, benzalkonium chloride, boric acid, dextrose, disodium phosphate, glycine, magnesium chloride, potassium chloride, purified water, sodium borate, sodium chloride, sodium citrate, and sodium lactate
Questions? call **1-888-734-7348**, weekdays, 9 AM – 5 PM EST
Caution: Do not use if Visine imprinted neckband on bottle is broken or missing.

How Supplied: In ½ FL OZ and 1 FL OZ plastic dispenser bottle.
Shown in Product Identification Guide, page 105

VISINE® PURE TEARS PORTABLES   OTC
Lubricant Eye Drops
Dry Eye Relief
Preservative Free Single-Use Vials

Description: Visine® Pure Tears Portables Preservative Free Lubricant Eye Drops cools and comforts your dry, scratchy irritated eyes, and helps them feel their best. It relieves the dryness caused by computer use, reading, wind, heat and air conditioning, while it protects your eyes from further irritation. Specially formulated for people whose eyes are sensitive to preservatives, Visine® Pure Tears Portables is sealed in convenient single-use vials and is safe to use as often as needed. This "natural tears formula" contains 10 important ingredients found in your own natural tears.

Active Ingredients:	Purpose:
Glycerin 0.2%	Lubricant
Hypromellose 0.2%	Lubricant
Polyethylene glycol 400 1%	Lubricant

Uses:
• for the temporary relief of burning and irritation due to dryness of the eye
• for protection against further irritation
Warnings:
When using this product
• remove contact lenses before using
• do not use if this solution changes color or becomes cloudy
• do not touch tip of container to any surface to avoid contamination
• do not reuse; once opened, discard
Stop use and ask a doctor if
• you feel eye pain
• changes in vision occur
• redness or irritation of the eye lasts
• condition worsens or lasts more than 72 hours
If pregnant or breast-feeding, ask a health professional before use.
Keep out of reach of children. If swallowed, get medical help or contact a Poison Control Center right away.
Directions:
• put 1 or 2 drops in the affected eye(s) as needed
• children under 6 years of age: ask a doctor
Other Information:
• store at 15° to 25°C (59° to 77°F)
Inactive Ingredients: ascorbic acid, dextrose, disodium phosphate, glycine, magnesium chloride, potassium chloride, purified water, sodium chloride, sodium citrate, sodium lactate, and sodium phosphate
Questions? call **1-888-734-7348**, weekdays, 9 AM - 5 PM EST
Caution: Use only if single-use container is intact.
How Supplied: 1 box contains 28 single-use containers, 0.01 FL OZ (0.4 mL) each
Shown in Product Identification Guide, page 105

VISINE® PURE TEARS   OTC
Lubricant Eye Drops
Dry Eye Relief
SINGLE-DROP DISPENSER

For the temporary relief of burning and irritation due to dryness of the eye and for use as a protectant against further irritation.

Continued on next page

Visine Pure Tears—Cont.

Description:
- Gets The Dry Out®.
- "Natural Tears Formula" contains 10 important ingredients found in your own natural tears. Refreshes tired eyes.
- An advanced alternative to single-use vials for frequent users of artificial tears
- Instead of adding preservatives to the formula, Visine Pure Tears uses an innovative dispenser with an antibacterial silver coil in the tip to help prevent contamination.
- Unique "one-click, one drop" dispenser is simple to use, with no mess or waste.

Active Ingredients:	Purpose:
Glycerin 0.2%	Lubricant
Hypromellose 0.2%	Lubricant
Polyethylene glycol 400 1%	Lubricant

Uses:
- for the temporary relief of burning and irritation due to dryness of the eye
- for protection against further irritation

Warnings:
When using this product
- remove contact lenses before using
- do not use if this solution changes color or becomes cloudy
- do not touch tip of container to any surface to avoid contamination
- replace cap after each use

Stop use and ask a doctor if
- you feel eye pain
- changes in vision occur
- redness or irritation of the eye lasts
- condition worsens or lasts more than 72 hours

If pregnant or breast-feeding, ask a health professional before use.

Keep out of reach of children. If swallowed, get medical help or contact a Poison Control Center right away.

Directions:
- put 1 or 2 drops in the affected eye(s) as needed
- children under 6 years of age: ask a doctor

Other Information:
- store at 15° to 25°C (59° to 77°F)

Inactive Ingredients: ascorbic acid, dextrose, disodium phosphate, glycine, magnesium chloride, potassium chloride, purified water, sodium chloride, sodium citrate, sodium lactate, and sodium phosphate

Questions? call **1-888-734-7348**, weekdays, 9 AM - 5PM EST

Caution: Do not use if Visine® imprinted seals on top or bottom flaps of carton are broken or missing.

How Supplied: 0.3 FL OZ bottle
Shown in Product Identification Guide, page 105

VISINE TEARS® LASTING RELIEF   OTC
Lubricant Eye Drops
Dry Eye Relief

Description: Visine Tears Lasting Relief Lubricant Eye Drops cools and comforts your dry, scratchy, irritated eyes, and helps them feel their best. It relieves the dryness caused by computer use, reading, wind, heat and air conditioning, while it protects your eyes from further irritation. Visine Tears Lasting Relief is an advanced dry eye formula made to stay on the eye longer. This "natural tears" formula contains 10 important ingredients found in your own natural tears.

Active Ingredients	Purpose
Glycerin 0.2%	Lubricant
Hypromellose 0.36%	Lubricant
Polyethylene glycol 400 1%	Lubricant

Uses:
- for the temporary relief of burning, irritation, and discomfort due to dryness of the eye or exposure to wind or sun
- for protection against further irritation

Warnings: **When using this product**
- remove contact lenses before using
- do not use if this solution changes color or becomes cloudy
- do not touch tip of container to any surface to avoid contamination
- replace cap after each use

Stop use and ask a doctor if
- you feel eye pain
- changes in vision occur
- redness or irritation of the eye lasts
- condition worsens or lasts more than 72 hours

If pregnant or breast-feeding, ask a health professional before use.

Keep out of reach of children. If swallowed, get medical help or contact a Poison Control Center right away.

Directions:
- put 1 or 2 drops in the affected eye(s) as needed
- children under 6 years of age: ask a doctor

Other Information
- store at 15° to 25°C (59° to 77°F)

Inactive Ingredients: ascorbic acid, benzalkonium chloride, boric acid, dextrose, glycine, magnesium chloride, potassium chloride, purified water, sodium borate, sodium chloride, sodium citrate dihydrate, sodium lactate, and sodium phosphate dibasic

Questions? call **1-888-734-7348**, weekdays, 9 AM – 5 PM EST

Date: 09/13/06 (Revised Final)
Shown in Product Identification Guide, page 105

King Pharmaceuticals, Inc.
501 FIFTH STREET
BRISTOL, TN 37620

Direct Inquiries:
Customer Service:
Telephone: 1 (888) 358-6436
Fax: 1 (866) 990-0545
To report an Adverse Drug Experience:
Telephone: 1 (800) 546-4905
Fax: 1 (423) 990-0519

CORTISPORIN®   ℞
Ophthalmic Suspension Sterile
[cŏrtĭ-spŏrin]
(neomycin and polymyxin B sulfates and hydrocortisone ophthalmicsuspension, USP)

Description: CORTISPORIN Ophthalmic Suspension (neomycin and polymyxin B sulfates and hydrocortisone ophthalmic suspension) is a sterile antimicrobial and anti-inflammatory suspension for ophthalmic use. Each mL contains: neomycin sulfate equivalent to 3.5 mg neomycin base, polymyxin B sulfate equivalent to 10,000 polymyxin B units, and hydrocortisone 10 mg (1%). The vehicle contains thimerosal 0.001% (added as a preservative) and the inactive ingredients cetyl alcohol, glyceryl monostearate, mineral oil, polyoxyl 40 stearate, propylene glycol, and Water for Injection. Sulfuric acid may be added to adjust pH.
Neomycin sulfate is the sulfate salt of neomycin B and C, which are produced by the growth of *Streptomyces fradiae* Waksman (Fam. Streptomycetaceae). It has a potency equivalent of not less than 600 µg of neomycin stan-

dard per mg, calculated on an anhydrous basis. The structural formulae are:

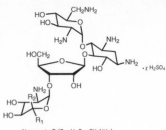

Neomycin B (R₁=H, R₂=CH₂NH₂)
Neomycin C (R₁=CH₂NH₂, R₂=H)

Polymyxin B sulfate is the sulfate salt of polymyxin B₁ and B₂, which are produced by the growth of *Bacillus polymyxa* (Prazmowski) Migula (Fam. Bacillaceae). It has a potency of not less than 6,000 polymyxin B units per mg, calculated on an anhydrous basis. The structural formulae are:

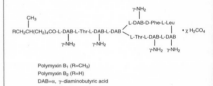

Polymyxin B₁ (R=CH₃)
Polymyxin B₂ (R=H)
DAB=α, γ-diaminobutyric acid

Hydrocortisone, 11β,17,21-trihydroxypregn-4-ene-3,20-dione, is an antiinflammatory hormone. Its structural formula is:

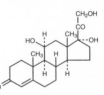

How Supplied: Plastic DROP DOSE® dispenser bottle of 7.5 mL (NDC 61570-036-75).
Rx only.
Store at 15° to 25°C (59° to 77°F).
Prescribing Information as of October 2003.
Monarch Pharmaceuticals®
Distributed by: Monarch Pharmaceuticals, Inc., Bristol, TN 37620
(A wholly owned subsidiary of King Pharmaceuticals, Inc.)
Manufactured by: DSM Pharmaceuticals, Inc., Greenville, NC   27834
     455232
Shown in Product Identification Guide, page 105

NEOSPORIN®   ℞
Ophthalmic Solution Sterile
(neomycin and polymyxin B sulfates and gramicidin ophthalmic solution, USP)

Description: NEOSPORIN Ophthalmic Solution (neomycin and polymyxin B sulfates and gramicidin ophthalmic solution) is a sterile antimicrobial solution for ophthalmic use. Each mL contains: neomycin sulfate equivalent to 1.75 mg neomycin base, polymyxin B sulfate equivalent to 10,000 polymyxin B units, and gramicidin 0.025 mg. The vehicle contains alcohol 0.5%, thimerosal 0.001% (added as a preservative), and the inactive ingredients propylene glycol, polyoxyethylene polyoxypropylene compound, sodium chloride, and Water for Injection. Neomycin sulfate is the sulfate salt of neomycin B and C, which are produced by the growth of *Streptomyces fradiae* Waksman (Fam. Streptomycetaceae). It has a potency equivalent of not less than 600 µg of neomycin standard per mg, calculated on an anhydrous basis. The structural formulae are:

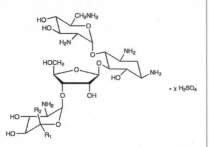

Neomycin B (R₁=H, R₂=CH₂NH₂)
Neomycin C (R₁=CH₂NH₂, R₂=H)

Polymyxin B sulfate is the sulfate salt of polymyxin B_1 and B_2 which are produced by the growth of *Bacillus polymyxa* (Prazmowski) Migula (Fam. Bacillaceae). It has a potency of not less than 6,000 polymyxin B units per mg, calculated on an anhydrous basis. The structural formulae are:

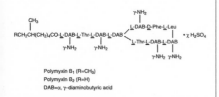

Polymyxin B_1 (R=CH₃)
Polymyxin B_2 (R=H)
DAB=α, γ-diaminobutyric acid

Gramicidin (also called Gramicidin D) is a mixture of three pairs of antibacterial substances (Gramicidin A, B, and C) produced by the growth of *Bacillus brevis* Dubos (Fam. Bacillaceae). It has a potency of not less than 900 µg of standard gramicidin per mg. The structural formulae are:

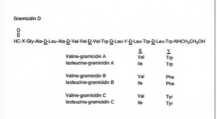

Gramicidin D

HC-X-Gly-Ala-D-Leu-Ala-D-Val-Val-D-Val-Trp-D-Leu-Y-D-Leu-Trp-D-Leu-Trp-NHCH₂CH₂OH

	X	Y
Valine-gramicidin A	Val	Trp
Isoleucine-gramicidin A	Ile	Trp
Valine-gramicidin B	Val	Phe
Isoleucine-gramicidin B	Ile	Phe
Valine-gramicidin C	Val	Tyr
Isoleucine-gramicidin C	Ile	Tyr

Clinical Pharmacology: A wide range of antibacterial action is provided by the overlapping spectra of neomycin, polymyxin B sulfate, and gramicidin.

Neomycin is bactericidal for many gram-positive and gram-negative organisms. It is an amino-glycoside antibiotic which inhibits protein synthesis by binding with ribosomal RNA and causing misreading of the bacterial genetic code.

Polymyxin B is bactericidal for a variety of gram-negative organisms. It increases the permeability of the bacterial cell membrane by interacting with the phospholipid components of the membrane.

Gramicidin is bactericidal for a variety of gram- positive organisms. It increases the permeability of the bacterial cell membrane to inorganic cations by forming a network of channels through the normal lipid bilayer of the membrane.

Microbiology: Neomycin sulfate, polymyxin B sulfate, and gramicidin together are considered active against the following microorganisms: *Staphylococcus aureus*, streptococci, including *Streptococcus pneumoniae*, *Escherichia coli*, *Haemophilus influenzae*, *Klebsiella / Enterobacter* species, *Neisseria* species, and *Pseudomonas aeruginosa*. The product does not provide adequate coverage against *Serratia marcescens*.

Indications and Usage: NEOSPORIN Ophthalmic Solution is indicated for the topical treatment of superficial infections of the external eye and its adnexa caused by susceptible bacteria. Such infections encompass conjunctivitis, keratitis and keratoconjunctivitis, blepharitis and blepharoconjunctivitis.

Contraindications: NEOSPORIN Ophthalmic Solution is contraindicated in individuals who have shown hypersensitivity to any of its components.

Warnings: NOT FOR INJECTION INTO THE EYE. NEOSPORIN Ophthalmic Solution should never be directly introduced into the anterior chamber of the eye or injected subconjunctivally.

Topical antibiotics, particularly neomycin sulfate, may cause cutaneous sensitization. A precise incidence of hypersensitivity reactions (primarily skin rash) due to topical antibiotics is not known. The manifestations of sensitization to topical antibiotics are usually itching, reddening, and edema of the conjunctiva and eyelid. A sensitization reaction may manifest simply as a failure to heal. During long-term use of topical antibiotic products, periodic examination for such signs is advisable, and the patient should be told to discontinue the product if they are observed. Symptoms usually subside quickly on withdrawing the medication. Application of products containing these ingredients should be avoided for the patient thereafter (see **PRECAUTIONS: General**).

Precautions:

General: As with other antibiotic preparations, prolonged use of NEOSPORIN Ophthalmic Solution may result in overgrowth of nonsusceptible organisms including fungi. If superinfection occurs, appropriate measures should be initiated.

Bacterial resistance to NEOSPORIN Ophthalmic Solution may also develop. If purulent discharge, inflammation, or pain becomes aggravated, the patient should discontinue use of the medication and consult a physician.

There have been reports of bacterial keratitis associated with the use of topical ophthalmic products in multiple-dose containers which have been inadvertently contaminated by patients, most of whom had a concurrent corneal disease or a disruption of the ocular epithelial surface (see **PRECAUTIONS: Information for Patients**).

Allergic cross-reactions may occur which could prevent the use of any or all of the following antibiotics for the treatment of future infections: kanamycin, paromomycin, streptomycin, and possibly gentamicin.

Information for Patients: Patients should be instructed to avoid allowing the tip of the dispensing container to contact the eye, eyelid, fingers, or any other surface. The use of this product by more than one person may spread infection.

Patients should also be instructed that ocular products, if handled improperly, can become contaminated by common bacteria known to cause ocular infections. Serious damage to the eye and subsequent loss of vision may result from using contaminated products (see **PRECAUTIONS: General**).

If the condition persists or gets worse, or if a rash or other allergic reaction develops, the patient should be advised to stop use and consult

a physician. Do not use this product if you are allergic to any of the listed ingredients.

Keep tightly closed when not in use. Keep out of reach of children.

Carcinogenesis, Mutagenesis, Impairment of Fertility: Long-term studies in animals to evaluate carcinogenic or mutagenic potential have not been conducted with polymyxin B sulfate or gramicidin. Treatment of cultured human lymphocytes in vitro with neomycin increased the frequency of chromosome aberrations at the highest concentration (80 µg/mL) tested. However, the effects of neomycin on carcinogenesis and mutagenesis in humans are unknown. Polymyxin B has been reported to impair the motility of equine sperm, but its effects on male or female fertility are unknown.

Pregnancy: *Teratogenic Effects:*   Teratogenic Effects: Pregnancy Category C. Animal reproduction studies have not been conducted with neomycin sulfate, polymyxin B sulfate, or gramicidin. It is also not known whether NEOSPORIN Ophthalmic Solution can cause fetal harm when administered to a pregnant woman or can affect reproduction capacity. NEOSPORIN Ophthalmic Solution should be given to a pregnant woman only if clearly needed.

Nursing Mothers: It is not known whether this drug is excreted in human milk. Because many drugs are excreted in human milk, caution should be exercised when NEOSPORIN Ophthalmic Solution is administered to a nursing woman.

Pediatric Use: Safety and effectiveness in pediatric patients have not been established.

Geriatric Use: Clinical studies of Neosporin® Ophthalmic Solution did not include sufficient numbers of subjects aged 65 and over to determine whether they respond differently from younger subjects. Other reported clinical experience has not identified differences in responses between the elderly and younger patients.

Adverse Reactions: Adverse reactions have occurred with the anti-infective components of NEOSPORIN Ophthalmic Solution. The exact incidence is not known. Reactions occurring most often are allergic sensitization reactions including itching, swelling, and conjunctival erythema (see **WARNINGS**). More serious hypersensitivity reactions, including anaphylaxis, have been reported rarely.

Local irritation on instillation has also been reported.

Dosage and Administration: Instill one or two drops into the affected eye every 4 hours for 7 to 10 days. In severe infections, dosage may be increased to as much as two drops every hour.

How Supplied: Drop Dose® of 10 mL (plastic dispenser bottle) (NDC 61570–045–10).

Rx only.

Store at 15° to 25°C (59° to 77°F) and protect from light.

Prescribing Information as of July 2004.

Distributed by: Monarch Pharmaceuticals, Inc., Bristol, TN 37620

(A wholly owned subsidiary of King Pharmaceuticals, Inc.)

Manufactured by: DSM Pharmaceuticals, Inc., Greenville, NC 27834

VIROPTIC®   ℞
Ophthalmic Solution, 1% Sterile
(trifluridine ophthalmic solution)

Description: VIROPTIC is the brand name for trifluridine (also known as trifluorothymidine, F_3TdR, F_3T), an antiviral drug for topical treatment of epithelial keratitis caused by her-

Continued on next page

Viroptic—Cont.

pes simplex virus. The chemical name of trifluridine is α,α,α-trifluorothymidine; it has the following structural formula:

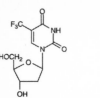

MW=296.21 $C_{10}H_{11}F_3N_2O_5$

VIROPTIC sterile ophthalmic solution contains 1% trifluridine in an aqueous solution with acetic acid and sodium acetate (buffers), sodium chloride, and thimerosal 0.001% (added as a preservative). The pH range is 5.5 to 6.0 and osmolality is approximately 283 mOsm.

Clinical Pharmacology: Trifluridine is a fluorinated pyrimidine nucleoside with *in vitro* and *in vivo* activity against herpes simplex virus, types 1 and 2 and vacciniavirus. Some strains of adenovirus are also inhibited *in vitro*. VIROPTIC is also effective in the treatment of epithelial keratitis that has not responded clinically to the topical administration of idoxuridine or when ocular toxicity or hypersensitivity to idoxuridine has occurred. In a smaller number of patients found to be resistant to topical vidarabine, VIROPTIC was also effective.

Trifluridine interferes with DNA synthesis in cultured mammalian cells. However, its antiviral mechanism of action is not completely known.

In vitro perfusion studies on excised rabbit corneas have shown that trifluridine penetrates the intact cornea as evidenced by recovery of parental drug and its major metabolite, 5-carboxy-2′-deoxyuridine, on the endothelial side of the cornea. Absence of the corneal epithelium enhances the penetration of trifluridine approximately two-fold.

Intraocular penetration of trifluridine occurs after topical instillation of VIROPTIC into human eyes. Decreased corneal integrity or stromal or uveal inflammation may enhance the penetration of trifluridine into the aqueous humor. Unlike the results of ocular penetration of trifluridine *in vitro*, 5-carboxy-2′- deoxyuridine was not found in detectable concentrations within the aqueous humor of the human eye. Systemic absorption of trifluridine following therapeutic dosing with VIROPTIC appears to be negligible. No detectable concentrations of trifluridine or 5-carboxy-2′-deoxyuridine were found in the sera of adult healthy normal subjects who had VIROPTIC instilled into their eyes seven times daily for 14 consecutive days.

Clinical Studies: During a controlled multicenter clinical trial, 92 of 97 (95%) patients (78 of 81 with dendritic and 14 of 16 with geographic ulcers) responded to therapy with VIROPTIC as evidenced by complete corneal re-epithelialization within the 14-day therapy period. Fifty-six of 75 (75%) patients (49 of 58 with dendritic and 7 of 17 with geographic ulcers) responded to idoxuridine therapy. The mean time to corneal re-epithelialization for dendritic ulcers (6 days) and geographic ulcers (7 days) was similar for both therapies.

In other clinical studies. VIROPTIC was evaluated in the treatment of herpes simplex virus keratitis in patients who were unresponsive or intolerant to the topical administration of idoxuridine or vidarabine. VIROPTIC was effective in 138 of 150 (92%) patients (109 of 114 with dendritic and 29 of 36 with geographic ulcers) as evidenced by corneal re-

epithelialization. The mean time to corneal re-epithelialization was 6 days for patients with dendritic ulcers and 12 days for patients with geographic ulcers.

The clinical efficacy of VIROPTIC in the treatment of stromal keratitis and uveitis due to herpes simplex virus or ophthalmic infections caused by vacciniavirus and adenovirus has not been established by well-controlled clinical trials. VIROPTIC has not been shown to be effective in the prophylaxis of herpes simplex virus keratoconjunctivitis and epithelial keratitis by well-controlled clinical trials. VIROPTIC is not effective against bacterial, fungal, or chlamydial infections of the cornea or nonviral trophic lesions.

Indications and Usage: VIROPTIC Ophthalmic Solution, 1% (trifluridine ophthalmic solution) is indicated for the treatment of primay keratoconjunctivitis and recurrent epithelial keratitis due to herpes simplex virus, types 1 and 2.

Contraindications: VIROPTIC Ophthalmic Solution, 1% is contraindicated for patients who develop hypersensitivity reactions or chemical intolerance to trifluridine.

Warnings: The recommended dosage and frequency of administration should not be exceeded (see **Dosage and Administration**).

Precautions:

General: VIROPTIC Ophthalmic Solution, 1% should be prescribed only for patients who have a clinical diagnosis of herpetic keratitis. VIROPTIC may cause mild local irritation of the conjunctiva and cornea when instilled, but these effects are usually transient.

Although documented *in vitro* viral resistance to trifluridine has not been reported following multiple exposures to VIROPTIC, the possibility of the development of viral resistance exists.

Carcinogenesis, Mutagenesis, Impairment of Fertility: *Mutagenic Potential:* Trifluridine has been shown to exert mutagenic, DNA-damaging and cell-transforming activities in various standard *in vitro* test systems, and clastogenic activity in *Vicia faba* cells. It did not induce chromosome aberrations in bone marrow cells of male or female rats following a single subcutaneous dose of 100 mg/ kg, but was weakly positive in female, but not in male, rats following daily subcutaneous administration at 700 mg/kg/day for 5 days.

Although the significance of these test results is not clear or fully understood, there exists the possibility that mutagenic agents may cause genetic damage in humans.

Oncogenic Potential: Lifetime carcinogenicity bioassays in rats and mice given daily subcutaneous doses of trifluridine have been performed. Rats tested at 1.5, 7.5, and 15 mg/ day had increased incidences of adenocarcinomas of the intestinal tract and mammary glands, hemangiosarcomas of the spleen and liver, carcinosarcomas of the prostate gland, and granulosa-thecal cell tumors of the ovary. Mice were tested at 1, 5, and 10 mg/kg/day; those given 10 mg/kg/day trifluridine had significantly increased incidences of adenocarcinomas of the intestinal tract and uterus. Those given 10 mg/kg/day also had a significantly increased incidence of testicular atrophy as compared to vehicle control mice.

Pregnancy: *Teratogenic Effects:* Pregnancy Category C. Trifluridine was not teratogenic at doses up to 5 mg/kg/day (23 times the estimated human exposure) when given subcutaneously to rats and rabbits. However, fetal toxicity consisting of delayed ossification of portions of the skeleton occurred at dose levels of 2.5 and 5 mg/kg/day in rats and at 2.5 mg/kg/day resorption in rabbits. In both rats and rabbits, 1 mg/ kg/day (5 times the estimated human exposure) was a no-effect level. There were no teratogenic or fetotoxic effects after topical application of VIROPTIC Ophthalmic Solution,

1% (approximately 5 times the estimated human exposure) to the eyes of rabbits on the 6th through the 18th days of pregnancy. In a non-standard test, trifluridine solution has been shown to be teratogenic when injected directly into the yolk sac of chicken eggs. There are no adequate and well-controlled studies in pregnant women. VIROPTIC Ophthalmic Solution, 1% should be used during pregnancy only if the potential benefit justifies the potential risk to the fetus.

Nursing Mothers: It is unlikely that trifluridine is excreted in human milk after ophthalmic instillation of VIROPTIC because of the relatively small dosage (≤5 mg/day), its dilution in body fluids and its extremely short half-life (approximately 12 minutes). The drug should not be prescribed for nursing mothers unless the potential benefits outweigh the potential risks.

Pediatric Use: Safety and effectiveness in pediatric patients below six years of age have not been established.

Adverse Reactions: The most frequent adverse reactions reported during controlled clinical trials were mild, transient burning or stinging upon instillation (4.6%) and palpebral edema (2.8%). Other adverse reactions in decreasing order of reported frequency were superficial punctate keratopathy, epithelial keratopathy, hypersensitivity reaction, stromal edema, irritation, keratitis sicca, hyperemia, and increased intraocular pressure.

Overdosage: Overdosage by ocular instillation is unlikely because any excess solution should be quickly expelled from the conjunctival sac.

Acute overdosage by accidental oral ingestion of VIROPTIC has not occurred. However, should such ingestion occur, the 75 mg dosage of trifluridine in a 7.5 mL bottle of VIROPTIC is not likely to produce adverse effects. Single intravenous doses of 1.5 to 30 mg/kg/day in children and adults with neoplastic disease produce reversible bone marrow depression as the only potentially serious toxic effect and only after three to five courses of therapy. The acute oral LD_{50} in the mouse and rat was 4379 mg/kg or higher.

Dosage and Administration: Instill one drop of VIROPTIC Ophthalmic Solution, 1% onto the cornea of the affected eye every 2 hours while awake for a maximum daily dosage of nine drops until the corneal ulcer has completely re-epithelialized. Following re-epithelialization, treatment for an additional 7 days of one drop every 4 hours while awake for a minimum daily dosage of five drops is recommended.

If there are no signs of improvement after 7 days of therapy or complete re-epithelialization has not occurred after 14 days of therapy, other forms of therapy should be considered. Continuous administration of VIROPTIC for periods exceeding 21 days should be avoided because of potential ocular toxicity.

How Supplied: VIROPTIC Ophthalmic Solution, 1% is supplied as a sterile ophthalmic solution in a plastic Drop Dose® dispenser bottle of 7.5 mL (NDC 61570-037-75).

Store under refrigeration 2° to 8°C (36° to 46°F).

Animal Pharmacology and Animal Toxicology: Corneal wound healing studies in rabbits showed that VIROPTIC did not significantly retard closure of epithelial wounds. However, mild toxic changes such as intracellular edema of the basal cell layer, mild thinning of the overlying epithelium and reduced strength of stromal wounds were observed.

Whereas instillation of VIROPTIC into rabbit eyes during a subchronic toxicity study produced some degree of corneal epithelial thinning, a 12-month chronic toxicity study in rabbits in which VIROPTIC was instilled into eyes in intermittent, multiple, full-therapy courses showed no drug-related changes in the cornea.

Distributed by: Monarch Pharmaceuticals®, Inc., Bristol, TN 37620
Manufactured by: Catalytica Pharmaceuticals, Inc., Greenville, NC 27835

Date of issue: 10/00
643141

Monarch Pharmaceuticals®

MedPointe Pharmaceuticals
MedPointe Healthcare Inc.
SOMERSET, NJ 08873

For Medical Information, Contact:
Generally:
Medical Information
800-526-3840
After Hours and Weekend Emergencies:
800-526-3840
MedPointe Pharmaceuticals
MedPointe Healthcare Inc.
Sales and Ordering
Somerset, NJ 08873

OPTIVAR®   ℞
(azelastine hydrochloride ophthalmic solution), 0.05%

Description: OPTIVAR® (azelastine hydrochloride ophthalmic solution), 0.05% is a sterile ophthalmic solution containing azelastine hydrochloride, a relatively selective H_1-receptor antagonist for topical administration to the eyes. Azelastine hydrochloride is a white crystalline powder with a molecular weight of 418.37. Azelastine hydrochloride is sparingly soluble in water, methanol and propylene glycol, and slightly soluble in ethanol, octanol, and glycerine. Azelastine hydrochloride is a racemic mixture with a melting point of 225°C. The chemical name for azelastine hydrochloride is (±)-1-(2H)-phthalazinone, 4-[(4-chlorophenyl) methyl]-2-(hexahydro-1-methyl-1H-azepin-4-yl)-, monohydrochloride and is represented by the following chemical structure:

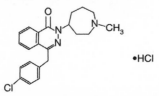

Empirical   chemical   structure: $C_{22}H_{24}ClN_3O \cdot HCl$
Each mL of OPTIVAR® contains: **Active:** 0.5 mg azelastine hydrochloride, equivalent to 0.457 mg of azelastine base; **Preservative:** 0.125 mg benzalkonium chloride; **Inactives:** disodium edetate dihydrate, hypromellose, sorbitol solution, sodium hydroxide and water for injection. It has a pH of approximately 5.0 to 6.5 and an osmolality of approximately 271 to 312 mOsmol/L.
Clinical Pharmacology: Azelastine hydrochloride is a relatively selective histamine H_1 antagonist and an inhibitor of the release of histamine and other mediators from cells (e.g. mast cells) involved in the allergic response. Based on *in-vitro* studies using human cell lines, inhibition of other mediators involved in allergic reactions (e.g. leukotrienes and PAF)

has been demonstrated with azelastine hydrochloride. Decreased chemotaxis and activation of eosinophils has also been demonstrated.

Pharmacokinetics and Metabolism
Absorption of azelastine following ocular administration was relatively low. A study in symptomatic patients receiving one drop of OPTIVAR® in each eye two to four times a day (0.06 to 0.12 mg azelastine hydrochloride) demonstrated plasma concentrations of azelastine hydrochloride to generally be between 0.02 and 0.25 ng/mL after 56 days of treatment. Three of nineteen patients had quantifiable amounts of N-desmethylazelastine that ranged from 0.25–0.87 ng/mL at Day 56.
Based on intravenous and oral administration, the elimination half-life, steady-state volume of distribution and plasma clearance were 22 hours, 14.5 L/kg and 0.5 L/h/kg, respectively. Approximately 75% of an oral dose of radiolabeled azelastine hydrochloride was excreted in the feces with less than 10% as unchanged azelastine. Azelastine hydrochloride is oxidatively metabolized to the principal metabolite, N-desmethylazelastine, by the cytochrome P450 enzyme system. *In-vitro* studies in human plasma indicate that the plasma protein binding of azelastine and N-desmethylazelastine are approximately 88% and 97%, respectively.

Clinical Trials
In a conjunctival antigen challenge study, OPTIVAR® was more effective than its vehicle in preventing itching associated with allergic conjunctivitis. OPTIVAR® had a rapid (within 3 minutes) onset of effect and a duration of effect of approximately 8 hours for the prevention of itching.
In environmental studies, adult and pediatric patients with seasonal allergic conjunctivitis were treated with OPTIVAR® for two to eight weeks. In these studies, OPTIVAR® was more effective than its vehicle in relieving itching associated with allergic conjunctivitis.
Indications and Usage: OPTIVAR® is indicated for the treatment of itching of the eye associated with allergic conjunctivitis.
Contraindications: OPTIVAR® is contraindicated in persons with known or suspected hypersensitivity to any of its components.
Warnings: OPTIVAR® is for ocular use only and not for injection or oral use.
Precautions:
Information for Patients:
To prevent contaminating the dropper tip and solution, care should be taken not to touch any surface, the eyelids, or surrounding areas with the dropper tip of the bottle. Keep bottle tightly closed when not in use. This product is sterile when packaged.
Patients should be advised not to wear a contact lens if their eye is red. OPTIVAR® should not be used to treat contact lens related irritation. The preservative in OPTIVAR®, benzalkonium chloride, may be absorbed by soft contact lenses. Patients who wear soft contact lenses and **whose eyes are not red**, should be instructed to wait at least ten minutes after instilling OPTIVAR® before they insert their contact lenses.
Carcinogenesis, Mutagenesis, Impairment of Fertility:
Azelastine hydrochloride administered orally for 24 months was not carcinogenic in rats and mice at doses up to 30 mg/kg/day and 25 mg/kg/day, respectively. Based on a 30 µL drop size, these doses were approximately 25,000 and 21,000 times higher than the maximum recommended ocular human use level of 0.001 mg/ kg/day for a 50 kg adult.
Azelastine hydrochloride showed no genotoxic effects in the Ames test, DNA repair test,

mouse lymphoma forward mutation assay, mouse micronucleus test, or chromosomal aberration test in rat bone marrow. Reproduction and fertility studies in rats showed no effects on male or female fertility at oral doses of up to 25,000 times the maximum recommended ocular human use level. At 68.6 mg/kg/day (57,000 times the maximum recommended ocular human use level), the duration of the estrous cycle was prolonged and copulatory activity and the number of pregnancies were decreased. The numbers of corpora lutea and implantations were decreased; however, the implantation ratio was not affected.
Pregnancy:
Teratogenic Effects: Pregnancy Category C. Azelastine hydrochloride has been shown to be embryotoxic, fetotoxic, and teratogenic (external and skeletal abnormalities) in mice at an oral dose of 68.6 mg/kg/day (57,000 times the recommended ocular human use level). At an oral dose of 30 mg/kg/day (25,000 times the recommended ocular human use level), delayed ossification (undeveloped metacarpus) and the incidence of 14th rib were increased in rats. At 68.6 mg/kg/day (57,000 times the maximum recommended ocular human use level) azelastine hydrochloride caused resorption and fetotoxic effects in rats. The relevance to humans of these skeletal findings noted at only high drug exposure levels is unknown.
There are no adequate and well-controlled studies in pregnant women. OPTIVAR® should be used during pregnancy only if the potential benefit justifies the potential risk to the fetus.
Nursing Mothers:
It is not known whether azelastine hydrochloride is excreted in human milk. Because many drugs are excreted in human milk, caution should be exercised when OPTIVAR® is administered to a nursing woman.
Pediatric Use:
Safety and effectiveness in pediatric patients below the age of 3 have not been established.
Geriatric Use:
No overall differences in safety or effectiveness have been observed between elderly and younger adult patients.
Adverse Reactions: In controlled multiple-dose studies where patients were treated for up to 56 days, the most frequently reported adverse reactions were transient eye burning/stinging (approximately 30%), headaches (approximately 15%) and bitter taste (approximately 10%). The occurrence of these events was generally mild.
The following events were reported in 1–10% of patients: asthma, conjunctivitis, dyspnea, eye pain, fatigue, influenza-like symptoms, pharyngitis, pruritus, rhinitis and temporary blurring. Some of these events were similar to the underlying disease being studied.
Dosage and Administration: The recommended dose is one drop instilled into each affected eye twice a day.
How Supplied: OPTIVAR® (azelastine hydrochloride ophthalmic solution), 0.05% is supplied as follows: 6 mL (NDC#0037-7025-60) solution in a translucent 10 mL HDPE container with a LDPE dropper tip, and a white HDPE screw cap.
Storage
Store UPRIGHT between 2° and 25°C (36° and 77°F)
Rx only
U.S. Patent 5,164,194
Manufactured by: Patheon UK Ltd., Swindon, United Kingdom
Distributed by:
MedPointe Pharmaceuticals
MedPointe Healthcare Inc.
Somerset, New Jersey 08873
Made in United Kingdom
Rev. 12/04

Merck & Co., Inc.
PO BOX 4 WP39-206
WEST POINT, PA 19486-0004

For Medical Information Contact:
Generally:
Product and service information:
Call the Merck National Service Center,
8:00 AM to 7:00 PM (ET), Monday through
Friday:
(800) NSC-MERCK
(800) 672-6372
FAX: (800) MERCK-68
FAX: (800) 637-2568
Adverse Drug Experiences:
Call the Merck National Service Center,
8:00 AM to 7:00 PM (ET), Monday through
Friday:
(800) NSC-MERCK
(800) 672-6372
Pregnancy Registries
(800) 986-8999
In Emergencies:
24-hour emergency information for healthcare
professionals:
(800) NSC-MERCK
(800) 672-6372
Sales and Ordering:
For product orders and direct account inquiries only, call the Order Management Center,
8:00 AM to 7:00 PM (ET), Monday through
Friday:
(800) MERCK RX
(800) 637-2579

COSOPT®   ℞
**(dorzolamide hydrochloride-timolol maleate
ophthalmic solution)**
Sterile Ophthalmic Solution

Description: COSOPT* (dorzolamide
hydrochloride-timolol maleate ophthalmic solution) is the combination of a topical carbonic anhydrase inhibitor and a topical beta-adrenergic
receptor blocking agent.
Dorzolamide hydrochloride is described
chemically as: (4S-trans)-4-(ethylamino)-5,6-
dihydro-6-methyl-4H-thieno[2,3-b] thiopyran-
2-sulfonamide 7,7-dioxide monohydrochloride.
Dorzolamide hydrochloride is optically active.
The specific rotation is:

$[\alpha]$ 25°C
        (C=1, water) = $\sim$ −17°.
    405 nm

Its empirical formula is $C_{10}H_{16}N_2O_4S_3 \bullet HCl$
and its structural formula is:

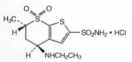

Dorzolamide hydrochloride has a molecular
weight of 360.91. It is a white to off-white,
crystalline powder, which is soluble in water
and slightly soluble in methanol and ethanol.
Timolol maleate is described chemically as:
(-)-1-(tert-butylamino)-3-[(4-morpholino-1,2,5-
thiadiazol-3-yl)oxy]-2-propanol maleate (1:1)
(salt). Timolol maleate possesses an asymmetric carbon atom in its structure and is provided
as the levo-isomer. The nominal optical rotation of timolol maleate is:

$[\alpha]$ 25°C
        in 1N HCl (C=5) = −12.2°
        (−11.7° to −12.5°).
    405 nm

Its molecular formula is
$C_{13}H_{24}N_4O_3S \bullet C_4H_4O_4$ and its structural formula is:

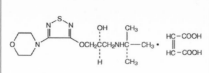

Timolol maleate has a molecular weight of
432.50. It is a white, odorless, crystalline powder which is soluble in water, methanol, and
alcohol. Timolol maleate is stable at room temperature.
COSOPT is supplied as a sterile, isotonic, buffered, slightly viscous, aqueous solution. The
pH of the solution is approximately 5.65, and
the osmolarity is 242-323 mOsM. Each mL of
COSOPT contains 20 mg dorzolamide
(22.26 mg of dorzolamide hydrochloride) and
5 mg timolol (6.83 mg timolol maleate). Inactive ingredients are sodium citrate, hydroxyethyl cellulose, sodium hydroxide, mannitol,
and water for injection. Benzalkonium chloride 0.0075% is added as a preservative.
*Registered trademark of MERCK & CO., Inc.

Clinical Pharmacology:
Mechanism of Action
COSOPT is comprised of two components:
dorzolamide hydrochloride and timolol maleate. Each of these two components decreases
elevated intraocular pressure, whether or not
associated with glaucoma, by reducing aqueous humor secretion. Elevated intraocular
pressure is a major risk factor in the pathogenesis of optic nerve damage and glaucomatous
visual field loss. The higher the level of intraocular pressure, the greater the likelihood of
glaucomatous field loss and optic nerve damage.
Dorzolamide hydrochloride is an inhibitor of
human carbonic anhydrase II. Inhibition of
carbonic anhydrase in the ciliary processes of
the eye decreases aqueous humor secretion,
presumably by slowing the formation of bicarbonate ions with subsequent reduction in sodium and fluid transport. Timolol maleate is a
beta$_1$ and beta$_2$ (non-selective) adrenergic receptor blocking agent that does not have significant intrinsic sympathomimetic, direct myocardial depressant, or local anesthetic
(membrane-stabilizing) activity. The combined
effect of these two agents administered as
COSOPT b.i.d. results in additional intraocular pressure reduction compared to either component administered alone, but the reduction
is not as much as when dorzolamide t.i.d. and
timolol b.i.d. are administered concomitantly
(see **Clinical Studies**).
Pharmacokinetics/Pharmacodynamics
Dorzolamide Hydrochloride
When topically applied, dorzolamide reaches
the systemic circulation. To assess the potential for systemic carbonic anhydrase inhibition
following topical administration, drug and metabolite concentrations in RBCs and plasma
and carbonic anhydrase inhibition in RBCs
were measured. Dorzolamide accumulates in
RBCs during chronic dosing as a result of binding to CA-II. The parent drug forms a single
N-desethyl metabolite, which inhibits CA-II
less potently than the parent drug but also inhibits CA-I. The metabolite also accumulates
in RBCs where it binds primarily to CA-I.
Plasma concentrations of dorzolamide and metabolite are generally below the assay limit of
quantitation (15nM). Dorzolamide binds moderately to plasma proteins (approximately
33%).
Dorzolamide is primarily excreted unchanged
in the urine; the metabolite also is excreted in
urine. After dosing is stopped, dorzolamide
washes out of RBCs nonlinearly, resulting in a

rapid decline of drug concentration initially,
followed by a slower elimination phase with a
half-life of about four months.
To simulate the systemic exposure after long-
term topical ocular administration,
dorzolamide was given orally to eight healthy
subjects for up to 20 weeks. The oral dose of
2 mg b.i.d. closely approximates the amount of
drug delivered by topical ocular administration of dorzolamide 2% t.i.d. Steady state was
reached within 8 weeks. The inhibition of
CA-II and total carbonic anhydrase activities
was below the degree of inhibition anticipated
to be necessary for a pharmacological effect on
renal function and respiration in healthy individuals.
Timolol Maleate
In a study of plasma drug concentrations in six
subjects, the systemic exposure to timolol was
determined following twice daily topical administration of timolol maleate ophthalmic solution 0.5%. The mean peak plasma concentration following morning dosing was 0.46 ng/mL.
Clinical Studies
Clinical studies of 3 to 15 months duration
were conducted to compare the IOP-lowering
effect over the course of the day of COSOPT
b.i.d. (dosed morning and bedtime) to
individually- and concomitantly-administered
0.5% timolol (b.i.d.) and 2.0% dorzolamide
(b.i.d. and t.i.d.). The IOP-lowering effect of
COSOPT b.i.d. was greater (1-3 mmHg) than
that of monotherapy with either 2.0%
dorzolamide t.i.d. or 0.5% timolol b.i.d. The
IOP-lowering effect of COSOPT b.i.d. was approximately 1 mmHg less than that of concomitant therapy with 2.0% dorzolamide t.i.d.
and 0.5% timolol b.i.d.
Open-label extensions of two studies were conducted for up to 12 months. During this period,
the IOP-lowering effect of COSOPT b.i.d. was
consistent during the 12 month follow-up period.
Indications and Usage: COSOPT is indicated for the reduction of elevated intraocular
pressure in patients with open-angle glaucoma
or ocular hypertension who are insufficiently responsive to beta-blockers (failed to achieve target IOP determined after multiple measurements over time). The IOP-lowering of COSOPT
b.i.d. was slightly less than that seen with the
concomitant administration of 0.5% timolol
b.i.d. and 2.0% dorzolamide t.i.d. (see **CLINI-
CAL PHARMACOLOGY, Clinical Studies**).
Contraindications: COSOPT is contraindicated in patients with (1) bronchial asthma; (2)
a history of bronchial asthma; (3) severe chronic
obstructive pulmonary disease (see **WARN-
INGS**); (4) sinus bradycardia; (5) second or
third degree atrioventricular block; (6) overt
cardiac failure (see **WARNINGS**); (7) cardiogenic shock; or (8) hypersensitivity to any component of this product.
Warnings:
Systemic Exposure
COSOPT contains dorzolamide, a sulfonamide, and timolol maleate, a beta-adrenergic
blocking agent; and although administered
topically, is absorbed systemically. Therefore,
the same types of adverse reactions that are
attributable to sulfonamides and/or systemic
administration of beta-adrenergic blocking
agents may occur with topical administration.
For example, severe respiratory reactions and
cardiac reactions, including death due to bronchospasm in patients with asthma, and rarely
death in association with cardiac failure, have
been reported following systemic or ophthalmic administration of timolol maleate (see
CONTRAINDICATIONS). Fatalities have
occurred, although rarely, due to severe reactions to sulfonamides including Stevens-

Johnson syndrome, toxic epidermal necrolysis, fulminant hepatic necrosis, agranulocytosis, aplastic anemia, and other blood dyscrasias. Sensitization may recur when a sulfonamide is readministered irrespective of the route of administration. If signs of serious reactions or hypersensitivity occur, discontinue the use of this preparation.

Cardiac Failure
Sympathetic stimulation may be essential for support of the circulation in individuals with diminished myocardial contractility, and its inhibition by beta-adrenergic receptor blockade may precipitate more severe failure.

In Patients Without a History of Cardiac Failure continued depression of the myocardium with beta-blocking agents over a period of time can, in some cases, lead to cardiac failure. At the first sign or symptom of cardiac failure, COSOPT should be discontinued.

Obstructive Pulmonary Disease
Patients with chronic obstructive pulmonary disease (e.g., chronic bronchitis, emphysema) of mild or moderate severity, bronchospastic disease, or a history of bronchospastic disease (other than bronchial asthma or a history of bronchial asthma, in which COSOPT is contraindicated [see **CONTRAINDICATIONS**]) should, in general, not receive beta-blocking agents, including COSOPT.

Major Surgery
The necessity or desirability of withdrawal of beta-adrenergic blocking agents prior to major surgery is controversial. Beta-adrenergic receptor blockade impairs the ability of the heart to respond to beta-adrenergically mediated reflex stimuli. This may augment the risk of general anesthesia in surgical procedures. Some patients receiving beta-adrenergic receptor blocking agents have experienced protracted severe hypotension during anesthesia. Difficulty in restarting and maintaining the heartbeat has also been reported. For these reasons, in patients undergoing elective surgery, some authorities recommend gradual withdrawal of beta-adrenergic receptor blocking agents.

If necessary during surgery, the effects of beta-adrenergic blocking agents may be reversed by sufficient doses of adrenergic agonists.

Diabetes Mellitus
Beta-adrenergic blocking agents should be administered with caution in patients subject to spontaneous hypoglycemia or to diabetic patients (especially those with labile diabetes) who are receiving insulin or oral hypoglycemic agents. Beta-adrenergic receptor blocking agents may mask the signs and symptoms of acute hypoglycemia.

Thyrotoxicosis
Beta-adrenergic blocking agents may mask certain clinical signs (e.g., tachycardia) of hyperthyroidism. Patients suspected of developing thyrotoxicosis should be managed carefully to avoid abrupt withdrawal of beta-adrenergic blocking agents that might precipitate a thyroid storm.

Precautions:
General
Dorzolamide has not been studied in patients with severe renal impairment (CrCl <30 mL/min). Because dorzolamide and its metabolite are excreted prodominantly by the kidney, COSOPT is not recommended in such patients. Dorzolamide has not been studied in patients with hepatic impairment and should therefore be used with caution in such patients.

While taking beta-blockers, patients with a history of atopy or a history of severe anaphylactic reactions to a variety of allergens may be more reactive to repeated accidental, diagnostic, or therapeutic challenge with such allergens. Such patients may be unresponsive to the usual doses of epinephrine used to treat anaphylactic reactions.

In clinical studies, local ocular adverse effects, primarily conjunctivitis and lid reactions, were reported with chronic administration of COSOPT. Many of these reactions had the clinical appearance and course of an allergic-type reaction that resolved upon discontinuation of drug therapy. If such reactions are observed, COSOPT should be discontinued and the patient evaluated before considering restarting the drug. (See **ADVERSE REACTIONS**.)

The management of patients with acute angle-closure glaucoma requires therapeutic interventions in addition to ocular hypotensive agents. COSOPT has not been studied in patients with acute angle-closure glaucoma.

Choroidal detachment after filtration procedures has been reported with the administration of aqueous suppressant therapy (e.g., timolol).

Beta-adrenergic blockade has been reported to potentiate muscle weakness consistent with certain myasthenic symptoms (e.g., diplopia, ptosis, and generalized weakness). Timolol has been reported rarely to increase muscle weakness in some patients with myasthenia gravis or myasthenic symptoms.

There have been reports of bacterial keratitis associated with the use of multiple dose containers of topical ophthalmic products. These containers had been inadvertently contaminated by patients who, in most cases, had a concurrent corneal disease or a disruption of the ocular epithelial surface. (See **PRECAUTIONS, Information for Patients**.)

Information for Patients
Patients with bronchial asthma, a history of bronchial asthma, severe chronic obstructive pulmonary disease, sinus bradycardia, second or third degree atrioventricular block, or cardiac failure should be advised not to take this product. (See **CONTRAINDICATIONS**.)

COSOPT contains dorzolamide (which is a sulfonamide) and although administered topically is absorbed systemically. Therefore the same types of adverse reactions that are attributable to sulfonamides may occur with topical administration. Patients should be advised that if serious or unusual reactions or signs of hypersensitivity occur, they should discontinue the use of the product (see **WARNINGS**).

Patients should be advised that if they develop any ocular reactions, particularly conjunctivitis and lid reactions, they should discontinue use and seek their physician's advice.

Patients should be instructed to avoid allowing the tip of the dispensing container to contact the eye or surrounding structures.

Patients should also be instructed that ocular solutions, if handled improperly or if the tip of the dispensing container contacts the eye or surrounding structures, can become contaminated by common bacteria known to cause ocular infections. Serious damage to the eye and subsequent loss of vision may result from using contaminated solutions. (See **PRECAUTIONS, General**.)

Patients also should be advised that if they have ocular surgery or develop an intercurrent ocular condition (e.g., trauma or infection), they should immediately seek their physician's advice concerning the continued use of the present multidose container.

If more than one topical ophthalmic drug is being used, the drugs should be administered at least ten minutes apart.

Patients should be advised that COSOPT contains benzalkonium chloride which may be absorbed by soft contact lenses. Contact lenses should be removed prior to administration of the solution. Lenses may be reinserted 15 minutes following administration of COSOPT.

Drug Interactions
Carbonic anhydrase inhibitors: There is a potential for an additive effect on the known systemic effects of carbonic anhydrase inhibition in patients receiving an oral carbonic anhydrase inhibitor and COSOPT. The concomitant administration of COSOPT and oral carbonic anhydrase inhibitors is not recommended.

Acid-base disturbances: Although acid-base and electrolyte disturbances were not reported in the clinical trials with dorzolamide hydrochloride ophthalmic solution, these disturbances have been reported with oral carbonic anhydrase inhibitors and have, in some instances, resulted in drug interactions (e.g., toxicity associated with high-dose salicylate therapy). Therefore, the potential for such drug interactions should be considered in patients receiving COSOPT.

Beta-adrenergic blocking agents: Patients who are receiving a beta-adrenergic blocking agent orally and COSOPT should be observed for potential additive effects of beta-blockade, both systemic and on intraocular pressure. The concomitant use of two topical beta-adrenergic blocking agents is not recommended.

Calcium antagonists: Caution should be used in the coadministration of beta-adrenergic blocking agents, such as COSOPT, and oral or intravenous calcium antagonists because of possible atrioventricular conduction disturbances, left ventricular failure, and hypotension. In patients with impaired cardiac function, coadministration should be avoided.

Catecholamine-depleting drugs: Close observation of the patient is recommended when a beta-blocker is administered to patients receiving catecholamine-depleting drugs such as reserpine, because of possible additive effects and the production of hypotension and/or marked bradycardia, which may result in vertigo, syncope, or postural hypotension.

Digitalis and calcium antagonists: The concomitant use of beta-adrenergic blocking agents with digitalis and calcium antagonists may have additive effects in prolonging atrioventricular conduction time.

CYP2D6 inhibitors: Potentiated systemic beta-blockade (e.g., decreased heart rate, depression) has been reported during combined treatment with CYP2D6 inhibitors (e.g., quinidine, SSRIs) and timolol.

Clonidine: Oral beta-adrenergic blocking agents may exacerbate the rebound hypertension which can follow the withdrawal of clonidine. There have been no reports of exacerbation of rebound hypertension with ophthalmic timolol maleate.

Injectable Epinephrine: (See **PRECAUTIONS, General, Anaphylaxis**.)

Carcinogenesis, Mutagenesis, Impairment of Fertility
In a two-year study of dorzolamide hydrochloride administered orally to male and female Sprague-Dawley rats, urinary bladder papillomas were seen in male rats in the highest dosage group of 20 mg/kg/day (250 times the recommended human ophthalmic dose). Papillomas were not seen in rats given oral doses equivalent to approximately 12 times the recommended human ophthalmic dose. No treatment-related tumors were seen in a 21-month study in female and male mice given oral doses up to 75 mg/kg/day (~900 times the recommended human ophthalmic dose).

The increased incidence of urinary bladder papillomas seen in the high-dose male rats is a class-effect of carbonic anhydrase inhibitors in rats. Rats are particularly prone to developing

Continued on next page

Information on the Merck & Co., Inc., products listed on these pages is from the prescribing information in use May 1, 2006. For information, please call 1-800-NSC-MERCK [1-800-672-6372].

Cosopt—Cont.

papillomas in response to foreign bodies, compounds causing crystalluria, and diverse sodium salts.

No changes in bladder urothelium were seen in dogs given oral dorzolamide hydrochloride for one year at 2 mg/kg/day (25 times the recommended human ophthalmic dose) or monkeys dosed topically to the eye at 0.4 mg/kg/day (~5 times the recommended human ophthalmic dose) for one year.

In a two-year study of timolol maleate administered orally to rats, there was a statistically significant increase in the incidence of adrenal pheochromocytomas in male rats administered 300 mg/kg/day (approximately 42,000 times the systemic exposure following the maximum recommended human ophthalmic dose). Similar differences were not observed in rats administered oral doses equivalent to approximately 14,000 times the maximum recommended human ophthalmic dose.

In a lifetime oral study of timolol maleate in mice, there were statistically significant increases in the incidence of benign and malignant pulmonary tumors, benign uterine polyps and mammary adenocarcinomas in female mice at 500 mg/kg/day, (approximately 71,000 times the systemic exposure following the maximum recommended human ophthalmic dose), but not at 5 or 50 mg/kg/day (approximately 700 or 7,000, respectively, times the systemic exposure following the maximum recommended human ophthalmic dose). In a subsequent study in female mice, in which postmortem examinations were limited to the uterus and the lungs, a statistically significant increase in the incidence of pulmonary tumors was again observed at 500 mg/kg/day.

The increased occurrence of mammary adenocarcinomas was associated with elevations in serum prolactin which occurred in female mice administered oral timolol at 500 mg/kg/day, but not at doses of 5 or 50 mg/kg/day. An increased incidence of mammary adenocarcinomas in rodents has been associated with administration of several other therapeutic agents that elevate serum prolactin, but no correlation between serum prolactin levels and mammary tumors has been established in humans. Furthermore, in adult human female subjects who received oral dosages of up to 60 mg of timolol maleate (the maximum recommended human oral dosage), there were no clinically meaningful changes in serum prolactin.

The following tests for mutagenic potential were negative for dorzolamide: (1) *in vivo* (mouse) cytogenetic assay; (2) *in vitro* chromosomal aberration assay; (3) alkaline elution assay; (4) V-79 assay; and (5) Ames test.

Timolol maleate was devoid of mutagenic potential when tested *in vivo* (mouse) in the micronucleus test and cytogenetic assay (doses up to 800 mg/kg) and *in vitro* in a neoplastic cell transformation assay (up to 100 µg/mL). In Ames tests the highest concentrations of timolol employed, 5,000 or 10,000 µg/plate, were associated with statistically significant elevations of revertants observed with tester strain TA100 (in seven replicate assays), but not in the remaining three strains. In the assays with tester strain TA100, no consistent dose response relationship was observed, and the ratio of test to control revertants did not reach 2. A ratio of 2 is usually considered the criterion for a positive Ames test.

Reproduction and fertility studies in rats with either timolol maleate or dorzolamide hydrochloride demonstrated no adverse effect on male or female fertility at doses up to approximately 100 times the systemic exposure following the maximum recommended human ophthalmic dose.

Pregnancy
Teratogenic Effects.
Pregnancy Category C. Developmental toxicity studies with dorzolamide hydrochloride in rabbits at oral doses of ≥2.5 mg/kg/day (31 times the recommended human ophthalmic dose) revealed malformations of the vertebral bodies. These malformations occurred at doses that caused metabolic acidosis with decreased body weight gain in dams and decreased fetal weights. No treatment-related malformations were seen at 1.0 mg/kg/day (13 times the recommended human ophthalmic dose).

Teratogenicity studies with timolol in mice, rats, and rabbits at oral doses up to 50 mg/kg/day (7,000 times the systemic exposure following the maximum recommended human ophthalmic dose) demonstrated no evidence of fetal malformations. Although delayed fetal ossification was observed at this dose in rats, there were no adverse effects on postnatal development of offspring. Doses of 1000 mg/kg/day (142,000 times the systemic exposure following the maximum recommended human ophthalmic dose) was maternotoxic in mice and resulted in an increased number of fetal resorptions. Increased fetal resorptions were also seen in rabbits at doses of 14,000 times the systemic exposure following the maximum recommended human ophthalmic dose, in this case without apparent maternotoxicity.

There are no adequate and well-controlled studies in pregnant women. COSOPT should be used during pregnancy only if the potential benefit justifies the potential risk to the fetus.

Nursing Mothers
It is not known whether dorzolamide is excreted in human milk. Timolol maleate has been detected in human milk following oral and ophthalmic drug administration. Because of the potential for serious adverse reactions from COSOPT in nursing infants, a decision should be made whether to discontinue nursing or to discontinue the drug, taking into account the importance of the drug to the mother.

Pediatric Use
Safety and effectiveness in pediatric patients have not been established.

Geriatric Use
No overall differences in safety or effectiveness have been observed between elderly and younger patients.

Adverse Reactions: COSOPT was evaluated for safety in 1035 patients with elevated intraocular pressure treated for open-angle-glaucoma or ocular hypertension. Approximately 5% of all patients discontinued therapy with COSOPT because of adverse reactions. The most frequently reported adverse events were taste perversion (bitter, sour, or unusual taste) or ocular burning and/or stinging in up to 30% of patients. Conjunctival hyperemia, blurred vision, superficial punctate keratitis or eye itching were reported between 5-15% of patients. The following adverse events were reported in 1-5% of patients: abdominal pain, back pain, blepharitis, bronchitis, cloudy vision, conjunctival discharge, conjunctival edema, conjunctival follicles, conjunctival injection, conjunctivitis, corneal erosion, corneal staining, cortical lens opacity, cough, dizziness, dryness of eyes, dyspepsia, eye debris, eye discharge, eye pain, eye tearing, eyelid edema, eyelid erythema, eyelid exudate/scales, eyelid pain or discomfort, foreign body sensation, glaucomatous cupping, headache, hypertension, influenza, lens nucleus coloration, lens opacity, nausea, nuclear lens opacity, pharyngitis, post-subcapsular cataract, sinusitis, upper respiratory infection, urinary tract infection, visual field defect, vitreous detachment. The following adverse events have occurred either at low incidence (<1%) during clinical trials or have been reported during the use of COSOPT in clinical practice where these

events were reported voluntarily from a population of unknown size and frequency of occurrence cannot be determined precisely. They have been chosen for inclusion based on factors such as seriousness, frequency of reporting, possible causal connection to COSOPT, or a combination of these factors: bradycardia, cardiac failure, cerebral vascular accident, chest pain, choroidal detachment following filtration surgery (see **PRECAUTIONS, General**), depression, diarrhea, dry mouth, dyspnea, heart block, hypotension, iridocyclitis, myocardial infarction, nasal congestion, paresthesia, photophobia, respiratory failure, skin rashes, urolithiasis, and vomiting.

Other adverse reactions that have been reported with the individual components are listed below:

Dorzolamide — Allergic/Hypersensitivity: Signs and symptoms of local reactions including palpebral reactions and systemic allergic reactions including angioedema, bronchospasm, pruritus, urticaria; *Body as a Whole:* Asthenia/fatigue; *Skin / Mucous Membranes:* Contact dermatitis, epistaxis, throat irritation; *Special Senses:* Eyelid crusting, signs and symptoms of ocular allergic reaction, and transient myopia.

Timolol (ocular administration)— Body as a Whole: Asthenia/fatigue; *Cardiovascular:* Arrhythmia, syncope, cerebral ischemia, worsening of angina pectoris, palpitation, cardiac arrest, pulmonary edema, edema, claudication, Raynaud's phenomenon, and cold hands and feet; *Digestive:* Anorexia; *Immunologic:* Systemic lupus erythematosus; *Nervous System / Psychiatric:* Increase in signs and symptoms of myasthenia gravis, somnolence, insomnia, nightmares, behavioral changes and psychic disturbances including confusion, hallucinations, anxiety, disorientation, nervousness, and memory loss; *Skin:* Alopecia, psoriasiform rash or exacerbation of psoriasis; *Hypersensitivity:* Signs and symptoms of systemic allergic reactions, including anaphylaxis, angioedema, urticaria, and localized and generalized rash; *Respiratory:* Bronchospasm (predominantly in patients with pre-existing bronchospastic disease); *Endocrine:* Masked symptoms of hypoglycemia in diabetic patients (see **WARNINGS**); *Special Senses:* Ptosis, decreased corneal sensitivity, cystoid macular edema, visual disturbances including refractive changes and diplopia, pseudopemphigoid, and tinnitus; *Urogenital:* Retroperitoneal fibrosis, decreased libido, impotence, and Peyronie's disease.

The following additional adverse effects have been reported in clinical experience with ORAL timolol maleate or other ORAL beta-blocking agents and may be considered potential effects of ophthalmic timolol maleate: *Allergic:* Erythematous rash, fever combined with aching and sore throat, laryngospasm with respiratory distress; *Body as a Whole:* Extremity pain, decreased exercise tolerance, weight loss; *Cardiovascular:* Worsening of arterial insufficiency, vasodilatation; *Digestive:* Gastrointestinal pain, hepatomegaly, mesenteric arterial thrombosis, ischemic colitis; *Hematologic:* Nonthrombocytopenic purpura; thrombocytopenic purpura, agranulocytosis; *Endocrine:* Hyperglycemia, hypoglycemia; *Skin:* Pruritus, skin irritation, increased pigmentation, sweating; *Musculoskeletal:* Arthralgia; *Nervous System / Psychiatric:* Vertigo, local weakness, diminished concentration, reversible mental depression progressing to catatonia, an acute reversible syndrome characterized by disorientation for time and place, emotional lability, slightly clouded sensorium, and decreased performance on neuropsychometrics; *Respiratory:* Rales, bronchial obstruction; *Urogenital:* Urination difficulties.

Overdosage: There are no human data available on overdosage with COSOPT.

Symptoms consistent with systemic administration of beta-blockers or carbonic anhydrase inhibitors may occur, including electrolyte imbalance, development of an acidotic state, dizziness, headache, shortness of breath, bradycardia, bronchospasm, cardiac arrest and possible central nervous system effects. Serum electrolyte levels (particularly potassium) and blood pH levels should be monitored (see also **ADVERSE REACTIONS**).

A study of patients with renal failure showed that timolol did not dialyze readily.

Dosage and Administration:

The dose is one drop of COSOPT in the affected eye(s) two times daily.

If more than one topical ophthalmic drug is being used, the drugs should be administered at least ten minutes apart (see also **PRECAUTIONS, Drug Interactions**).

How Supplied: COSOPT Ophthalmic Solution is a clear, colorless to nearly colorless, slightly viscous solution.

No. 3628 — COSOPT Ophthalmic Solution is supplied in an OCUMETER * PLUS container, a white, translucent, HDPE plastic ophthalmic dispenser with a controlled drop tip and a white polystyrene cap with dark blue label as follows:

NDC 0006-3628-35, 5 mL in a 7.5 mL capacity bottle

NDC 0006-3628-36, 10 mL in an 18 mL capacity bottle

Storage

Store COSOPT at 15–30°C (59–86°F). Protect from light.

*Registered trademark of MERCK & CO., Inc.

Instructions for Use:

Please follow these instructions carefully when using COSOPT*. Use COSOPT as prescribed by your doctor.

1. If you use other topically applied ophthalmic medications, they should be administered at least 10 minutes before or after COSOPT.
2. Wash hands before each use.
3. Before using the medication for the first time, be sure the Safety Strip on the front of the bottle is unbroken. A gap between the bottle and the cap is normal for an unopened bottle.

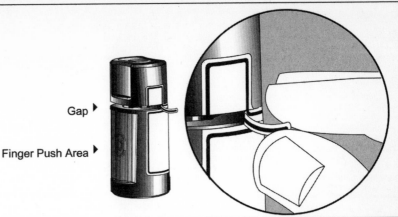

Gap ▶

Finger Push Area ▶

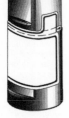

Opening Arrows ▶

Safety Strip ▶

4. Tear off the Safety Strip to break the seal. [See first figure above]
5. To open the bottle, unscrew the cap by turning as indicated by the arrows on the top of the cap. Do not pull the cap directly up and away from the bottle. Pulling the cap directly up will prevent your dispenser from operating properly. [See first figure at top of next column]
6. Tilt your head back and pull your lower eyelid down slightly to form a pocket between your eyelid and your eye. [See second figure at top of next column]
7. Invert the bottle, and press lightly with the thumb or index finger over the "Finger Push Area" (as shown) until a single drop is dispensed into the eye as directed by your doctor. [See second figure above] DO NOT TOUCH YOUR EYE OR EYELID WITH THE DROPPER TIP.

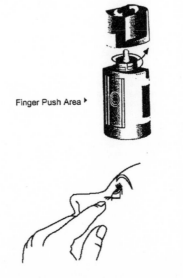

Finger Push Area ▶

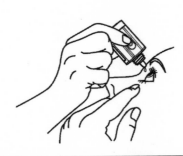

Finger Push Area ▶

OPHTHALMIC MEDICATIONS, IF HANDLED IMPROPERLY, CAN BECOME CONTAMINATED BY COMMON BACTERIA KNOWN TO CAUSE EYE INFECTIONS. SERIOUS DAMAGE TO THE EYE AND SUBSEQUENT LOSS OF VISION MAY RESULT FROM USING CONTAMINATED OPHTHALMIC MEDICATIONS. IF YOU THINK YOUR MEDICATION MAY BE CONTAMINATED, OR IF YOU DEVELOP AN EYE INFECTION, CONTACT YOUR DOCTOR IMMEDIATELY CONCERNING CONTINUED USE OF THIS BOTTLE.

8. If drop dispensing is difficult after opening for the first time, replace the cap on the bottle and tighten (DO NOT OVERTIGHTEN) and then remove by turning the cap in the opposite direction as indicated by the arrows on the top of the cap.
9. Repeat steps 6 & 7 with the other eye if instructed to do so by your doctor.
10. Replace the cap by turning until it is firmly touching the bottle. The arrow on the left side of the cap must be aligned with the arrow on the left side of the bottle label for proper closure. Do not overtighten or you may damage the bottle and/or cap.
11. The dispenser tip is designed to provide a single drop; therefore, do NOT enlarge the hole of the dispenser tip.
12. After you have used all doses, there will be some COSOPT left in the bottle. You should not be concerned since an extra amount of COSOPT has been added and you will get the full amount of COSOPT that your doctor prescribed. Do not attempt to remove the excess medicine from the bottle.

WARNING: Keep out of reach of children.

If you have any questions about the use of COSOPT, please consult your doctor.

* Registered trademark of MERCK & CO., Inc.

Manuf. for:

Merck & Co., Inc., Whitehouse Station, NJ 08889, USA

By: Laboratories Merck Sharp & Dohme-Chibret

63963 Clermont-Ferrand Cedex 9, France

9711301   Issued January 2006

Continued on next page

Information on the Merck & Co., Inc., products listed on these pages is from the prescribing information in use May 1, 2006. For information, please call 1-800-NSC-MERCK [1-800-672-6372].

Cosopt—Cont.

Patient Information about
COSOPT®* (dorzolamide hydrochloride–
timolol maleate ophthalmic solution)
COSOPT (pronounced "CO-sopt")
Read this information before you start using
COSOPT and each time you refill your prescription. This is in case any information has
changed. This leaflet provides a summary of
certain information about COSOPT. Your doctor or pharmacist can give you more complete
information about COSOPT. This leaflet does
not take the place of careful discussions with
your doctor. You and your doctor should discuss COSOPT when you start using your medicine and at regular checkups. Only your doctor can prescribe COSOPT for you.

What is COSOPT?
COSOPT is an eyedrop. It contains
dorzolamide hydrochloride, which is an ophthalmic carbonic anhydrase inhibiting drug. It
also contains timolol maleate, which is a beta-
blocking drug. Both drugs work to lower pressure in the eye, but in different ways.
COSOPT is a medicine for lowering pressure
in the eye in people with open-angle glaucoma
or ocular hypertension. It is used when a beta-
blocker eyedrop alone is not adequate to control eye pressure.

What should I know about high pressure in the eye?
People with open-angle glaucoma or ocular hypertension have pressures in one or both of
their eye(s) that are too high for them.
High pressure in the eye may damage the optic
nerve. This may lead to loss of vision and possible blindness. There generally are few symptoms that you can feel to tell you whether you
have high pressure within your eye. Your doctor needs to examine your eyes to determine
this. If you have high pressure in your eye, you
will need your pressure checked and your eyes
examined regularly.

Who should not use COSOPT?
Do not use COSOPT if you have:
• asthma or have ever had asthma,
• severe lung problems,
• slow or irregular heartbeat or heart failure,
• allergies to any of its ingredients. See the list
  at the end of the leaflet.
If you are not sure whether you should use
COSOPT, contact your doctor or pharmacist.

What should I tell my doctor before and during treatment with COSOPT?
Tell your doctor:
• if you are pregnant or plan to become pregnant,
• if you are breast-feeding or intend to breast-
  feed,
• about any medical problems you have now or
  had in the past, especially heart problems or
  breathing problems including asthma,
• if you now have or had in the past kidney or
  liver problems,
• if you have diabetes, thyroid disease or muscle weakness,
• about all medicines that you are taking or
  plan to take, including those you can get
  without a prescription,
• about any allergies including allergies to any
  medications, especially sulfa drugs,
• if you develop an eye infection, develop a red
  or swollen eye or eyelid, receive an eye injury, have eye surgery, or develop new or
  worsening eye symptoms,
• if you plan on having any type of surgery.

How should I use COSOPT?
COSOPT is an eyedrop. The usual dose is one
drop in the morning and one drop in the evening. Your doctor will tell you if just one or
both eyes are to be treated.
If you are using COSOPT with another eyedrop, the eyedrops should be used at least 10
minutes apart. It is very important to use your
medication exactly as directed by your doctor.

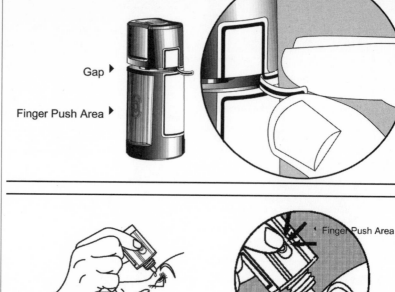

Gap ▶

Finger Push Area ▶

◄ Finger Push Area

If you stop using your medicine, contact your
doctor immediately.
COSOPT contains a preservative called benzalkonium chloride. This preservative may be
absorbed by soft contact lenses. Contact lenses
should be removed before using COSOPT. The
lenses can be placed back into your eyes 15
minutes after using the eyedrops.
Do not allow the tip of the bottle to touch the
eye or areas around the eye. The bottle may
become contaminated with bacteria. This can
cause eye infections leading to serious damage
to the eye, even loss of vision. Keep the tip of
the bottle away from contact with any surface
to avoid contamination.
*Registered trademark of MERCK & CO., Inc.
COPYRIGHT © 2005 MERCK & CO., Inc.
All rights reserved

Instructions for Use
Please follow these instructions carefully when
using COSOPT. Use COSOPT as prescribed by
your doctor.
1. If you use other topically applied ophthalmic medications, they should be administered at least 10 minutes before or after
   COSOPT.
2. Wash hands before each use.
3. Before using the medication for the first
   time, be sure the Safety Strip on the front
   of the bottle is unbroken. A gap between
   the bottle and the cap is normal for an unopened bottle.
   [See first figure at top of next column]
4. Tear off the Safety Strip to break the seal.
   [See first figure above]
5. To open the bottle, unscrew the cap by
   turning as indicated by the arrows on the
   top of the cap. Do not pull the cap directly
   up and away from the bottle. Pulling the
   cap directly up will prevent your dispenser
   from operating properly.
   [See second figure at top of next column]
6. Tilt your head back and pull your lower
   eyelid down slightly to form a pocket between your eyelid and your eye.
   [See third figure at top of next column]

Opening Arrows ▶

Safety Strip ▶

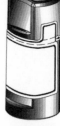

Finger Push Area ▶

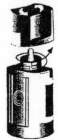

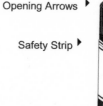

7. Invert the bottle, and press lightly with the
   thumb or index finger over the "Finger

Push Area" (as shown) until a single drop is dispensed into the eye as directed by your doctor.
[See second figure at top of previous page]
DO NOT TOUCH YOUR EYE OR EYELID WITH THE DROPPER TIP.
OPHTHALMIC MEDICATIONS, IF HANDLED IMPROPERLY, CAN BECOME CONTAMINATED BY COMMON BACTERIA KNOWN TO CAUSE EYE INFECTIONS. SERIOUS DAMAGE TO THE EYE AND SUBSEQUENT LOSS OF VISION MAY RESULT FROM USING CONTAMINATED OPHTHALMIC MEDICATIONS. IF YOU THINK YOUR MEDICATION MAY BE CONTAMINATED, OR IF YOU DEVELOP AN EYE INFECTION, CONTACT YOUR DOCTOR IMMEDIATELY CONCERNING CONTINUED USE OF THIS BOTTLE.

8. If drop dispensing is difficult after opening for the first time, replace the cap on the bottle and tighten (DO NOT OVERTIGHTEN) and then remove by turning the cap in the opposite direction as indicated by the arrows on the top of the cap.
9. Repeat steps 6 & 7 with the other eye if instructed to do so by your doctor.
10. Replace the cap by turning until it is firmly touching the bottle. The arrow on the left side of the cap must be aligned with the arrow on the left side of the bottle label for proper closure. Do not overtighten or you may damage the bottle and cap.
11. The dispenser tip is designed to provide a single drop; therefore, do NOT enlarge the hole of the dispenser tip.
12. After you have used all doses, there will be some COSOPT left in the bottle. You should not be concerned since an extra amount of COSOPT has been added and you will get the full amount of COSOPT that your doctor prescribed. Do not attempt to remove the excess medicine from the bottle.

Can I use COSOPT with other medicines?
Tell your doctor or pharmacist about all drugs that you are using or plan to use. This includes other eyedrops and drugs obtained without a prescription. This is particularly important if you are taking medicine to lower blood pressure or to treat heart disease, or if you are taking large doses of aspirin.
Ask your doctor's advice about taking COSOPT if you are also using:
- oral carbonic anhydrase inhibitors (for example, acetazolamide, Diamox®)
- oral beta-blockers (for example, propranolol, Inderal®)
- calcium antagonists (for example, nifedipine, Procardia®)
- catecholamine-depleting drugs (for example, reserpine)
- digitalis in combination with calcium antagonists (for example, Lanoxin® with Procardia®)
- quinidine (for example, Cardioquin®)
- clonidine (for example, Catapres®)
- injectable epinephrine (for example, EpiPen®).
- SSRI's (for example Prozac®)

Your doctor or pharmacist can tell you if any of the drugs you are using are in the above list.
What are the possible side effects of COSOPT?
Any medicine may have unintended or undesirable effects. These are called side effects. Side effects may not occur, but if they do occur, you may need medical attention. The most common side effects you may experience are:
- eye symptoms such as burning and stinging, redness of the eye(s), blurred vision, tearing or itching.
- a bitter, sour or unusual taste after putting in your eyedrops.

Other side effects may occur rarely, and some of these may be serious. Tell your doctor right away if you experience:
- shortness of breath
- visual changes
- an irregular heartbeat and/or a slowing of your heart rate.
The above list is NOT a complete list of side effects reported with COSOPT. Your doctor can discuss with you a more complete list of side effects. Please tell your doctor [or pharmacist] promptly about any of these or any other unusual symptom.
What should I do in case of an overdose?
If you swallow the contents of the bottle, contact your doctor immediately. Among other effects, you may feel light-headed, have difficulty breathing, or feel your heart rate has slowed.
How should I store COSOPT?
Keep your medicine in a safe place where children cannot reach it. Store COSOPT at room temperature (59-86°F, 15-30°C). Protect the bottle from light. Do not use your medicine after the expiration date on the bottle.
What else should I know about COSOPT?
Do not use COSOPT for a condition for which it was not prescribed. Do not give COSOPT to other people, even if they have the same condition you have. It may harm them.
Inactive ingredients:
The inactive ingredients of COSOPT are sodium citrate, hydroxyethylcellulose, sodium hydroxide, mannitol, water for injection and benzalkonium chloride added as a preservative.
Issued January 2006   MERCK & CO., Inc.
541A-12/05 511880Z Whitehouse Station, NJ
08889, USA
Shown in Product Identification Guide, page 105

TIMOPTIC®   ℞
0.25% and 0.5%
(Timolol Maleate Ophthalmic Solution)
Sterile Ophthalmic Solution
Description:
TIMOPTIC* (timolol maleate ophthalmic solution) is a non-selective beta-adrenergic receptor blocking agent. Its chemical name is (-)-1-(*tert*-butylamino)-3-[(4 morpholino-1, 2, 5-thiadiazol-3-yl) oxy]-2-propanol maleate (1:1) (salt). Timolol maleate possesses an asymmetric carbon atom in its structure and is provided as the levo-isomer. The nominal optical rotation of timolol maleate is:

$$[\alpha] \begin{array}{l} 25° \\ \\ 405\ nm \end{array} \text{in 1.0N HCl (C = 5\%)} = -12.2° \\ (-11.7° \text{ to } -12.5°).$$

Its molecular formula is $C_{13}H_{24}N_4O_3S \cdot C_4H_4O_4$ and its structural formula is:

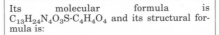
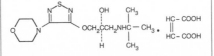

Timolol maleate has a molecular weight of 432.50. It is a white, odorless, crystalline powder which is soluble in water, methanol, and alcohol. TIMOPTIC is stable at room temperature.
TIMOPTIC Ophthalmic Solution is supplied as a sterile, isotonic, buffered, aqueous solution of timolol maleate in two dosage strengths: Each mL of TIMOPTIC 0.25% contains 2.5 mg of timolol (3.4 mg of timolol maleate). The pH of the solution is approximately 7.0, and the osmolarity is 274-328 mOsm.

Each mL of TIMOPTIC 0.5% contains 5 mg of timolol (6.8 mg of timolol maleate). Inactive ingredients: monobasic and dibasic sodium phosphate, sodium hydroxide to adjust pH, and water for injection. Benzalkonium chloride 0.01% is added as preservative.

* Registered trademark of MERCK & CO., INC.
Clinical Pharmacology:
Mechanism of Action
Timolol maleate is a $beta_1$ and $beta_2$(nonselective) adrenergic receptor blocking agent that does not have significant intrinsic sympathomimetic, direct myocardial depressant, or local anesthetic (membrane-stabilizing) activity.
Beta-adrenergic receptor blockade reduces cardiac output in both healthy subjects and patients with heart disease. In patients with severe impairment of myocardial function, beta-adrenergic receptor blockade may inhibit the stimulatory effect of the sympathetic nervous system necessary to maintain adequate cardiac function.
Beta-adrenergic receptor blockade in the bronchi and bronchioles results in increased airway resistance from unopposed parasympathetic activity. Such an effect in patients with asthma or other bronchospastic conditions is potentially dangerous.
TIMOPTIC Ophthalmic Solution, when applied topically on the eye, has the action of reducing elevated as well as normal intraocular pressure, whether or not accompanied by glaucoma. Elevated intraocular pressure is a major risk factor in the pathogenesis of glaucomatous visual field loss. The higher the level of intraocular pressure, the greater the likelihood of glaucomatous visual field loss and optic nerve damage.
The onset of reduction in intraocular pressure following administration of TIMOPTIC can usually be detected within one-half hour after a single dose. The maximum effect usually occurs in one to two hours and significant lowering of intraocular pressure can be maintained for periods as long as 24 hours with a single dose. Repeated observations over a period of one year indicate that the intraocular pressure-lowering effect of TIMOPTIC is well maintained.
The precise mechanism of the ocular hypotensive action of TIMOPTIC is not clearly established at this time. Tonography and fluorophotometry studies in man suggest that its predominant action may be related to reduced aqueous formation. However, in some studies a slight increase in outflow facility was also observed.
Pharmacokinetics
In a study of plasma drug concentration in six subjects, the systemic exposure to timolol was determined following twice daily administration of TIMOPTIC 0.5%. The mean peak plasma concentration following morning dosing was 0.46 ng/mL and following afternoon dosing was 0.35 ng/mL.
Clinical Studies
In controlled multiclinic studies in patients with untreated intraocular pressures of 22 mmHg or greater, TIMOPTIC 0.25 percent or 0.5 percent administered twice a day produced a greater reduction in intraocular pressure than 1, 2, 3, or 4 percent pilocarpine solu-

Continued on next page

Information on the Merck & Co., Inc., products listed on these pages is from the prescribing information in use May 1, 2006. For information, please call 1-800-NSC-MERCK [1-800-672-6372].

Timoptic—Cont.

tion administered four times a day or 0.5, 1, or 2 percent epinephrine hydrochloride solution administered twice a day.

In these studies, TIMOPTIC was generally well tolerated and produced fewer and less severe side effects than either pilocarpine or epinephrine. A slight reduction of resting heart rate in some patients receiving TIMOPTIC (mean reduction 2.9 beats/minute standard deviation 10.2) was observed.

Indications and Usage:
Timoptic Ophthalmic Solution is indicated in the treatment of elevated intraocular pressure in patients with ocular hypertension or open-angle glaucoma.

Contraindications:
TIMOPTIC is contraindicated in patients with (1) bronchial asthma; (2) a history of bronchial asthma; (3) severe chronic obstructive pulmonary disease (see **WARNINGS**); (4) sinus bradycardia; (5) second or third degree atrioventricular block; (6) overt cardiac failure (see **WARNINGS**); (7) cardiogenic shock; or (8) hypersensitivity to any component of this product.

Warnings:
As with many topically applied ophthalmic drugs, this drug is absorbed systemically.

The same adverse reactions found with systemic administration of beta-adrenergic blocking agents may occur with topical administration. For example, severe respiratory reactions and cardiac reactions, including death due to bronchospasm in patients with asthma, and rarely death in association with cardiac failure, have been reported following systemic or ophthalmic administration of timolol maleate (see CONTRAINDICATIONS).

Cardiac Failure
Sympathetic stimulation may be essential for support of the circulation in individuals with diminished myocardial contractility, and its inhibition by beta-adrenergic receptor blockade may precipitate more severe failure.

In Patients Without a History of Cardiac Failure continued depression of the myocardium with beta-blocking agents over a period of time can, in some cases, lead to cardiac failure. At the first sign or symptom of cardiac failure TIMOPTIC should be discontinued.

Obstructive Pulmonary Disease
Patients with chronic obstructive pulmonary disease (e.g., chronic bronchitis, emphysema) of mild or moderate severity, bronchospastic disease, or a history of bronchospastic disease (other than bronchial asthma or a history of bronchial asthma, in which TIMOPTIC is contraindicated [see **CONTRAINDICATIONS**]) should, in general, not receive beta-blockers, including TIMOPTIC.

Major Surgery
The necessity or desirability of withdrawal of beta-adrenergic blocking agents prior to major surgery is controversial. Beta-adrenergic receptor blockade impairs the ability of the heart to respond to beta-adrenergically mediated reflex stimuli. This may augment the risk of general anesthesia in surgical procedures. Some patients receiving beta-adrenergic receptor blocking agents have experienced protracted severe hypotension during anesthesia. Difficulty in restarting and maintaining the heartbeat has also been reported. For these reasons, in patients undergoing elective surgery, some authorities recommend gradual withdrawal of beta-adrenergic receptor blocking agents.

If necessary during surgery, the effects of beta-adrenergic blocking agents may be reversed by sufficient doses of adrenergic agonists.

Diabetes Mellitus
Beta-adrenergic blocking agents should be administered with caution in patients subject to spontaneous hypoglycemia or to diabetic pa-

tients (especially those with labile diabetes) who are receiving insulin or oral hypoglycemic agents. Beta-adrenergic receptor blocking agents may mask the signs and symptoms of acute hypoglycemia.

Thyrotoxicosis
Beta-adrenergic blocking agents may mask certain clinical signs (e.g., tachycardia) of hyperthyroidism. Patients suspected of developing thyrotoxicosis should be managed carefully to avoid abrupt withdrawal of beta-adrenergic blocking agents that might precipitate a thyroid storm.

Precautions:
General
Because of potential effects of beta-adrenergic blocking agents on blood pressure and pulse, these agents should be used with caution in patients with cerebrovascular insufficiency. If signs or symptoms suggesting reduced cerebral blood flow develop following initiation of therapy with TIMOPTIC, alternative therapy should be considered.

There have been reports of bacterial keratitis associated with the use of multiple-dose containers of topical ophthalmic products. These containers had been inadvertently contaminated by patients who, in most cases, had a concurrent corneal disease or a disruption of the ocular epithelial surface. (See **PRECAUTIONS, Information for Patients**.)

Choroidal detachment after filtration procedures has been reported with the administration of aqueous suppressant therapy (e.g. timolol).

Angle-closure glaucoma: In patients with angle-closure glaucoma, the immediate objective of treatment is to reopen the angle. This requires constricting the pupil. Timolol maleate has little or no effect on the pupil. TIMOPTIC should not be used alone in the treatment of angle-closure glaucoma.

Anaphylaxis: While taking beta-blockers, patients with a history of atopy or a history of severe anaphylactic reactions to a variety of allergens may be more reactive to repeated accidental, diagnostic, or therapeutic challenge with such allergens. Such patients may be unresponsive to the usual doses of epinephrine used to treat anaphylactic reactions.

Muscle Weakness: Beta-adrenergic blockade has been reported to potentiate muscle weakness consistent with certain myasthenic symptoms (e.g., diplopia, ptosis, and generalized weakness). Timolol has been reported rarely to increase muscle weakness in some patients with myasthenia gravis or myasthenic symptoms.

Information for Patients
Patients should be instructed to avoid allowing the tip of the dispensing container to contact the eye or surrounding structures.

Patients should also be instructed that ocular solutions, if handled improperly, can become contaminated by common bacteria known to cause ocular infections. Serious damage to the eye and subsequent loss of vision may result from using contaminated solutions. (See **PRECAUTIONS, General**.)

Patients should also be advised that if they have ocular surgery or develop an intercurrent ocular condition (e.g., trauma or infection), they should immediately seek their physician's advice concerning the continued use of the present multidose container.

Patients with bronchial asthma, a history of bronchial asthma, severe chronic obstructive pulmonary disease, sinus bradycardia, second or third degree atrioventricular block, or cardiac failure should be advised not to take this product. (See **CONTRAINDICATIONS**.)

Patients should be advised that TIMOPTIC contains benzalkonium chloride which may be absorbed by soft contact lenses. Contact lenses should be removed prior to administration of the solution. Lenses may be reinserted 15 minutes following TIMOPTIC administration.

Drug Interactions
Although TIMOPTIC used alone has little or no effect on pupil size, mydriasis resulting from concomitant therapy with TIMOPTIC and epinephrine has been reported occasionally.

Beta-adrenergic blocking agents: Patients who are receiving a beta-adrenergic blocking agent orally and TIMOPTIC should be observed for potential additive effects of beta-blockade, both systemic and on intraocular pressure. The concomitant use of two topical beta-adrenergic blocking agents is not recommended.

Calcium antagonists: Caution should be used in the coadministration of beta-adrenergic blocking agents, such as TIMOPTIC, and oral or intravenous calcium antagonists because of possible atrioventricular conduction disturbances, left ventricular failure, and hypotension. In patients with impaired cardiac function, coadministration should be avoided.

Catecholamine-depleting drugs: Close observation of the patient is recommended when a beta blocker is administered to patients receiving catecholamine-depleting drugs such as reserpine, because of possible additive effects and the production of hypotension and/or marked bradycardia, which may result in vertigo, syncope, or postural hypotension.

Digitalis and calcium antagonists: The concomitant use of beta-adrenergic blocking agents with digitalis and calcium antagonists may have additive effects in prolonging atrioventricular conduction time.

CYP2D6 inhibitors: Potentiated systemic beta-blockade (e.g., decreased heart rate, depression) has been reported during combined treatment with CYP2D6 inhibitors (e.g. quinidine, SSRIs) and timolol.

Clonidine: Oral beta-adrenergic blocking agents may exacerbate the rebound hypertension which can follow the withdrawal of clonidine. There have been no reports of exacerbation of rebound hypertension with ophthalmic timolol maleate.

Injectable epinephrine: (See **PRECAUTIONS, General**, Anaphylaxis)

Carcinogenesis, Mutagenesis, Impairment of Fertility
In a two-year oral study of timolol maleate administered orally to rats, there was a statistically significant increase in the incidence of adrenal pheochromocytomas in male rats administered 300 mg/kg/day (approximately 42,000 times the systemic exposure following the maximum recommended human ophthalmic dose). Similar difference were not observed in rats administered oral doses equivalent to approximately 14,000 times the maximum recommended human ophthalmic dose.

In a lifetime oral study in mice, there were statistically significant increases in the incidence of benign and malignant pulmonary tumors, benign uterine polyps and mammary adenocarcinomas in female mice at 500 mg/kg/day, (approximately 71,000 times the systemic exposure following the maximum recommended human ophthalmic dose), but not at 5 or 50 mg/kg/day (approximately 700 or 7,000, respectively, times the systemic exposure following the maximum recommended human ophthalmic dose). In a subsequent study in female mice, in which post-mortem examinations were limited to the uterus and the lungs, a statistically significant increase in the incidence of pulmonary tumors was again observed at 500 mg/kg/day.

The increased occurrence of mammary adenocarcinomas was associated with elevations in serum prolactin which occurred in female mice administered oral timolol at 500 mg/kg/day, but not at doses of 5 or 50 mg/kg/day. An increased incidence of mammary adenocarcinomas in rodents has been associated with administration of several other therapeutic agents that elevate serum prolactin, but no correlation between serum prolactin levels and mammary tumors has been established in humans. Furthermore, in adult human female subjects who received oral dosages of up to 60 mg of timolol maleate (the maximum recommended human oral dosage), there were no clinically meaningful changes in serum prolactin.

Timolol maleate was devoid of mutagenic potential when tested *in vivo* (mouse) in the micronucleus test and cytogenetic assay (doses up to 800 mg/kg) and *in vitro* in a neoplastic-cell transformation assay (up to 100 mcg/mL). In Ames tests the highest concentrations of timolol employed, 5000 or 10,000 mcg/plate, were associated with statistically significant elevations of revertants observed with tester strain TA100 (in seven replicate assays), but not in the remaining three strains. In the assays with tester strain TA100, no consistent dose response relationship was observed, and the ratio of test to control revertants did not reach 2. A ratio of 2 is usually considered the criterion for a positive Ames test.

Reproduction and fertility studies in rats demonstrated no adverse effect on male or female fertility at doses up to 21,000 times the systemic exposure following the maximum recommended human ophthalmic dose.

Pregnancy:
Teratogenic Effects— Pregnancy Category C. Teratogenicity studies with timolol in mice, rats, and rabbits at oral doses up to 50 mg/kg/ day (7,000 times the systemic exposure following the maximum recommended human ophthalmic dose) demonstrated no evidence of fetal malformations. Although delayed fetal ossification was observed at this dose in rats, there were no adverse effects on postnatal development of offspring. Doses of 1000 mg/kg/day (142,000 times the systemic exposure following the maximum recommended human ophthalmic dose) were maternotoxic in mice and resulted in an increased number of fetal resorptions. Increased fetal resorptions were also seen in rabbits at doses of 14,000 times the systemic exposure following the maximum recommended human ophthalmic dose, in this case without apparent maternotoxicity.

There are no adequate and well-controlled studies in pregnant women. TIMOPTIC should be used during pregnancy only if the potential benefit justifies the potential risk to the fetus.

Nursing Mothers
Timolol maleate has been detected in human milk following oral and ophthalmic drug administration. Because of the potential for serious adverse reactions from TIMOPTIC in nursing infants, a decision should be made whether to discontinue nursing or to discontinue the drug, taking into account the importance of the drug to the mother.

Pediatric Use
Safety and effectiveness in pediatric patients have not been established.

Geriatric Use
No overall differences in safety or effectiveness have been observed between elderly and younger patients.

Adverse Reactions:
The most frequently reported adverse experiences have been burning and stinging upon instillation (approximately one in eight patients).

The following additional adverse experiences have been reported less frequently with ocular administration of this or other timolol maleate formulations:

BODY AS A WHOLE
Headache, asthenia/fatigue, and chest pain.

CARDIOVASCULAR
Bradycardia, arrhythmia, hypotension, hypertension, syncope, heart block, cerebral vascular accident, cerebral ischemia, cardiac failure, worsening of angina pectoris, palpitation, car-

diac arrest, pulmonary edema, edema, claudication, Raynaud's phenomenon, and cold hands and feet.

DIGESTIVE
Nausea, diarrhea, dyspepsia, anorexia, and dry mouth.

IMMUNOLOGIC
Systemic lupus erythematosus.

NERVOUS SYSTEM/PSYCHIATRIC
Dizziness, increase in signs and symptoms of myasthenia gravis, paresthesia, somnolence, insomnia, nightmares, behavioral changes and psychic disturbances including depression, confusion, hallucinations, anxiety, disorientation, nervousness, and memory loss.

SKIN
Alopecia and psoriasiform rash or exacerbation of psoriasis.

HYPERSENSITIVITY
Signs and symptoms of systemic allergic reactions, including anaphylaxis, angioedema, urticaria, and localized and generalized rash.

RESPIRATORY
Bronchospasm (predominantly in patients with pre-existing bronchospastic disease), respiratory failure, dyspnea, nasal congestion, cough and upper respiratory infections.

ENDOCRINE
Masked symptoms of hypoglycemia in diabetic patients (see **WARNINGS**).

SPECIAL SENSES
Signs and symptoms of ocular irritation including conjunctivitis, blepharitis, keratitis, ocular pain, discharge (e.g., crusting), foreign body sensation, itching and tearing, and dry eyes; ptosis; decreased corneal sensitivity; cystoid macular edema; visual disturbances including refractive changes and diplopia; pseudopemphigoid; choroidal detachment following filtration surgery (see **PRECAUTIONS, General**); and tinnitus.

UROGENITAL
Retroperitoneal fibrosis, decreased libido, impotence, and Peyronie's disease.

The following additional adverse effects have been reported in clinical experience with ORAL timolol maleate or other ORAL beta-blocking agents and may be considered potential effects of ophthalmic timolol maleate: *Allergic:* Erythematous rash, fever combined with aching and sore throat, laryngospasm with respiratory distress; *Body as a Whole:* Extremity pain, decreased exercise tolerance, weight loss; *Cardiovascular:* Worsening of arterial insufficiency, vasodilatation; *Digestive:* Gastrointestinal pain, hepatomegaly, vomiting, mesenteric arterial thrombosis, ischemic colitis; *Hematologic:* Nonthrombocytopenic purpura; thrombocytopenic purpura, agranulocytosis; *Endocrine:* Hyperglycemia, hypoglycemia; *Skin:* Pruritus, skin irritation, increased pigmentation, sweating; *Musculoskeletal:* Arthralgia; *Nervous System/ Psychiatric:* Vertigo, local weakness, diminished concentration, reversible mental depression progressing to catatonia, and acute reversible syndrome characterized by disorientation for time and place, emotional lability, slightly clouded sensorium, and decreased performance on neuropsychometrics; *Respiratory:* Rales, bronchial obstruction; *Urogenital:* Urination difficulties.

Overdosage:
There have been reports of inadvertent overdosage with TIMOPTIC Ophthalmic Solution resulting in systemic effects similar to those seen with systemic beta-adrenergic blocking agents such as dizziness, headache, shortness of breath, bradycardia, bronchospasm, and cardiac arrest (see also ADVERSE REACTIONS).

Overdosage has been reported with Tablets BLOCADREN* (timolol maleate tablets). A 30-year-old female ingested 650 mg of BLOCADREN (maximum recommended oral daily dose is 60 mg) and experienced second

and third degree heart block. She recovered without treatment but approximately two months later developed irregular heartbeat, hypertension, dizziness, tinnitus, faintness, increased pulse rate, and borderline first degree heart block.

An *in vitro* hemodialysis study, using ^{14}C timolol added to human plasma or whole blood, showed that timolol was readily dialyzed from these fluids; however, a study of patients with renal failure showed that timolol did not dialyze readily.

* Registered trademark of MERCK & CO., INC.

Dosage and Administration:
TIMOPTIC Ophthalmic Solution is available in concentrations of 0.25 and 0.5 percent. The usual starting dose is one drop of 0.25 percent TIMOPTIC in the affected eye(s) twice a day. If the clinical response is not adequate, the dosage may be changed to one drop of 0.5 percent solution in the affected eye(s) twice a day. Since in some patients the pressure-lowering response to TIMOPTIC may require a few weeks to stabilize, evaluation should include a determination of intraocular pressure after approximately 4 weeks of treatment with TIMOPTIC.

If the intraocular pressure is maintained at satisfactory levels, the dosage schedule may be changed to one drop once a day in the affected eye(s). Because of diurnal variations in intraocular pressure, satisfactory response to the once-a-day dose is best determined by measuring the intraocular pressure at different times during the day.

Dosages above one drop of 0.5 percent TIMOPTIC twice a day generally have not been shown to produce further reduction in intraocular pressure. If the patient's intraocular pressure is still not at a satisfactory level on this regimen, concomitant therapy with other agent(s) for lowering intraocular pressure can be instituted. The concomitant use of two topical beta-adrenergic blocking agents is not recommended. (See PRECAUTIONS, Drug Interactions, Beta-adrenergic blocking agents.)

How Supplied:
Sterile Ophthalmic Solution TIMOPTIC is a clear, colorless to light yellow solution.
No. 8895—TIMOPTIC Ophthalmic Solution, 0.25% timolol equivalent, is supplied in an OCUMETER®* PLUS container, a white, translucent HDPE plastic ophthalmic dispenser with a controlled drop tip and a white polystyrene cap with yellow label as follows:
NDC 0006-8895-35, 5 mL in a 7.5 mL capacity bottle
No. 8896—TIMOPTIC Ophthalmic Solution, 0.5% timolol equivalent, is supplied in an OCUMETER®* PLUS container, a white translucent, HDPE plastic ophthalmic dispenser with a controlled drop tip and a white polystyrene cap with yellow label as follows:
NDC 0006-8896-35, 5 mL in a 7.5 mL capacity bottle
NDC 0006-8896-36, 10 mL in an 18 mL capacity bottle.

Storage:
Store at room temperature, 15–30°C (59–86°F). Protect from freezing. Protect from light.

---

* Registered trademark of MERCK & CO., INC.

Continued on next page

Information on the Merck & Co., Inc., products listed on these pages is from the prescribing information in use May 1, 2006. For information, please call 1-800-NSC-MERCK [1-800-672-6372].

Timoptic—Cont.

INSTRUCTIONS FOR USE

Please follow these instructions carefully when using TIMOPTIC*. Use TIMOPTIC as prescribed by your doctor.

1. If you use other topically applied ophthalmic medications, they should be administered at least 10 minutes before or after TIMOPTIC.
2. Wash hands before each use.
3. Before using the medication for the first time, be sure the Safety Strip on the front of the bottle is unbroken. A gap between the bottle and the cap is normal for an unopened bottle.

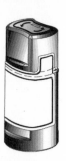

Opening Arrows ▶

Safety Strip ▶

4. Tear off the Safety Strip to break the seal. [See first figure above]
5. To open the bottle, unscrew the cap by turning as indicated by the arrows on the top of the cap. Do not pull the cap directly up and away from the bottle. Pulling the cap directly up will prevent your container from opening properly.

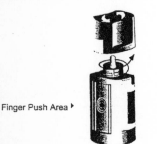

Finger Push Area ▶

6. Tilt your head back and pull your lower eyelid down slightly to form a pocket between your eyelid and your eye.

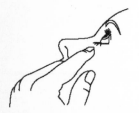

7. Invert the bottle, and press lightly with the thumb or index finger over the "Finger Push Area" (as shown) until a single drop is dispensed into the eye as directed by your doctor.
   [See second figure above]
   DO NOT TOUCH YOUR EYE OR EYELID WITH THE DROPPER TIP.
   OPHTHALMIC MEDICATIONS, IF HANDLED IMPROPERLY, CAN BECOME CONTAMINATED BY COMMON BACTERIA KNOWN TO CAUSE EYE INFECTIONS. SERIOUS DAMAGE TO THE

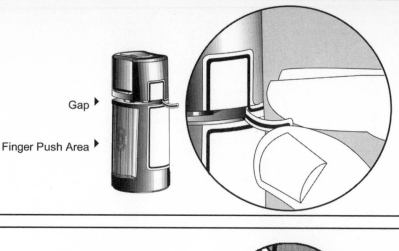

Gap ▶

Finger Push Area ▶

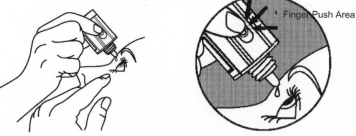

◀ Finger Push Area

EYE AND SUBSEQUENT LOSS OF VISION MAY RESULT FROM USING CONTAMINATED OPHTHALMIC MEDICATIONS. IF YOU THINK YOUR MEDICATION MAY BE CONTAMINATED, OR IF YOU DEVELOP AN EYE INFECTION, CONTACT YOUR DOCTOR IMMEDIATELY CONCERNING CONTINUED USE OF THIS BOTTLE.

8. If drop dispensing is difficult after opening for the first time, replace the cap on the bottle and tighten (DO NOT OVERTIGHTEN) and then remove by turning the cap in the opposite direction as indicated by the arrows on the top of the cap.
9. Repeat steps 6 & 7 with the other eye if instructed to do so by your doctor.
10. Replace the cap by turning until it is firmly touching the bottle. The arrow on the left side of the cap must be aligned with the arrow on the left side of the bottle label for proper closure. Do not overtighten or you may damage the bottle and cap.
11. The dispenser tip is designed to provide a single drop; therefore, do NOT enlarge the hole of the dispenser tip.
12. After you have used all doses, there will be some TIMOPTIC left in the bottle. You should not be concerned since an extra amount of TIMOPTIC has been added and you will get the full amount of TIMOPTIC that your doctor prescribed. Do not attempt to remove excess medicine from the bottle.

WARNING: Keep out of reach of children.
If you have any questions about the use of TIMOPTIC, please consult your doctor.

* Registered trademark of MERCK & CO., Inc.
Manuf. for:
Merck & Co., Inc., Whitehouse Station, NJ 08889, USA
By: Laboratories Merck Sharp & Dohme-Chibret
63963 Clermont-Ferrand Cedex 9, France
  9391006   Issued September 2005

Shown in Product Identification Guide, page 105

TIMOPTIC®   ℞
0.25% and 0.5%
(timolol maleate ophthalmic solution)
in OCUDOSE® (dispenser)
Preservative-Free Sterile Ophthalmic Solution in a Sterile Ophthalmic Unit Dose Dispenser

Description:

Timolol maleate is a non-selective beta-adrenergic receptor blocking agent. Its chemical name is (-) - 1 - (*tert* - butylamino) - 3 - [(4 - morpholino - 1, 2, 5 - thiadiazol - 3 - yl) oxy] - 2 - propanol maleate (1:1) (salt). Timolol maleate possesses an asymmetric carbon atom in its structure and is provided as the levoisomer. The nominal optical rotation of timolol maleate is

$$[\alpha]^{25°}_{405\ nm} \text{ in } 1.0N\ HCl\ (C = 5\%) = -12.2° \ (-11.7° \text{ to } -12.5°).$$

Its molecular formula is $C_{13}H_{24}N_4O_3S \cdot C_4H_4O_4$ and its structural formula is:

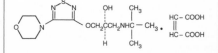

Timolol maleate has a molecular weight of 432.50. It is a white, odorless, crystalline powder which is soluble in water, methanol, and alcohol. Timolol maleate is stable at room temperature. Timolol maleate ophthalmic solution is supplied in two formulations: Ophthalmic Solution TIMOPTIC* (timolol maleate ophthalmic solution), which contains the preservative benzalkonium chloride; and Ophthalmic Solution TIMOPTIC* (timolol maleate ophthalmic solution), the preservative-free formulation. Preservative-free Ophthalmic Solution The pH of the solution is approximately 7.0, and the osmolarity is 252–328 mOsm. TIMOPTIC is supplied in OCUDOSE*, a unit dose container, as a sterile, isotonic, buffered, aqueous solution of timolol maleate in two dosage strengths: Each mL of Preservative-free TIMOPTIC in OCUDOSE 0.25% contains 2.5 mg of timolol (3.4 mg of timolol maleate). Each mL of Preservative-free TIMOPTIC in OCUDOSE 0.5% contains 5 mg of timolol (6.8 mg of timolol maleate). Inactive ingredients: monobasic and dibasic sodium phosphate, sodium hydroxide to adjust pH, and water for injection.

---

* Registered trademark of MERCK & CO., INC.

Clinical Pharmacology:

Mechanism of Action

Timolol maleate is a beta$_1$ and beta$_2$ (non-lective) adrenergic receptor blocking agent that does not have significant intrinsic sympathomimetic, direct myocardial depressant, or local anesthetic (membrane-stabilizing) activity.

Beta-adrenergic receptor blockade reduces cardiac output in both healthy subjects and patients with heart disease. In patients with severe impairment of myocardial function beta-adrenergic receptor blockade may inhibit the stimulatory effect of the sympathetic nervous system necessary to maintain adequate cardiac function.

Beta-adrenergic receptor blockade in the bronchi and bronchioles results in increased airway resistance from unopposed parasympathetic activity. Such an effect in patients with asthma or other bronchospastic conditions is potentially dangerous.

TIMOPTIC (timolol maleate ophthalmic solution), when applied topically on the eye, has the action of reducing elevated as well as normal intraocular pressure, whether or not accompanied by glaucoma. Elevated intraocular pressure is a major risk factor in the pathogenesis of glaucomatous visual field loss. The higher the level of intraocular pressure, the greater the likelihood of glaucomatous visual field loss and optic nerve damage.

The onset of reduction in intraocular pressure following administration of TIMOPTIC (timolol maleate ophthalmic solution) can usually be detected within one-half hour after a single dose. The maximum effect usually occurs in one to two hours and significant lowering of intraocular pressure can be maintained for periods as long as 24 hours with a single dose. Repeated observations over a period of one year indicate that the intraocular pressure-lowering effect of TIMOPTIC (timolol maleate ophthalmic solution) is well maintained.

The precise mechanism of the ocular hypotensive action of TIMOPTIC (timolol maleate ophthalmic solution) is not clearly established at this time. Tonography and fluorophotometry studies in man suggest that its predominant action may be related to reduced aqueous formation. However, in some studies a slight increase in outflow facility was also observed.

Pharmacokinetics

In a study of plasma drug concentration in six subjects, the systemic exposure to timolol was determined following twice daily administration of TIMOPTIC 0.5%. The mean peak plasma concentration following morning dosing was 0.46 ng/mL and following afternoon dosing was 0.35 ng/mL.

Clinical Studies

In controlled multiclinic studies in patients with untreated intraocular pressures of 22 mmHg or greater, TIMOPTIC (timolol maleate ophthalmic solution) 0.25 percent or 0.5 percent administered twice a day produced a greater reduction in intraocular pressure than 1,2,3, or 4 percent pilocarpine solution administered four times a day or 0.5, 1, or 2 percent epinephrine hydrochloride solution administered twice a day.

In these studies, TIMOPTIC (timolol maleate ophthalmic solution) was generally well tolerated and produced fewer and less severe side effects than either pilocarpine or epinephrine. A slight reduction of resting heart rate in some patients receiving TIMOPTIC (timolol maleate ophthalmic solution) (mean reduction 2.9 beats/minute standard deviation 10.2) was observed.

Indications and Usage:

Preservative-free TIMOPTIC in OCUDOSE is indicated in the treatment of elevated intraocular pressure in patients with ocular hypertension or open-angle glaucoma.

Preservative-free TIMOPTIC in OCUDOSE may be used when a patient is sensitive to the preservative in TIMOPTIC (timolol maleate ophthalmic solution), benzalkonium chloride, or when use of a preservative-free topical medication is advisable.

Contraindications:

Preservative-free TIMOPTIC in OCUDOSE is contraindicated in patients with (1) bronchial asthma; (2) a history of bronchial asthma; (3) severe chronic obstructive pulmonary disease (see **WARNINGS**); (4) sinus bradycardia; (5) second or third degree atrioventricular block; (6) overt cardiac failure (see **WARNINGS**); (7) cardiogenic shock; or (8) hypersensitivity to any component of this product.

Warnings:

As with many topically applied ophthalmic drugs, this drug is absorbed systemically.

The same adverse reactions found with systemic administration of beta-adrenergic blocking agents may occur with topical administration. For example, severe respiratory reactions and cardiac reactions, including death due to bronchospasm in patients with asthma, and rarely death in association with cardiac failure, have been reported following systemic or ophthalmic administration of timolol maleate (see CONTRAINDICATIONS).

Cardiac Failure

Sympathetic stimulation may be essential for support of the circulation in individuals with diminished myocardial contractility, and its inhibition by beta-adrenergic receptor blockade may precipitate more severe failure.

In Patients Without a History of Cardiac Failure continued depression of the myocardium with beta-blocking agents over a period of time can, in some cases, lead to cardiac failure. At the first sign or symptom of cardiac failure Preservative-free TIMOPTIC in OCUDOSE should be discontinued.

Obstructive Pulmonary Disease

Patients with chronic obstructive pulmonary disease (e.g., chronic bronchitis, emphysema) of mild or moderate severity, bronchospastic disease, or a history of bronchospastic disease (other than bronchial asthma or a history of bronchial asthma, in which TIMOPTIC in OCUDOSE is contraindicated [see **CONTRAINDICATIONS**]) should, in general, not receive beta-blockers, including Preservative-free TIMOPTIC in OCUDOSE.

Major Surgery

The necessity or desirability of withdrawal of beta-adrenergic blocking agents prior to major surgery is controversial. Beta-adrenergic receptor blockade impairs the ability of the heart to respond to beta-adrenergically mediated reflex stimuli. This may augment the risk of general anesthesia in surgical procedures. Some patients receiving beta-adrenergic receptor blocking agents have experienced protracted severe hypotension during anesthesia. Difficulty in restarting and maintaining the heartbeat has also been reported. For these reasons, in patients undergoing elective surgery, some authorities recommend gradual withdrawal of beta-adrenergic receptor blocking agents.

If necessary during surgery, the effects of beta-adrenergic blocking agents may be reversed by sufficient doses of adrenergic agonists.

Diabetes Mellitus

Beta-adrenergic blocking agents should be administered with caution in patients subject to spontaneous hypoglycemia or to diabetic patients (especially those with labile diabetes) who are receiving insulin or oral hypoglycemic agents. Beta-adrenergic receptor blocking agents may mask the signs and symptoms of acute hypoglycemia.

Thyrotoxicosis

Beta-adrenergic blocking agents may mask certain clinical signs (e.g., tachycardia) of hyperthyroidism. Patients suspected of developing thyrotoxicosis should be managed carefully to avoid abrupt withdrawal of beta-adrenergic blocking agents that might precipitate a thyroid storm.

Precautions:

General

Because of potential effects of beta-adrenergic blocking agents on blood pressure and pulse, these agents should be used with caution in patients with cerebrovascular insufficiency. If signs or symptoms suggesting reduced cerebral blood flow develop following initiation of therapy with Preservative-free TIMOPTIC in OCUDOSE, alternative therapy should be considered.

Choroidal detachment after filtration procedures has been reported with the administration of aqueous suppressant therapy (e.g. timolol).

Angle-closure glaucoma: In patients with angle-closure glaucoma, the immediate objective of treatment is to reopen the angle. This requires constricting the pupil. Timolol maleate has little or no effect on the pupil. TIMOPTIC in OCUDOSE should not be used alone in the treatment of angle-closure glaucoma.

Anaphylaxis: While taking beta-blockers, patients with a history of atopy or a history of severe anaphylactic reactions to a variety of allergens may be more reactive to repeated accidental, diagnostic, or therapeutic challenge with such allergens. Such patients may be unresponsive to the usual doses of epinephrine used to treat anaphylactic reactions.

Muscle Weakness: Beta-adrenergic blockade has been reported to potentiate muscle weakness consistent with certain myasthenic symptoms (e.g., diplopia, ptosis, and generalized weakness). Timolol has been reported rarely to increase muscle weakness in some patients with myasthenia gravis or myasthenic symptoms.

Information for Patients

Patients should be instructed about the use of Preservative-free TIMOPTIC in OCUDOSE.

Since sterility cannot be maintained after the individual unit is opened, patients should be instructed to use the product immediately after opening, and to discard the individual unit and any remaining contents immediately after use.

Continued on next page

Information on the Merck & Co., Inc., products listed on these pages is from the prescribing information in use May 1, 2006. For information, please call 1-800-NSC-MERCK [1-800-672-6372].

Timoptic in Ocudose—Cont.

Patients with bronchial asthma, a history of bronchial asthma, severe chronic obstructive pulmonary disease, sinus bradycardia, second or third degree atrioventricular block, or cardiac failure should be advised not to take this product. (See **CONTRAINDICATIONS**.)

Drug Interactions

Although TIMOPTIC (timolol maleate ophthalmic solution) used alone has little or no effect on pupil size, mydriasis resulting from concomitant therapy with TIMOPTIC (timolol maleate ophthalmic solution) and epinephrine has been reported occasionally.

Beta-adrenergic blocking agents: Patients who are receiving a beta-adrenergic blocking agent orally and Preservative-free TIMOPTIC in OCUDOSE should be observed for potential additive effects of beta-blockade, both systemic and on intraocular pressure. The concomitant use of two topical beta-adrenergic blocking agents is not recommended.

Calcium antagonists: Caution should be used in the coadministration of beta-adrenergic blocking agents, such as Preservative-free TIMOPTIC in OCUDOSE, and oral or intravenous calcium antagonists, because of possible atrioventricular conduction disturbances, left ventricular failure, and hypotension. In patients with impaired cardiac function, coadministration should be avoided.

Catecholamine-depleting drugs: Close observation of the patient is recommended when a beta blocker is administered to patients receiving catecholamine-depleting drugs such as reserpine, because of possible additive effects and the production of hypotension and/or marked bradycardia, which may result in vertigo, syncope, or postural hypotension.

Digitalis and calcium antagonists: The concomitant use of beta-adrenergic blocking agents with digitalis and calcium antagonists may have additive effects in prolonging atrioventricular conduction time.

CYP2D6 inhibitors: Potentiated systemic beta-blockade (e.g., decreased heart rate, depression) has been reported during combined treatment with CYP2D6 inhibitors (e.g., quinidine, SSRIs) and timolol.

Clonidine: Oral beta-adrenergic blocking agents may exacerbate the rebound hypertension which can follow the withdrawal of clonidine. There have been no reports of exacerbation of rebound hypertension with ophthalmic timolol maleate.

Injectable epinephrine: (See **PRECAUTIONS, General**, Anaphylaxis)

Carcinogenesis, Mutagenesis, Impairment of Fertility

In a two-year oral study of timolol maleate administered orally to rats, there was a statistically significant increase in the incidence of adrenal pheochromocytomas in male rats administered 300 mg/kg/day (approximately 42,000 times the systemic exposure following the maximum recommended human ophthalmic dose). Similar differences were not observed in rats administered oral doses equivalent to approximately 14,000 times the maximum recommended human ophthalmic dose.

In a lifetime oral study in mice, there were statistically significant increases in the incidence of benign and malignant pulmonary tumors, benign uterine polyps and mammary adenocarcinomas in female mice at 500 mg/kg/day (approximately 71,000 times the systemic exposure following the maximum recommended human ophthalmic dose), but not at 5 or 50 mg/kg/day (approximately 700 or 7,000 times, respectively, the systemic exposure following the maximum recommended human ophthalmic dose). In a subsequent study in female mice, in which post-mortem examina-

tions were limited to the uterus and the lungs, a statistically significant increase in the incidence of pulmonary tumors was again observed at 500 mg/kg/day.

The increased occurrence of mammary adenocarcinomas was associated with elevations in serum prolactin which occurred in female mice administered oral timolol at 500 mg/kg/day, but not at doses of 5 or 50 mg/kg/day. An increased incidence of mammary adenocarcinomas in rodents has been associated with administration of several other therapeutic agents that elevate serum prolactin, but no correlation between serum prolactin levels and mammary tumors has been established in humans. Furthermore, in adult human female subjects who received oral timolol at doses of up to 60 mg of timolol maleate (the maximum recommended human oral dosage), there were no clinically meaningful changes in serum prolactin.

Timolol maleate was devoid of mutagenic potential when tested *in vivo* (mouse) in the micronucleus test and cytogenetic assay (doses up to 800 mg/kg) and *in vitro* in a neoplastic cell transformation assay (up to 100 mcg/mL). In Ames tests the highest concentrations of timolol employed, 5000 or 10,000 mcg/plate, were associated with statistically significant elevations of revertants observed with tester strain TA 100 (in seven replicate assays), but not in the remaining three strains. In the assays with tester strain TA 100, no consistent dose response relationship was observed, and the ratio of test to control revertants did not reach 2. A ratio of 2 is usually considered the criterion for a positive Ames test.

Reproduction and fertility studies in rats demonstrated no adverse effect on male or female fertility at doses up to 21,000 times the systemic exposure following the maximum recommended human ophthalmic dose.

Pregnancy:

Teratogenic Effects—Pregnancy Category C. Teratogenicity studies with timolol in mice, rats and rabbits at oral doses up to 50 mg/kg/day (7,000 times the systemic exposure following the maximum recommended human ophthalmic dose) demonstrated no evidence of fetal malformations. Although delayed fetal ossification was observed at this dose in rats, there were no adverse effects on postnatal development of offspring. Doses of 1000 mg/kg/day (142,000 times the systemic exposure following the maximum recommended human ophthalmic dose) were maternotoxic in mice and resulted in an increased number of fetal resorptions. Increased fetal resorptions were also seen in rabbits at doses of 14,000 times the systemic exposure following the maximum recommended human ophthalmic dose, in this case without apparent maternotoxicity.

There are no adequate and well-controlled studies in pregnant women. Preservative-free TIMOPTIC in OCUDOSE should be used during pregnancy only if the potential benefit justifies the potential risk to the fetus.

Nursing Mothers

Timolol maleate has been detected in human milk following oral and ophthalmic drug administration. Because of the potential for serious adverse reactions from timolol in nursing infants, a decision should be made whether to discontinue nursing or to discontinue the drug, taking into account the importance of the drug to the mother.

Pediatric Use

Safety and effectiveness in pediatric patients have not been established.

Geriatric Use

No overall differences in safety or effectiveness have been observed between elderly and younger patients.

Adverse Reactions:

The most frequently reported adverse experiences have been burning and stinging upon instillation (approximately one in eight patients).

The following additional adverse experiences have been reported less frequently with ocular administration of this or other timolol maleate formulations:

BODY AS A WHOLE
Headache, asthenia/fatigue, chest pain.

CARDIOVASCULAR
Bradycardia, arrhythmia, hypotension, hypertension, syncope, heart block, cerebral vascular accident, cerebral ischemia, cardiac failure, worsening of angina pectoris, palpitation, cardiac arrest, pulmonary edema, edema, claudication, Raynaud's phenomenon, and cold hands and feet.

DIGESTIVE
Nausea, diarrhea. dyspepsia, anorexia, and dry mouth.

IMMUNOLOGIC
Systemic lupus erythematosus.

NERVOUS SYSTEM/PSYCHIATRIC
Dizziness, increase in signs and symptoms of myasthenia gravis, paresthesia, somnolence, insomnia, nightmares, behavioral changes and psychic disturbances including depression, confusion, hallucinations, anxiety, disorientation, nervousness, and memory loss.

SKIN
Alopecia and psoriasiform rash or exacerbation of psoriasis.

HYPERSENSITIVITY
Signs and symptoms of systemic allergic reactions, including anaphylaxis, angioedema, urticaria, and localized and generalized rash.

RESPIRATORY
Bronchospasm (predominantly in patients with pre-existing bronchospastic disease), respiratory failure, dyspnea, nasal congestion, cough and upper respiratory infections.

ENDOCRINE
Masked symptoms of hypoglycemia in diabetic patients (see **WARNINGS**).

SPECIAL SENSES
Signs and symptoms of ocular irritation including conjunctivitis, blepharitis, keratitis, ocular pain, discharge (e.g., crusting), foreign body sensation, itching and tearing, and dry eyes; ptosis; decreased corneal sensitivity; cystoid macular edema; visual disturbances including refractive changes and diplopia; pseudopemphigoid; choroidal detachment following filtration surgery (see **PRECAUTIONS, General**); and tinnitus.

UROGENITAL
Retroperitoneal fibrosis, decreased libido, impotence, and Peyronie's disease.

The following additional adverse effects have been reported in clinical experience with ORAL timolol maleate or other ORAL beta blocking agents, and may be considered potential effects of ophthalmic timolol maleate: *Allergic:* Erythematous rash, fever combined with aching and sore throat, laryngospasm with respiratory distress; *Body as a Whole:* Extremity pain, decreased exercise tolerance, weight loss; *Cardiovascular:* Worsening of arterial insufficiency, vasodilatation; *Digestive:* Gastrointestinal pain, hepatomegaly, vomiting, mesenteric arterial thrombosis, ischemic colitis; *Hematologic:* Nonthrombocytopenic purpura; thrombocytopenic purpura; agranulocytosis; *Endocrine:* Hyperglycemia, hypoglycemia; *Skin:* Pruritus, skin irritation, increased pigmentation, sweating; *Musculoskeletal:* Arthralgia; *Nervous System/Psychiatric:* Vertigo, local weakness, diminished concentration, reversible mental depression progressing to catatonia, an acute reversible syndrome characterized by disorientation for time and place, emotional lability, slightly clouded sensorium, and decreased performance on neuropsychometrics; *Respiratory:* Rales, bronchial obstruction; *Urogenital:* Urination difficulties.

Overdosage:

There have been reports of inadvertent overdosage with Ophthalmic Solution TIMOPTIC (timolol maleate ophthalmic solution) resulting in systemic effects similar to those seen with systemic beta-adrenergic blocking agents such as dizziness, headache, shortness of breath, bradycardia, bronchospasm, and cardiac arrest (see also **ADVERSE REACTIONS**).

Overdosage has been reported with Tablets BLOCADREN* (timolol maleate tablets). A 30 year old female ingested 650 mg of BLOCADREN (maximum recommended oral daily dose is 60 mg) and experienced second and third degree heart block. She recovered without treatment but approximately two months later developed irregular heartbeat, hypertension, dizziness, tinnitus, faintness, increased pulse rate, and borderline first degree heart block.

An *in vitro* hemodialysis study, using ^{14}C timolol added to human plasma or whole blood, showed that timolol was readily dialyzed from these fluids; however, a study of patients with renal failure showed that timolol did not dialyze readily.

---

* Registered trademark of MERCK & CO., INC.

Dosage and Administration:

Preservative-free TIMOPTIC in OCUDOSE is a sterile solution that does not contain a preservative. The solution from one individual unit is to be used immediately after opening for administration to one or both eyes. Since sterility cannot be guaranteed after the individual unit is opened, the remaining contents should be discarded immediately after administration.

Preservative-free TIMOPTIC in OCUDOSE is available in concentrations of 0.25 and 0.5 percent. The usual starting dose is one drop of 0.25 percent Preservative-free TIMOPTIC in OCUDOSE in the affected eye(s) administered twice a day. Apply enough gentle pressure on the individual container to obtain a single drop of solution. If the clinical response is not adequate, the dosage may be changed to one drop of 0.5 percent solution in the affected eye(s) administered twice a day.

Since in some patients the pressure-lowering response to Preservative-free TIMOPTIC in OCUDOSE may require a few weeks to stabilize, evaluation should include a determination of intraocular pressure after approximately 4 weeks of treatment with Preservative-free TIMOPTIC in OCUDOSE.

If the intraocular pressure is maintained at satisfactory levels, the dosage schedule may be changed to one drop once a day in the affected eye(s). Because of diurnal variations in intraocular pressure, satisfactory response to the once-a-day dose is best determined by measuring the intraocular pressure at different times during the day.

Dosages above one drop of 0.5 percent TIMOPTIC (timolol maleate ophthalmic solution) twice a day generally have not been shown to produce further reduction in intraocular pressure. If the patient's intraocular pressure is still not at a satisfactory level on this regimen, concomitant therapy with other agent(s) for lowering intraocular pressure can be instituted taking into consideration that the preparation(s) used concomitantly may contain one or more preservatives. The concomitant use of two topical beta-adrenergic blocking agents is not recommended. (See **PRECAUTIONS, Drug Interactions, Beta-adrenergic blocking agents**.)

How Supplied:

Preservative-free Sterile Ophthalmic Solution TIMOPTIC in OCUDOSE is a clear, colorless to light yellow solution.

No. 9689—Preservative-free TIMOPTIC, 0.25% timolol equivalent, is supplied in OCUDOSE, a clear low density polyethylene unit dose container. Each individual unit contains 0.2 mL of solution, and is available in a foil laminate overwrapped pouch as follows:

NDC 0006-9689-60; 60 Individual Unit Doses

No. 9690—Preservative-free TIMOPTIC, 0.5% timolol equivalent, is supplied in OCUDOSE, a clear low density polyethylene unit dose container. Each individual unit contains 0.2 mL of solution, and is available in a foil laminate overwrapped pouch as follows:

NDC 0006-9690-60; 60 Individual Unit Doses

Storage

Store at room temperature, 15–30°C (59–86°F). Protect from freezing. Protect from light.

Because evaporation can occur through the unprotected polyethylene unit dose container and prolonged exposure to direct light can modify the product, the unit dose container should be kept in the protective foil overwrap and used within one month after the foil package has been opened.

Manuf. for:

Merck & Co., Inc., Whitehouse Station, NJ 08889, USA

By: Laboratories Merck Sharp & Dohme-Chibret

63963 Clermont-Ferrand Cedex 9, France

9351205   Issued July 2005

COPYRIGHT © 1986, 1995 MERCK & CO., INC.

All rights reserved

Shown in Product Identification Guide, page 105

TIMOPTIC-XE®

℞

0.25% and 0.5%

(timolol maleate ophthalmic gel forming solution)

Sterile Ophthalmic Gel Forming Solution

Description:

TIMOPTIC-XE* (timolol maleate ophthalmic gel forming solution) is a non-selective beta-adrenergic receptor blocking agent. Its chemical name is (-)-1-(*tert*-butyl-amino)-3-[(4-morpholino - 1,2,5 - thiadiazol - 3 - yl)oxy] - 2 - propanol maleate (1:1) (salt). Timolol maleate possesses an asymmetric carbon atom in its structure and is provided as the levo-isomer. The optical rotation of timolol maleate is:

$$[\alpha]_{405\ nm}^{25°} \text{ in 1.0N HCl (C = 5\%) = } -12.2°$$
$$(-11.7° \text{ to } -12.5°).$$

Its molecular formula is $C_{13}H_{24}N_4O_3S \cdot C_4H_4O_4$ and its structural formula is:

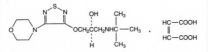

Timolol maleate has a molecular weight of 432.50. It is a white, odorless, crystalline powder which is soluble in water, methanol, and alcohol.

TIMOPTIC-XE Sterile Ophthalmic Gel Forming Solution is supplied as a sterile, isotonic, buffered, aqueous solution of timolol maleate in two dosage strengths. The pH of the solution is approximately 7.0, and the osmolarity is 260– 330 mOsm. Each mL of TIMOPTIC-XE 0.25% contains 2.5 mg of timolol (3.4 mg of timolol maleate). Each mL of TIMOPTIC-XE 0.5% contains 5 mg of timolol (6.8 mg of timolol maleate). Inactive ingredients: GELRITE gellan gum, tromethamine, mannitol, and water for injection. Preservative: benzododecinium bromide 0.012%.

GELRITE is a purified anionic heteropolysaccharide derived from gellan gum. An aqueous solution of GELRITE, in the presence of a cation, has the ability to gel. Upon contact with the precorneal tear film, TIMOPTIC-XE forms a gel that is subsequently removed by the flow of tears.

---

* Registered trademark of MERCK & CO., INC.

Clinical Pharmacology:

Mechanism of Action

Timolol maleate is a beta$_1$ and beta$_2$ (non-selective) adrenergic receptor blocking agent that does not have significant intrinsic sympathomimetic, direct myocardial depressant, or local anesthetic (membrane-stabilizing) activity.

TIMOPTIC-XE, when applied topically on the eye, has the action of reducing elevated, as well as normal intraocular pressure, whether or not accompanied by glaucoma. Elevated intraocular pressure is a major risk factor in the pathogenesis of glaucomatous visual field loss and optic nerve damage.

The precise mechanism of the ocular hypotensive action of TIMOPTIC-XE is not clearly established at this time. Tonography and fluorophotometry studies of TIMOPTIC* (timolol maleate ophthalmic solution) in man suggest that its predominant action may be related to reduced aqueous formation. However, in some studies, a slight increase in outflow facility was also observed.

Beta-adrenergic receptor blockade reduces cardiac output in both healthy subjects and patients with heart disease. In patients with severe impairment of myocardial function beta-adrenergic receptor blockade may inhibit the stimulatory effect of the sympathetic nervous system necessary to maintain adequate cardiac function.

Beta-adrenergic receptor blockade in the bronchi and bronchioles results in increased airway resistance from unopposed parasympathetic activity. Such an effect in patients with asthma or other bronchospastic conditions is potentially dangerous.

Pharmacokinetics

In a study of plasma drug concentration in six subjects, the systemic exposure to timolol was determined following once daily administration of TIMOPTIC-XE 0.5% in the morning. The mean peak plasma concentration following this morning dose was 0.28 ng/mL.

Clinical Studies

In controlled, double-masked, multicenter clinical studies, comparing TIMOPTIC-XE 0.25% to TIMOPTIC 0.25% and TIMOPTIC-XE 0.5% to TIMOPTIC 0.5%, TIMOPTIC-XE administered once a day was shown to be equally effective in lowering intraocular pressure as the equivalent concentration of TIMOPTIC administered twice a day. The effect of timolol in lowering intraocular pressure was evident for 24 hours with a single dose of TIMOPTIC-XE. Repeated observations over a period of six months indicate that the intraocular pressure-lowering effect of TIMOPTIC-XE was consistent. The results from the largest U.S. and international clinical

---

Continued on next page

Information on the Merck & Co., Inc., products listed on these pages is from the prescribing information in use May 1, 2006. For information, please call 1-800-NSC-MERCK [1-800-672-6372].

Timoptic-XE—Cont.

trials comparing TIMOPTIC-XE 0.5% to TIMOPTIC 0.5% are shown in Figure 1. TIMOPTIC-XE administered once daily had a safety profile similar to that of an equivalent concentration of TIMOPTIC administered twice daily. Due to the physical characteristics of the formulation, there was a higher incidence of transient blurred vision in patients administered TIMOPTIC-XE. A slight reduction in resting heart rate was observed in some patients receiving TIMOPTIC-XE 0.5% (mean reduction 24 hours post-dose 0.8 beats/minute, mean reduction 2 hours post-dose 3.8 beats/minute). (See **ADVERSE REACTIONS**.) TIMOPTIC-XE has not been studied in patients wearing contact lenses.

* Registered trademark of MERCK & CO., INC.

Indications and Usage:
TIMOPTIC-XE Sterile Ophthalmic Gel Forming Solution is indicated in the treatment of elevated intraocular pressure in patients with ocular hypertension or open-angle glaucoma.

Figure 1

Mean IOP and Std Deviation (mm Hg) by Treatment Group

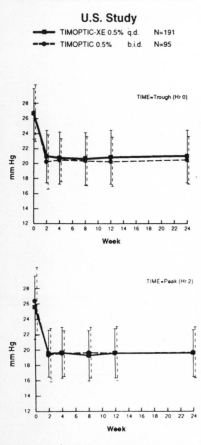

U.S. Study

[See figures at top of next column]

Contraindications:
TIMOPTIC-XE is contraindicated in patients with (1) bronchial asthma; (2) a history of

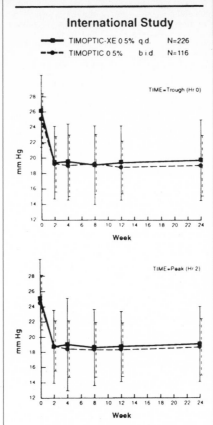

International Study

bronchial asthma; (3) severe chronic obstructive pulmonary disease (see **WARNINGS**); (4) sinus bradycardia; (5) second or third degree atrioventricular block; (6) overt cardiac failure (see **WARNINGS**); (7) cardiogenic shock; or (8) hypersensitivity to any component of this product.

Warnings:
As with many topically applied ophthalmic drugs, this drug is absorbed systemically.

The same adverse reactions found with systemic administration of beta-adrenergic blocking agents may occur with topical ophthalmic administration. For example, severe respiratory reactions and cardiac reactions, including death due to bronchospasm in patients with asthma, and rarely death in association with cardiac failure, have been reported following systemic or ophthalmic administration of timolol maleate. (See CONTRAINDICATIONS.)

Cardiac Failure
Sympathetic stimulation may be essential for support of the circulation in individuals with diminished myocardial contractility, and its inhibition by beta-adrenergic receptor blockade may precipitate more severe failure.
In Patients Without a History of Cardiac Failure, continued depression of the myocardium with beta-blocking agents over a period of time can, in some cases, lead to cardiac failure. At the first sign or symptom of cardiac failure, TIMOPTIC-XE should be discontinued.

Obstructive Pulmonary Disease
Patients with chronic obstructive pulmonary disease (e.g., chronic bronchitis, emphysema) of mild or moderate severity, bronchospastic disease, or a history of bronchospastic disease (other than bronchial asthma or a history of bronchial asthma, in which TIMOPTIC-XE is contraindicated [see **CONTRAINDICATIONS**]) should, in general, not receive beta-blockers, including TIMOPTIC-XE.

Major Surgery
The necessity or desirability of withdrawal of beta-adrenergic blocking agents prior to major surgery is controversial. Beta-adrenergic receptor blockade impairs the ability of the heart to respond to beta-adrenergically mediated reflex stimuli. This may augment the risk of general anesthesia in surgical procedures. Some patients receiving beta-adrenergic receptor blocking agents have experienced protracted, severe hypotension during anesthesia. Difficulty in restarting and maintaining the heartbeat has also been reported. For these reasons, in patients undergoing elective surgery, some authorities recommend gradual withdrawal of beta-adrenergic receptor blocking agents.
If necessary during surgery, the effects of beta-adrenergic blocking agents may be reversed by sufficient doses of adrenergic agonists.

Diabetes Mellitus
Beta-adrenergic blocking agents should be administered with caution in patients subject to spontaneous hypoglycemia or to diabetic patients (especially those with labile diabetes) who are receiving insulin or oral hypoglycemic agents. Beta-adrenergic receptor blocking agents may mask the signs and symptoms of acute hypoglycemia.

Thyrotoxicosis
Beta-adrenergic blocking agents may mask certain clinical signs (e.g., tachycardia) of hyperthyroidism. Patients suspected of developing thyrotoxicosis should be managed carefully to avoid abrupt withdrawal of beta-adrenergic blocking agents that might precipitate a thyroid storm.

Precautions:

General
Because of potential effects of beta-adrenergic blocking agents on blood pressure and pulse, these agents should be used with caution in patients with cerebrovascular insufficiency. If signs or symptoms suggesting reduced cerebral blood flow develop following initiation of therapy with TIMOPTIC-XE, alternative therapy should be considered.
There have been reports of bacterial keratitis associated with the use of multiple-dose containers of topical ophthalmic products. These containers had been inadvertently contaminated by patients who, in most cases, had a concurrent corneal disease or a disruption of the ocular epithelial surface. (See **PRECAUTIONS, Information for Patients**.)
Choroidal detachment after filtration procedures has been reported with the administration of aqueous suppressant therapy (e.g. timolol).
Angle-closure glaucoma: In patients with angle-closure glaucoma, the immediate objective of treatment is to reopen the angle. This may require constricting the pupil. Timolol maleate has little or no effect on the pupil. TIMOPTIC-XE should not be used alone in the treatment of angle-closure glaucoma.
Anaphylaxis: While taking beta-blockers, patients with a history of atopy or a history of severe anaphylactic reactions to a variety of allergens may be more reactive to repeated accidental, diagnostic, or therapeutic challenge with such allergens. Such patients may be unresponsive to the usual doses of epinephrine used to treat anaphylactic reactions.
Muscle Weakness: Beta-adrenergic blockade has been reported to potentiate muscle weakness consistent with certain myasthenic symptoms (e.g., diplopia, ptosis, and generalized weakness). Timolol has been reported rarely to increase muscle weakness in some patients with myasthenia gravis or myasthenic symptoms.

Information for Patients
Patients should be instructed to avoid allowing the tip of the dispensing container to contact the eye or surrounding structures.

Patients should also be instructed that ocular solutions, if handled improperly or if the tip of the dispensing container contacts the eye or surrounding structures, can become contaminated by common bacteria known to cause ocular infections. Serious damage to the eye and subsequent loss of vision may result from using contaminated solutions. (See **PRECAUTIONS, General**.)

Patients should also be advised that if they have ocular surgery or develop an intercurrent ocular condition (e.g., trauma or infection), they should immediately seek their physician's advice concerning the continued use of the present multidose container.

Patients should be instructed to invert the closed container and shake once before each use. It is not necessary to shake the container more than once.

Patients requiring concomitant topical ophthalmic medications should be instructed to administer them at least 10 minutes before instilling TIMOPTIC-XE.

Patients with bronchial asthma, a history of bronchial asthma, severe chronic obstructive pulmonary disease, sinus bradycardia, second or third degree atrioventricular block, or cardiac failure should be advised not to take this product. (See **CONTRAINDICATIONS**.)

Transient blurred vision, generally lasting from 30 seconds to 5 minutes, following instillation, and potential visual disturbances may impair the ability to perform hazardous tasks such as operating machinery or driving a motor vehicle.

Drug Interactions

Beta-adrenergic blocking agents: Patients who are receiving a beta-adrenergic blocking agent orally and TIMOPTIC-XE should be observed for potential additive effects of beta-blockade, both systemic and on intraocular pressure. The concomitant use of two topical beta-adrenergic blocking agents is not recommended.

Calcium antagonists: Caution should be used in the coadministration of beta-adrenergic blocking agents, such as TIMOPTIC-XE, and oral or intravenous calcium antagonists because of possible atrioventricular conduction disturbances, left ventricular failure, or hypotension. In patients with impaired cardiac function, coadministration should be avoided.

Catecholamine-depleting drugs: Close observation of the patient is recommended when a beta blocker is administered to patients receiving catecholamine-depleting drugs such as reserpine, because of possible additive effects and the production of hypotension and/or marked bradycardia, which may result in vertigo, syncope, or postural hypotension.

Digitalis and calcium antagonists: The concomitant use of beta-adrenergic blocking agents with digitalis and calcium antagonists may have additive effects in prolonging atrioventricular conduction time.

CYP2D6 inhibitors: Potentiated systemic beta-blockade (e.g., decreased heart rate, depression) has been reported during combined treatment with CYP2D6 inhibitors (e.g. quinidine, SSRIs) and timolol.

Clonidine: Oral beta-adrenergic blocking agents may exacerbate the rebound hypertension which can follow the withdrawal of clonidine. There have been no reports of exacerbation of rebound hypertension with ophthalmic timolol maleate.

Injectable epinephrine: (See **PRECAUTIONS, General**, Anaphylaxis)

Carcinogenesis, Mutagenesis, Impairment of Fertility

In a two-year study of timolol maleate administered orally to rats, there was a statistically significant increase in the incidence of adrenal pheochromocytomas in male rats administered 300 mg/kg/day (approximately 42,000 times

the systemic exposure following the maximum recommended human ophthalmic dose). Similar differences were not observed in rats administered oral doses equivalent to approximately 14,000 times the maximum recommended human ophthalmic dose.

In a lifetime oral study in mice, there were statistically significant increases in the incidence of benign and malignant pulmonary tumors, benign uterine polyps, and mammary adenocarcinomas in female mice at 500 mg/kg/day (approximately 71,000 times the systemic exposure following the maximum recommended human ophthalmic dose), but not at 5 or 50 mg/kg/day (approximately 700 or 7,000, respectively, times the systemic exposure following the maximum recommended human ophthalmic dose). In a subsequent study in female mice, in which post-mortem examinations were limited to the uterus and the lungs, a statistically significant increase in the incidence of pulmonary tumors was again observed at 500 mg/kg/day.

The increased occurrence of mammary adenocarcinomas was associated with elevations in serum prolactin, which occurred in female mice administered oral timolol at 500 mg/kg/day, but not at oral doses of 5 or 50 mg/kg/day. An increased incidence of mammary adenocarcinomas in rodents has been associated with administration of several other therapeutic agents that elevate serum prolactin, but no correlation between serum prolactin levels and mammary tumors has been established in humans. Furthermore, in adult human female subjects who received oral dosages of up to 60 mg of timolol maleate (the maximum recommended human oral dosage), there were no clinically meaningful changes in serum prolactin.

Timolol maleate was devoid of mutagenic potential when tested *in vivo* (mouse) in the micronucleus test and cytogenetic assay (doses up to 800 mg) and *in vitro* in a neoplastic cell transformation assay (up to 100 mcg/mL). In Ames tests, the highest concentrations of timolol employed, 5,000 or 10,000 mcg/plate, were associated with statistically significant elevations of revertants observed with tester strain TA100 (in seven replicate assays), but not in the remaining three strains. In the assays with tester strain TA100, no consistent dose response relationship was observed, and the ratio of test to control revertants did not reach 2. A ratio of 2 is usually considered the criterion for a positive Ames test.

Reproduction and fertility studies in rats demonstrated no adverse effect on male or female fertility at doses up to 21,000 times the systemic exposure following the maximum recommended human ophthalmic dose.

Pregnancy:

Teratogenic Effects—Pregnancy Category C. Teratogenicity studies with timolol in mice and rabbits at oral doses up to 50 mg/kg/day (7,000 times the systemic exposure following the maximum recommended human ophthalmic dose) demonstrated no evidence of fetal malformations. Although delayed fetal ossification was observed at this dose in rats, there were no adverse effects on postnatal development of offspring. Doses of 1000 mg/kg/day (142,000 times the systemic exposure following the maximum recommended human ophthalmic dose) were maternotoxic in mice and resulted in an increased number of fetal resorptions. Increased fetal resorptions were also seen in rabbits at doses of 14,000 times the systemic exposure following the maximum recommended human ophthalmic dose, in this case without apparent maternotoxicity.

There are no adequate and well-controlled studies in pregnant women. TIMOPTIC-XE should be used during pregnancy only if the potential benefit justifies the potential risk to the fetus.

Nursing Mothers

Timolol maleate has been detected in human milk following oral and ophthalmic drug administration. Because of the potential for serious adverse reactions from TIMOPTIC-XE in nursing infants, a decision should be made whether to discontinue nursing or to discontinue the drug, taking into account the importance of the drug to the mother.

Pediatric Use

Safety and effectiveness in pediatric patients have not been established.

Geriatric Use

No overall differences in safety or effectiveness have been observed between elderly and younger patients.

Adverse Reactions:

In clinical trials, transient blurred vision upon instillation of the drop was reported in approximately one in three patients (lasting from 30 seconds to 5 minutes). Less than 1% of patients discontinued from the studies due to blurred vision. The frequency of patients reporting burning and stinging upon instillation was comparable between TIMOPTIC-XE and TIMOPTIC (approximately one in eight patients).

Adverse experiences reported in 1–5% of patients were:

Ocular: Pain, conjunctivitis, discharge (e.g. crusting), foreign body sensation, itching and tearing;

Systemic: Headache, dizziness, and upper respiratory infections.

The following additional adverse experiences have been reported with the ocular administration of this or other timolol maleate formulations:

BODY AS A WHOLE

Asthenia/fatigue, and chest pain.

CARDIOVASCULAR

Bradycardia, arrhythmia, hypotension, hypertension, syncope, heart block, cerebral vascular accident, cerebral ischemia, cardiac failure, worsening of angina pectoris, palpitation, cardiac arrest, pulmonary edema, edema, claudication, Raynaud's phenomenon, and cold hands and feet.

DIGESTIVE

Nausea, diarrhea, dyspepsia, anorexia, and dry mouth.

IMMUNOLOGIC

Systemic lupus erythematosus.

NERVOUS SYSTEM/PSYCHIATRIC

Increase in signs and symptoms of myasthenia gravis, paresthesia, somnolence, insomnia, nightmares, behavioral changes and psychic disturbances including depression, confusion, hallucinations, anxiety, disorientation, nervousness, and memory loss.

SKIN

Alopecia and psoriasiform rash or exacerbation of psoriasis.

HYPERSENSITIVITY

Signs and symptoms of systemic allergic reactions including anaphylaxis, angioedema, urticaria, localized and generalized rash.

RESPIRATORY

Bronchospasm (predominantly in patients with preexisting bronchospastic disease), respiratory failure, dyspnea, nasal congestion, and cough.

ENDOCRINE

Masked symptoms of hypoglycemia in diabetic patients (see **WARNINGS**).

Continued on next page

Information on the Merck & Co., Inc., products listed on these pages is from the prescribing information in use May 1, 2006. For information, please call 1-800-NSC-MERCK [1-800-672-6372].

Timoptic-XE—Cont.

SPECIAL SENSES
Signs and symptoms of ocular irritation including blepharitis, keratitis, and dry eyes; ptosis; decreased corneal sensitivity; cystoid macular edema; visual disturbances including refractive changes and diplopia; pseudopemphigoid; choroidal detachment following filtration surgery (see **PRECAUTIONS, General**); and tinnitus.

UROGENITAL
Retroperitoneal fibrosis, decreased libido, impotence, and Peyronie's disease.

The following additional adverse effects have been reported in clinical experience with ORAL timolol maleate or other ORAL beta-blocking agents and may be considered potential effects of ophthalmic timolol maleate: *Allergic:* Erythematous rash, fever combined with aching and sore throat, laryngospasm with respiratory distress; *Body as a Whole:* Extremity pain, decreased exercise tolerance, weight loss; *Cardiovascular:* Worsening of arterial insufficiency, vasodilatation; *Digestive:* Gastrointestinal pain, hepatomegaly, vomiting, mesenteric arterial thrombosis, ischemic colitis; *Hematologic:* Nonthrombocytopenic purpura, thrombocytopenic purpura, agranulocytosis; *Endocrine:* Hyperglycemia, hypoglycemia; *Skin:* Pruritus, skin irritation, increased pigmentation, sweating; *Musculoskeletal:* Arthralgia; *Nervous System / Psychiatric:* Vertigo, local weakness, diminished concentration, reversible mental depression progressing to catatonia, an acute reversible syndrome characterized by disorientation for time and place, emotional lability, slightly clouded sensorium, and decreased performance on neuropsychometrics; *Respiratory:* Rales, bronchial obstruction; *Urogenital:* Urination difficulties.

Overdosage:
No data are available in regard to human overdosage with or accidental oral ingestion of TIMOPTIC-XE.

There have been reports of inadvertent overdosage with TIMOPTIC Ophthalmic Solution resulting in systemic effects similar to those seen with systemic beta-adrenergic blocking agents such as dizziness, headache, shortness of breath, bradycardia, bronchospasm, and cardiac arrest (see also **ADVERSE REACTIONS**).

Overdosage has been reported with Tablets BLOCADREN* (timolol maleate tablets). A 30-year-old female ingested 650 mg of BLOCADREN (maximum recommended oral daily dose is 60 mg) and experienced second and third degree heart block. She recovered without treatment but approximately two months later developed irregular heartbeat, hypertension, dizziness, tinnitus, faintness, increased pulse rate, and borderline first degree heart block.

An *in vitro* hemodialysis study, using ^{14}C timolol added to human plasma or whole blood, showed that timolol was readily dialyzed from these fluids; however, a study of patients with renal failure showed that timolol did not dialyze readily.

*Registered trademark of MERCK & CO., Inc.

Dosage and Administration:
Patients should be instructed to invert the closed container and shake once before each use. It is not necessary to shake the container more than once. Other topically applied ophthalmic medications should be administered at least 10 minutes before TIMOPTIC-XE. (See **PRECAUTIONS, Information for Patients** and accompanying INSTRUCTIONS FOR USE.)
TIMOPTIC-XE Sterile Ophthalmic Gel Forming Solution is available in concentrations of

0.25% and 0.5%. The dose is one drop of TIMOPTIC-XE (either 0.25% or 0.5%) in the affected eye(s) once a day.
Because in some patients the pressure-lowering response to TIMOPTIC-XE may require a few weeks to stabilize, evaluation should include a determination of intraocular pressure after approximately 4 weeks of treatment with TIMOPTIC-XE.
Dosages higher than one drop of 0.5% TIMOPTIC-XE once a day have not been studied. If the patient's intraocular pressure is still not at a satisfactory level on this regimen, concomitant therapy can be considered. The concomitant use of two topical beta-adrenergic blocking agents is not recommended. (See **PRECAUTIONS, Drug Interactions, Beta-adrenergic blocking agents**.)
When patients have been switched from therapy with TIMOPTIC administered twice daily to TIMOPTIC-XE administered once daily, the ocular hypotensive effect has remained consistent.

How Supplied:
TIMOPTIC-XE Sterile Ophthalmic Gel Forming Solution is a colorless to nearly colorless, slightly opalescent, and slightly viscous solution.
No. 3557—TIMOPTIC-XE Sterile Ophthalmic Gel Forming Solution, 0.25% timolol equivalent, is supplied in an OCUMETER®* PLUS container, a white, translucent, HDPE plastic ophthalmic dispenser with a controlled drop tip and a white polystyrene cap with yellow label as follows:
NDC 0006-3557-35, 5 mL in a 7.5 mL capacity bottle.
No. 3558—TIMOPTIC-XE Sterile Ophthalmic Gel Forming Solution, 0.5% timolol equivalent, is supplied in an OCUMETER PLUS container, a white, translucent, HDPE plastic ophthalmic dispenser with a controlled drop tip and a white polystyrene cap with yellow label as follows:
NDC 0006-3558-35, 5 mL in a 7.5 mL capacity bottle.
Storage
Store at 15-30°C (59-86°F). **AVOID FREEZING.** Protect from light.

---

* Registered trademark of MERCK & CO., INC.
    9611903   Issued September 2005
COPYRIGHT© 1995, 2003 MERCK & CO., Inc.
All rights reserved

**TIMOPTIC-XE® 0.25% AND 0.5%
(timolol maleate ophthalmic
gel forming solution)**
INSTRUCTIONS FOR USE
Please follow these instructions carefully when using TIMOPTIC-XE*. Use TIMOPTIC-XE as prescribed by your doctor.
1. If you use other topically applied ophthalmic medications, they should be administered at least 10 minutes before TIMOPTIC-XE.
2. Wash hands before each use.
3. Before using the medication for the first time, be sure the Safety Strip on the front of the bottle is unbroken. A gap between the bottle and the cap is normal for an unopened bottle.

Opening Arrows ›

Safety Strip ›

4. Tear off the safety strip to break the seal.

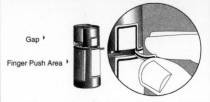
Gap ›

Finger Push Area ›

5. Invert the closed bottle and shake ONCE before each use. (It is not necessary to shake the bottle more than once.)
6. To open the bottle, unscrew the cap by turning as indicated by the arrows on the top of the cap. Do not pull the cap directly up and away from the bottle. Pulling the cap directly up will prevent your dispenser from operating properly.

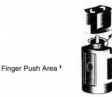
Finger Push Area ›

7. Tilt your head back and pull your lower eyelid down slightly to form a pocket between your eyelid and your eye.

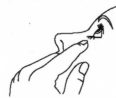

8. Invert the bottle, and press lightly with the thumb or index finger over the "Finger Push Area" (as shown) until a single drop is dispensed into the eye as directed by your doctor.

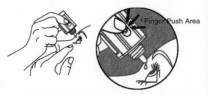
Finger Push Area

DO NOT TOUCH YOUR EYE OR EYELID WITH THE DROPPER TIP.

OPHTHALMIC MEDICATIONS, IF HANDLED IMPROPERLY, CAN BECOME CONTAMINATED BY COMMON BACTERIA KNOWN TO CAUSE EYE INFECTIONS. SERIOUS DAMAGE TO THE EYE AND SUBSEQUENT LOSS OF VISION MAY RESULT FROM USING CONTAMINATED OPHTHALMIC MEDICATIONS. IF YOU THINK YOUR MEDICATION MAY BE CONTAMINATED, OR YOU DEVELOP AN EYE INFECTION, CONTACT YOUR DOCTOR IMMEDIATELY CONCERNING CONTINUED USE OF THIS BOTTLE.
9. If drop dispensing is difficult after opening for the first time, replace the cap on the bottle and tighten (DO NOT OVERTIGHTEN) and then remove by turning the cap in the opposite direction as indicated by the arrows on the top of the cap.
10. Repeat steps 7 & 8 with the other eye if instructed to do so by your doctor.
11. Replace the cap by turning until it is firmly touching the bottle. The arrow on the left

side of the cap must be aligned with the arrow on the left side of the bottle label for proper closure. Do not overtighten or you may damage the bottle and cap.

12. The dispenser tip is designed to provide a single drop; therefore, do NOT enlarge the hole of the dispenser tip.

13. After you have used all doses, there will be some TIMOPTIC-XE left in the bottle. You should not be concerned since an extra amount of TIMOPTIC-XE has been added and you will get the full amount of TIMOPTIC-XE that your doctor prescribed. Do not attempt to remove excess medicine from the bottle.

WARNING: Keep out of reach of children. If you have any questions about the use of TIMOPTIC-XE, please consult your doctor.

* Registered trademark of MERCK & CO., Inc.
COPYRIGHT © 1995, 2003 MERCK & CO., Inc.
All rights reserved
Issued September 2005
Manuf. for:
MERCK & CO., Inc.
Whitehouse Station, NJ 08889, USA
By: Laboratories Merck Sharp & Dohme-Chibret
63963 Clermont-Ferrand Cedex 9, France
Shown in Product Identification Guide, page 105

TRUSOPT®   ℞
Sterile Ophthalmic Solution 2%
(dorzolamide hydrochloride ophthalmic solution)

Description: TRUSOPT* (dorzolamide hydrochloride ophthalmic solution) is a carbonic anhydrase inhibitor formulated for topical ophthalmic use.

Dorzolamide hydrochloride is described chemically as: (4S-trans)-4-(ethylamino)-5,6-dihydro-6-methyl-4H-thieno [2,3-b] thiopyran-2-sulfonamide 7,7-dioxide monohydrochloride. Dorzolamide hydrochloride is optically active. The specific rotation is

$$[\alpha]^{25°}_{405} \quad (C = 1, \text{water}) = \sim -17°.$$

Its empirical formula is $C_{10}H_{16}N_2O_4S_3 \cdot HCl$ and its structural formula is:

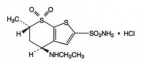

Dorzolamide hydrochloride has a molecular weight of 360.9 and a melting point of about 264°C. It is a white to off-white, crystalline powder, which is soluble in water and slightly soluble in methanol and ethanol.

TRUSOPT Sterile Ophthalmic Solution is supplied as a sterile, isotonic, buffered, slightly viscous, aqueous solution of dorzolamide hydrochloride. The pH of the solution is approximately 5.6, and the osmolarity is 260–330 mOsM. Each mL of TRUSOPT 2% contains 20 mg dorzolamide (22.3 mg of dorzolamide hydrochloride). Inactive ingredients are hydroxyethyl cellulose, mannitol, sodium citrate dihydrate, sodium hydroxide (to adjust pH) and water for injection. Benzalkonium chloride 0.0075% is added as a preservative.

* Registered trademark of MERCK & CO., Inc.

Clinical Pharmacology:
Mechanism of Action

Carbonic anhydrase (CA) is an enzyme found in many tissues of the body including the eye. It catalyzes the reversible reaction involving the hydration of carbon dioxide and the dehydration of carbonic acid. In humans, carbonic anhydrase exists as a number of isoenzymes, the most active being carbonic anhydrase II (CA-II), found primarily in red blood cells (RBCs), but also in other tissues. Inhibition of carbonic anhydrase in the ciliary processes of the eye decreases aqueous humor secretion, presumably by slowing the formation of bicarbonate ions with subsequent reduction in sodium and fluid transport. The result is a reduction in intraocular pressure (IOP).

TRUSOPT Ophthalmic Solution contains dorzolamide hydrochloride, an inhibitor of human carbonic anhydrase II. Following topical ocular administration, TRUSOPT reduces elevated intraocular pressure. Elevated intraocular pressure is a major risk factor in the pathogenesis of optic nerve damage and glaucomatous visual field loss.

Pharmacokinetics/Pharmacodynamics

When topically applied, dorzolamide reaches the systemic circulation. To assess the potential for systemic carbonic anhydrase inhibition following topical administration, drug and metabolite concentrations in RBCs and plasma and carbonic anhydrase inhibition in RBCs were measured. Dorzolamide accumulates in RBCs during chronic dosing as a result of binding to CA-II. The parent drug forms a single N-desethyl metabolite, which inhibits CA-II less potently than the parent drug but also inhibits CA-I. The metabolite also accumulates in RBCs where it binds primarily to CA-I. Plasma concentrations of dorzolamide and metabolite are generally below the assay limit of quantitation (15nM). Dorzolamide binds moderately to plasma proteins (approximately 33%). Dorzolamide is primarily excreted unchanged in the urine; the metabolite also is excreted in urine. After dosing is stopped, dorzolamide washes out of RBCs nonlinearly, resulting in a rapid decline of drug concentration initially, followed by a slower elimination phase with a half-life of about four months.

To simulate the systemic exposure after long-term topical ocular administration, dorzolamide was given orally to eight healthy subjects for up to 20 weeks. The oral dose of 2 mg b.i.d. closely approximates the amount of drug delivered by topical ocular administration of TRUSOPT 2% t.i.d. Steady state was reached within 8 weeks. The inhibition of CA-II and total carbonic anhydrase activities was below the degree of inhibition anticipated to be necessary for a pharmacological effect on renal function and respiration in healthy individuals.

Clinical Studies

The efficacy of TRUSOPT was demonstrated in clinical studies in the treatment of elevated intraocular pressure in patients with glaucoma or ocular hypertension (baseline IOP ≥23 mmHg). The IOP-lowering effect of TRUSOPT was approximately 3 to 5 mmHg throughout the day and this was consistent in clinical studies of up to one year duration.

The efficacy of TRUSOPT when dosed less frequently than three times a day (alone or in combination with other products) has not been established.

In a one year clinical study, the effect of TRUSOPT 2% t.i.d. on the corneal endothelium was compared to that of betaxolol ophthalmic solution b.i.d. and timolol maleate ophthalmic solution 0.5% b.i.d. There were no statistically significant differences between groups in corneal endothelial cell counts or in corneal thickness measurements. There was a mean loss of approximately 4% in the endothe-

lial cell counts for each group over the one year period.

Indications and Usage: TRUSOPT Ophthalmic Solution is indicated in the treatment of elevated intraocular pressure in patients with ocular hypertension or open- angle glaucoma.

Contraindications: TRUSOPT is contraindicated in patients who are hypersensitive to any component of this product.

Warnings: TRUSOPT is a sulfonamide and although administered topically is absorbed systemically. Therefore, the same types of adverse reactions that are attributable to sulfonamides may occur with topical administration with TRUSOPT. Fatalities have occurred, although rarely, due to severe reactions to sulfonamides including Stevens-Johnson syndrome, toxic epidermal necrolysis, fulminant hepatic necrosis, agranulocytosis, aplastic anemia, and other blood dyscrasias. Sensitization may recur when a sulfonamide is readministered irrespective of the route of administration. If signs of serious reactions or hypersensitivity occur, discontinue the use of this preparation.

Precautions:
General

The management of patients with acute angle-closure glaucoma requires therapeutic interventions in addition to ocular hypotensive agents. TRUSOPT has not been studied in patients with acute angle-closure glaucoma.

TRUSOPT has not been studied in patients with severe renal impairment (CrCl < 30 mL/min). Because TRUSOPT and its metabolite are excreted predominantly by the kidney, TRUSOPT is not recommended in such patients.

TRUSOPT has not been studied in patients with hepatic impairment and should therefore be used with caution in such patients.

In clinical studies, local ocular adverse effects, primarily conjunctivitis and lid reactions, were reported with chronic administration of TRUSOPT. Many of these reactions had the clinical appearance and course of an allergic-type reaction that resolved upon discontinuation of drug therapy. If such reactions are observed, TRUSOPT should be discontinued and the patient evaluated before considering restarting the drug. (See **ADVERSE REACTIONS**.)

There is a potential for an additive effect on the known systemic effects of carbonic anhydrase inhibition in patients receiving an oral carbonic anhydrase inhibitor and TRUSOPT. The concomitant administration of TRUSOPT and oral carbonic anhydrase inhibitors is not recommended.

There have been reports of bacterial keratitis associated with the use of multiple-dose containers of topical ophthalmic products. These containers had been inadvertently contaminated by patients who, in most cases, had a concurrent corneal disease or a disruption of the ocular epithelial surface.

Choroidal detachment has been reported with administration of aqueous suppressant therapy (e.g., dorzolamide) after filtration procedures.

Information for Patients

TRUSOPT is a sulfonamide and although administered topically is absorbed systemically.

Continued on next page

Information on the Merck & Co., Inc., products listed on these pages is from the prescribing information in use May 1, 2006. For information, please call 1-800-NSC-MERCK [1-800-672-6372].

Trusopt—Cont.

Therefore the same types of adverse reactions that are attributable to sulfonamides may occur with topical administration. Patients should be advised that if serious or unusual reactions or signs of hypersensitivity occur, they should discontinue the use of the product (see **WARNINGS**).

Patients should be advised that if they develop any ocular reactions, particularly conjunctivitis and lid reactions, they should discontinue use and seek their physician's advice.

Patients should be instructed to avoid allowing the tip of the dispensing container to contact the eye or surrounding structures.

Patients should also be instructed that ocular solutions, if handled improperly or if the tip of the dispensing container contacts the eye or surrounding structures, can become contaminated by common bacteria known to cause ocular infections. Serious damage to the eye and subsequent loss of vision may result from using contaminated solutions.

Patients also should be advised that if they have ocular surgery or develop an intercurrent ocular condition (e.g., trauma or infection), they should immediately seek their physician's advice concerning the continued use of the present multidose container.

If more than one topical ophthalmic drug is being used, the drugs should be administered at least ten minutes apart.

Patients should be advised that TRUSOPT contains benzalkonium chloride which may be absorbed by soft contact lenses. Contact lenses should be removed prior to administration of the solution. Lenses may be reinserted 15 minutes following TRUSOPT administration.

Drug Interactions

Although acid-base and electrolyte disturbances were not reported in the clinical trials with TRUSOPT, these disturbances have been reported with oral carbonic anhydrase inhibitors and have, in some instances, resulted in drug interactions (e.g., toxicity associated with high-dose salicylate therapy). Therefore, the potential for such drug interactions should be considered in patients receiving TRUSOPT.

Carcinogenesis, Mutagenesis, Impairment of Fertility

In a two-year study of dorzolamide hydrochloride administered orally to male and female Sprague-Dawley rats, urinary bladder papillomas were seen in male rats in the highest dosage group of 20 mg/kg/day (250 times the recommended human ophthalmic dose). Papillomas were not seen in rats given oral doses equivalent to approximately 12 times the recommended human ophthalmic dose. No treatment-related tumors were seen in a 21-month study in female and male mice given oral doses up to 75 mg/kg/day (900 times the recommended human ophthalmic dose).

The increased incidence of urinary bladder papillomas seen in the high-dose male rats is a class-effect of carbonic anhydrase inhibitors in rats. Rats are particularly prone to developing papillomas in response to foreign bodies, compounds causing crystalluria, and diverse sodium salts.

No changes in bladder urothelium were seen in dogs given oral dorzolamide hydrochloride for one year at 2 mg/kg/day (25 times the recommended human ophthalmic dose) or monkeys dosed topically to the eye at 0.4 mg/kg/day (5 times the recommended human ophthalmic dose) for one year.

The following tests for mutagenic potential were negative: (1) *in vivo* (mouse) cytogenetic assay; (2) *in vitro* chromosomal aberration assay; (3) alkaline elution assay; (4) V-79 assay; and (5) Ames test.

In reproduction studies of dorzolamide hydrochloride in rats, there were no adverse effects on the reproductive capacity of males or females at doses up to 188 or 94 times, respectively, the recommended human ophthalmic dose.

Pregnancy

Teratogenic Effects. Pregnancy Category C. Developmental toxicity studies with dorzolamide hydrochloride in rabbits at oral doses of ≥2.5 mg/kg/day (31 times the recommended human ophthalmic dose) revealed malformations of the vertebral bodies. These malformations occurred at doses that caused metabolic acidosis with decreased body weight gain in dams and decreased fetal weights. No treatment-related malformations were seen at 1.0 mg/kg/day (13 times the recommended human ophthalmic dose). There are no adequate and well-controlled studies in pregnant women. TRUSOPT should be used during pregnancy only if the potential benefit justifies the potential risk to the fetus.

Nursing Mothers

In a study of dorzolamide hydrochloride in lactating rats, decreases in body weight gain of 5 to 7% in offspring at an oral dose of 7.5 mg/kg/day (94 times the recommended human ophthalmic dose) were seen during lactation. A slight delay in postnatal development (incisor eruption, vaginal canalization and eye openings), secondary to lower fetal body weight, was noted.

It is not known whether this drug is excreted in human milk. Because many drugs are excreted in human milk and because of the potential for serious adverse reactions in nursing infants from TRUSOPT, a decision should be made whether to discontinue nursing or to discontinue the drug, taking into account the importance of the drug to the mother.

Pediatric Use

Safety and IOP-lowering effects of TRUSOPT have been demonstrated in pediatric patients in a 3-month, multicenter, double-masked, active-treatment-controlled trial.

Geriatric Use

No overall differences in safety and effectiveness have been observed between elderly and younger patients.

Adverse Reactions:

Controlled clinical trials: The most frequent adverse events associated with TRUSOPT were ocular burning, stinging, or discomfort immediately following ocular administration (approximately one-third of patients). Approximately one-quarter of patients noted a bitter taste following administration. Superficial punctate keratitis occurred in 10–15% of patients and signs and symptoms of ocular allergic reaction in approximately 10%. Events occurring in approximately 1–5% of patients were conjunctivitis and lid reactions (see PRECAUTIONS, General), blurred vision, eye redness, tearing, dryness, and photophobia. Other ocular events and systemic events were reported infrequently, including headache, nausea, asthenia/fatigue; and, rarely, skin rashes, urolithiasis, and iridocyclitis.

In a 3-month, double-masked, active-treatment-controlled, multicenter study in pediatric patients, the adverse experience profile of TRUSOPT was comparable to that seen in adult patients.

Clinical practice: The following adverse events have occurred either at low incidence (<1%) during clinical trials or have been reported during the use of TRUSOPT in clinical practice where these events were reported voluntarily from a population of unknown size and frequency of occurrence cannot be determined precisely. They have been chosen for inclusion based on factors such as seriousness, frequency of reporting, possible causal connection to TRUSOPT, or a combination of these factors: signs and symptoms of systemic allergic reactions including angioedema, bronchospasm, pruritus, and urticaria; dizziness, paresthesia; ocular pain, transient myopia, choroidal detachment following filtration surgery, eyelid crusting; dyspnea; contact dermatitis, epistaxis, dry mouth and throat irritation.

Overdosage: Electrolyte imbalance, development of an acidotic state, and possible central nervous system effects may occur. Serum electrolyte levels (particularly potassium) and blood pH levels should be monitored.

Dosage and Administration: The dose is one drop of TRUSOPT Ophthalmic Solution in the affected eyes(s) three times daily.

TRUSOPT may be used concomitantly with other topical ophthalmic drug products to lower intraocular pressure. If more than one topical ophthalmic drug is being used, the drugs should be administered at least ten minutes apart.

How Supplied: TRUSOPT Ophthalmic Solution is a slightly opalescent, nearly colorless, slightly viscous solution.

No. 3519—TRUSOPT Ophthalmic Solution 2% is supplied in an OCUMETER®* PLUS container, a white, translucent, HDPE plastic ophthalmic dispenser with a controlled drop tip and a white polystyrene cap with orange label as follows:

NDC 0006-3519-35, 5 mL, in a 7.5 mL capacity bottle

NDC 0006-3519-36, 10 mL, in an 18 mL capacity bottle.

Storage
Store TRUSOPT Ophthalmic Solution at 15–30°C (59–86°F). Protect from light.

Rx only

* Registered trademark of MERCK & CO., Inc.

Instructions for Use:
Please follow these instructions carefully when using TRUSOPT*. Use TRUSOPT as prescribed by your doctor.

1. If you use other topically applied ophthalmic medications, they should be administered at least 10 minutes before or after TRUSOPT.
2. Wash hands before each use.
3. Before using the medication for the first time, be sure the Safety Strip on the front of the bottle is unbroken. A gap between the bottle and the cap is normal for an unopened bottle.

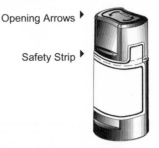

Opening Arrows ▸

Safety Strip ▸

4. Tear off the Safety Strip to break the seal. [See first figure at top of next page]
5. To open the bottle, unscrew the cap by turning as indicated by the arrows on the top of the cap. Do not pull the cap directly up and away from the bottle. Pulling the cap directly up will prevent your dispenser from operating properly. [See first figure at top of next column]
6. Tilt your head back and pull your lower eyelid down slightly to form a pocket between your eyelid and your eye. [See second figure at top of next column]
7. Invert the bottle, and press lightly with the thumb or index finger over the "Finger Push Area" (as shown) until a single drop

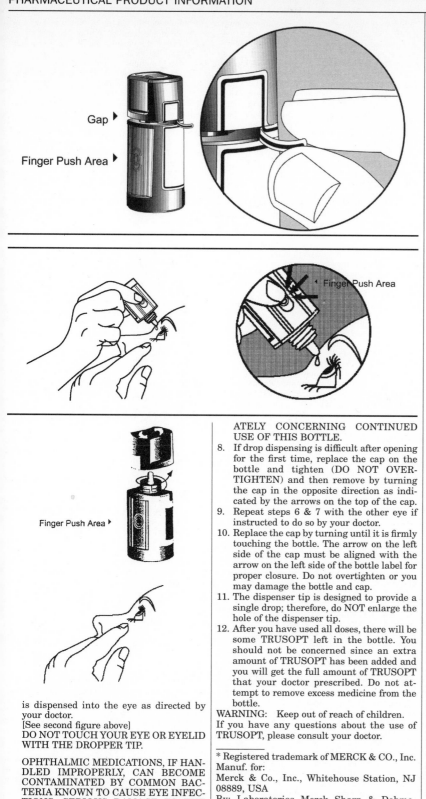

Gap ▶

Finger Push Area ▶

Finger Push Area ▶

Finger Push Area ▶

ATELY CONCERNING CONTINUED USE OF THIS BOTTLE.

8. If drop dispensing is difficult after opening for the first time, replace the cap on the bottle and tighten (DO NOT OVER-TIGHTEN) and then remove by turning the cap in the opposite direction as indicated by the arrows on the top of the cap.

9. Repeat steps 6 & 7 with the other eye if instructed to do so by your doctor.

10. Replace the cap by turning until it is firmly touching the bottle. The arrow on the left side of the cap must be aligned with the arrow on the left side of the bottle label for proper closure. Do not overtighten or you may damage the bottle and cap.

11. The dispenser tip is designed to provide a single drop; therefore, do NOT enlarge the hole of the dispenser tip.

12. After you have used all doses, there will be some TRUSOPT left in the bottle. You should not be concerned since an extra amount of TRUSOPT has been added and you will get the full amount of TRUSOPT that your doctor prescribed. Do not attempt to remove excess medicine from the bottle.

WARNING: Keep out of reach of children.

If you have any questions about the use of TRUSOPT, please consult your doctor.

is dispensed into the eye as directed by your doctor.

[See second figure above]

DO NOT TOUCH YOUR EYE OR EYELID WITH THE DROPPER TIP.

OPHTHALMIC MEDICATIONS, IF HANDLED IMPROPERLY, CAN BECOME CONTAMINATED BY COMMON BACTERIA KNOWN TO CAUSE EYE INFECTIONS. SERIOUS DAMAGE TO THE EYE AND SUBSEQUENT LOSS OF VISION MAY RESULT FROM USING CONTAMINATED OPHTHALMIC MEDICATIONS. IF YOU THINK YOUR MEDICATION MAY BE CONTAMINATED, OR IF YOU DEVELOP AN EYE INFECTION, CONTACT YOUR DOCTOR IMMEDI-

* Registered trademark of MERCK & CO., Inc.

Manuf. for:

Merck & Co., Inc., Whitehouse Station, NJ 08889, USA

By: Laboratories Merck Sharp & Dohme-Chibret

63963 Clermont-Ferrand Cedex 9, France

9368207   Issued September 2005

Shown in Product Identification Guide, page 105

Monarch Pharmaceuticals

Please see
King Pharmaceuticals, Inc.

Pharmacia & Upjohn

A division of Pfizer
235 EAST 42ND STREET
NEW YORK, NY 10017

For Medical Information, Contact:
(800) 438-1985
24 hours a day, 7 days a week

XALATAN®   ℞
[ză-lă-tăn]
(latanoprost ophthalmic solution)
0.005% (50 µg/mL)

Description: Latanoprost is a prostaglandin $F_{2\alpha}$ analogue. Its chemical name is isopropyl-(Z)-7[(1R,2R,3R,5S)3,5-dihydroxy-2-[(3R)-3-hydroxy-5-phenylpentyl]cyclopentyl]-5-heptenoate. Its molecular formula is $C_{26}H_{40}O_5$ and its chemical structure is:

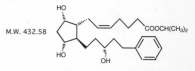

M.W. 432.58

Latanoprost is a colorless to slightly yellow oil that is very soluble in acetonitrile and freely soluble in acetone, ethanol, ethyl acetate, isopropanol, methanol and octanol. It is practically insoluble in water.

XALATAN Sterile Ophthalmic Solution (latanoprost ophthalmic solution) is supplied as a sterile, isotonic, buffered aqueous solution of latanoprost with a pH of approximately 6.7 and an osmolality of approximately 267 mOsmol/kg. Each mL of XALATAN contains 50 micrograms of latanoprost. Benzalkonium chloride, 0.02% is added as a preservative. The inactive ingredients are: sodium chloride, sodium dihydrogen phosphate monohydrate, disodium hydrogen phosphate anhydrous and water for injection. One drop contains approximately 1.5 µg of latanoprost.

Clinical Pharmacology:

Mechanism of Action

Latanoprost is a prostanoid selective FP receptor agonist that is believed to reduce the intraocular pressure (IOP) by increasing the outflow of aqueous humor. Studies in animals and man suggest that the main mechanism of action is increased uveoscleral outflow. Elevated IOP represents a major risk factor for glaucomatous field loss. The higher the level of IOP, the greater the likelihood of optic nerve damage and visual field loss.

Pharmacokinetics/Pharmacodynamics

Absorption: Latanoprost is absorbed through the cornea where the isopropyl ester prodrug is hydrolyzed to the acid form to become biologically active. Studies in man indicate that the peak concentration in the aqueous humor is reached about two hours after topical administration.

Distribution: The distribution volume in humans is 0.16 ± 0.02 L/kg. The acid of latanoprost can be measured in aqueous humor during the first 4 hours, and in plasma only during the first hour after local administration.

Metabolism: Latanoprost, an isopropyl ester prodrug, is hydrolyzed by esterases in the cor-

Continued on next page

Xalatan—Cont.

nea to the biologically active acid. The active acid of latanoprost reaching the systemic circulation is primarily metabolized by the liver to the 1,2-dinor and 1,2,3,4-tetranor metabolites via fatty acid β-oxidation.

Excretion: The elimination of the acid of latanoprost from human plasma is rapid ($t_{1/2}$ = 17 min) after both intravenous and topical administration. Systemic clearance is approximately 7 mL/min/kg. Following hepatic β-oxidation, the metabolites are mainly eliminated via the kidneys. Approximately 88% and 98% of the administered dose is recovered in the urine after topical and intravenous dosing, respectively.

Animal Studies

In monkeys, latanoprost has been shown to induce increased pigmentation of the iris. The mechanism of increased pigmentation seems to be stimulation of melanin production in melanocytes of the iris, with no proliferative changes observed. The change in iris color may be permanent.

Ocular administration of latanoprost at a dose of 6 μg/eye/ day (4 times the daily human dose) to cynomolgus monkeys has also been shown to induce increased palpebral fissure. This effect was reversible upon discontinuation of the drug.

Indications and Usage: XALATAN Sterile Ophthalmic Solution is indicated for the reduction of elevated intraocular pressure in patients with open-angle glaucoma or ocular hypertension.

Clinical Studies: Patients with mean baseline intraocular pressure of 24 – 25 mmHg who were treated for 6 months in multi-center, randomized, controlled trials demonstrated 6–8 mmHg reductions in intraocular pressure. This IOP reduction with XALATAN Sterile Ophthalmic Solution 0.005% dosed once daily was equivalent to the effect of timolol 0.5% dosed twice daily.

A 3-year open-label, prospective safety study with a 2-year extension phase was conducted to evaluate the progression of increased iris pigmentation with continuous use of XALATAN once-daily as adjunctive therapy in 519 patients with open-angle glaucoma. The analysis was based on observed-cases population of the 380 patients who continued in the extension phase.

Results showed that the onset of noticeable increased iris pigmentation occurred within the first year of treatment for the majority of the patients who developed noticeable increased iris pigmentation. Patients continued to show signs of increasing iris pigmentation throughout the five years of the study. Observation of increased iris pigmentation did not affect the incidence, nature or severity of adverse events (other than increased iris pigmentation) recorded in the study. IOP reduction was similar regardless of the development of increased iris pigmentation during the study.

Contraindications: Known hypersensitivity to latanoprost, benzalkonium chloride or any other ingredients in this product.

Warnings: XALATAN Sterile Ophthalmic Solution has been reported to cause changes to pigmented tissues. The most frequently reported changes have been increased pigmentation of the iris, periorbital tissue (eyelid) and eyelashes, and growth of eyelashes. Pigmentation is expected to increase as long as XALATAN is administered. After discontinuation of XALATAN, pigmentation of the iris is likely to be permanent while pigmentation of the periorbital tissue and eyelash changes have been reported to be reversible in some patients. Patients who receive treatment should be

informed of the possibility of increased pigmentation. The effects of increased pigmentation beyond 5 years are not known.

Precautions:

General: XALATAN Sterile Ophthalmic Solution may gradually increase the pigmentation of the iris. The eye color change is due to increased melanin content in the stromal melanocytes of the iris rather than to an increase in the number of melanocytes. This change may not be noticeable for several months to years (see **WARNINGS**). Typically, the brown pigmentation around the pupil spreads concentrically towards the periphery of the iris and the entire iris or parts of the iris become more brownish. Neither nevi nor freckles of the iris appear to be affected by treatment. While treatment with XALATAN can be continued in patients who develop noticeably increased iris pigmentation, these patients should be examined regularly.

During clinical trials, the increase in brown iris pigment has not been shown to progress further upon discontinuation of treatment, but the resultant color change may be permanent. Eyelid skin darkening, which may be reversible, has been reported in association with the use of XALATAN (see **WARNINGS**).

XALATAN may gradually change eyelashes and vellus hair in the treated eye; these changes include increased length, thickness, pigmentation, the number of lashes or hairs, and misdirected growth of eyelashes. Eyelash changes are usually reversible upon discontinuation of treatment.

XALATAN should be used with caution in patients with a history of intraocular inflammation (iritis/uveitis) and should generally not be used in patients with active intraocular inflammation.

Macular edema, including cystoid macular edema, has been reported during treatment with XALATAN. These reports have mainly occurred in aphakic patients, in pseudophakic patients with a torn posterior lens capsule, or in patients with known risk factors for macular edema. XALATAN should be used with caution in patients who do not have an intact posterior capsule or who have known risk factors for macular edema.

There is limited experience with XALATAN in the treatment of angle closure, inflammatory or neovascular glaucoma.

There have been reports of bacterial keratitis associated with the use of multiple-dose containers of topical ophthalmic products. These containers had been inadvertently contaminated by patients who, in most cases, had a concurrent corneal disease or a disruption of the ocular epithelial surface (see **PRECAUTIONS**, Information for Patients).

Contact lenses should be removed prior to the administration of XALATAN, and may be reinserted 15 minutes after administration (see **PRECAUTIONS**, Information for Patients).

Information for Patients (see **WARNINGS** and **PRECAUTIONS**): Patients should be advised about the potential for increased brown pigmentation of the iris, which may be permanent. Patients should also be informed about the possibility of eyelid skin darkening, which may be reversible after discontinuation of XALATAN.

Patients should also be informed of the possibility of eyelash and vellus hair changes in the treated eye during treatment with XALATAN. These changes may result in a disparity between eyes in length, thickness, pigmentation, number of eyelashes or vellus hairs, and/or direction of eyelash growth. Eyelash changes are usually reversible upon discontinuation of treatment.

Patients should be instructed to avoid allowing the tip of the dispensing container to contact the eye or surrounding structures because this could cause the tip to become contaminated by

common bacteria known to cause ocular infections. Serious damage to the eye and subsequent loss of vision may result from using contaminated solutions.

Patients also should be advised that if they develop an intercurrent ocular condition (e.g., trauma, or infection) or have ocular surgery, they should immediately seek their physician's advice concerning the continued use of the multiple-dose container.

Patients should be advised that if they develop any ocular reactions, particularly conjunctivitis and lid reactions, they should immediately seek their physician's advice.

Patients should also be advised that XALATAN contains benzalkonium chloride, which may be absorbed by contact lenses. Contact lenses should be removed prior to administration of the solution. Lenses may be reinserted 15 minutes following administration of XALATAN.

If more than one topical ophthalmic drug is being used, the drugs should be administered at least five (5) minutes apart.

Drug Interactions: *In vitro* studies have shown that precipitation occurs when eye drops containing thimerosal are mixed with XALATAN. If such drugs are used they should be administered at least five (5) minutes apart.

Carcinogenesis, Mutagenesis, Impairment of Fertility: Latanoprost was not mutagenic in bacteria, in mouse lymphoma or in mouse micronucleus tests. Chromosome aberrations were observed *in vitro* with human lymphocytes.

Latanoprost was not carcinogenic in either mice or rats when administered by oral gavage at doses of up to 170 μg/kg/day (approximately 2,800 times the recommended maximum human dose) for up to 20 and 24 months, respectively.

Additional *in vitro* and *in vivo* studies on unscheduled DNA synthesis in rats were negative. Latanoprost has not been found to have any effect on male or female fertility in animal studies.

Pregnancy: Teratogenic Effects: Pregnancy Category C.

Reproduction studies have been performed in rats and rabbits. In rabbits an incidence of 4 of 16 dams had no viable fetuses at a dose that was approximately 80 times the maximum human dose, and the highest nonembryocidal dose in rabbits was approximately 15 times the maximum human dose. There are no adequate and well-controlled studies in pregnant women. XALATAN should be used during pregnancy only if the potential benefit justifies the potential risk to the fetus.

Nursing Mothers: It is not known whether this drug or its metabolites are excreted in human milk. Because many drugs are excreted in human milk, caution should be exercised when XALATAN is administered to a nursing woman.

Pediatric Use: Safety and effectiveness in pediatric patients have not been established.

Geriatric Use: No overall differences in safety or effectiveness have been observed between elderly and younger patients.

Adverse Reactions: Adverse events referred to in other sections of this insert:
Eyelash changes (increased length, thickness, pigmentation, and number of lashes); eyelid skin darkening; intraocular inflammation (iritis/uveitis); iris pigmentation changes; and macular edema, including cystoid macular edema (see **WARNINGS** and **PRECAUTIONS**).

Controlled Clinical Trials:
The ocular adverse events and ocular signs and symptoms reported in 5 to 15% of the patients on XALATAN Sterile Ophthalmic Solution in the three 6-month, multi-center, double-masked, active-controlled trials were blurred vision, burning and stinging, conjunc-

tival hyperemia, foreign body sensation, itching, increased pigmentation of the iris, and punctuate epithelial keratopathy.

Local conjunctival hyperemia was observed; however, less than 1% of the patients treated with XALATAN required discontinuation of therapy because of intolerance to conjunctival hyperemia.

In addition to the above listed ocular events/signs and symptoms, the following were reported in 1 to 4% of the patients: dry eye, excessive tearing, eye pain, lid crusting, lid discomfort/pain, lid edema, lid erythema, and photophobia.

The following events were reported in less than 1% of the patients: conjunctivitis, diplopia and discharge from the eye.

During clinical studies, there were extremely rare reports of the following: retinal artery embolus, retinal detachment, and vitreous hemorrhage from diabetic retinopathy.

The most common systemic adverse events seen with XALATAN were upper respiratory tract infection/cold/flu, which occurred at a rate of approximately 4%. Chest pain/angina pectoris, muscle/joint/back pain, and rash/allergic skin reaction each occurred at a rate of 1 to 2%.

Clinical Practice:

The following events have been identified during postmarketing use of XALATAN in clinical practice. Because they are reported voluntarily from a population of unknown size, estimates of frequency cannot be made. The events, which have been chosen for inclusion due to either their seriousness, frequency of reporting, possible causal connection to XALATAN, or a combination of these factors, include: asthma and exacerbation of asthma; corneal edema and erosions; dyspnea; eyelash and vellus hair changes (increased length, thickness, pigmentation, and number); eyelid skin darkening; herpes keratitis; intraocular inflammation (iritis/uveitis); keratitis; macular edema, including cystoid macular edema; misdirected eyelashes sometimes resulting in eye irritation; dizziness, headache, and toxic epidermal necrolysis.

Overdosage: Apart from ocular irritation and conjunctival or episcleral hyperemia, the ocular effects of latanoprost administered at high doses are not known. Intravenous administration of large doses of latanoprost in monkeys has been associated with transient bronchoconstriction; however, in 11 patients with bronchial asthma treated with latanoprost, bronchoconstriction was not induced. Intravenous infusion of up to 3 µg/kg in healthy volunteers produced mean plasma concentrations 200 times higher than during clinical treatment and no adverse reactions were observed. Intravenous dosages of 5.5 to 10 µg/kg caused abdominal pain, dizziness, fatigue, hot flushes, nausea and sweating.

If overdosage with XALATAN Sterile Ophthalmic Solution occurs, treatment should be symptomatic.

Dosage and Administration: The recommended dosage is one drop (1.5 µg) in the affected eye(s) once daily in the evening. If one dose is missed, treatment should continue with the next dose as normal.

The dosage of XALATAN Sterile Ophthalmic Solution should not exceed once daily; the combined use of two or more prostaglandins, or prostaglandin analogs including XALATAN Sterile Ophthalmic Solution is not recommended. It has been shown that administration of these prostaglandin drug products more than once daily may decrease the intraocular pressure lowering effect or cause paradoxical elevations in IOP.

Reduction of the intraocular pressure starts approximately 3 to 4 hours after administration and the maximum effect is reached after 8 to 12 hours.

XALATAN may be used concomitantly with other topical ophthalmic drug products to lower intraocular pressure. If more than one topical ophthalmic drug is being used, the drugs should be administered at least five (5) minutes apart.

How Supplied: XALATAN Sterile Ophthalmic Solution is a clear, isotonic, buffered, preserved colorless solution of latanoprost 0.005% (50 µg/mL). It is supplied as a 2.5 mL solution in a 5 mL clear low density polyethylene bottle with a clear low density polyethylene dropper tip, a turquoise high density polyethylene screw cap, and a tamper-evident clear low density polyethylene overcap.

2.5 mL fill, 0.005% (50 µg/mL)
Package of 1 bottle   NDC 0013-8303-04
Storage: Protect from light. Store unopened bottle(s) under refrigeration at 2° to 8°C (36° to 46°F). During shipment to the patient, the bottle may be maintained at temperatures up to 40°C (104°F) for a period not exceeding 8 days. Once a bottle is opened for use, it may be stored at room temperature up to 25°C (77°F) for 6 weeks.

2.5 mL fill, 0.005% (50 µg/mL)
Multi-Pack of 3 bottles   NDC 0013-8303-01
Storage: Protect from light. Store unopened bottle(s) under refrigeration at 2° to 8°C (36° to 46°F). Once a bottle is opened for use, it may be stored at room temperature up to 25°C (77°C) for 6 weeks.

Rx only
Distributed by
Pharmacia & Upjohn Company
Division of Pfizer Inc, NY, NY 10017
Manufactured By:
Cardinal Health
Woodstock, IL 60098, USA
LAB-0135-7.0/LAB-0137-5.0
Revised November 2006
Shown in Product Identification Guide, page 105

Santen Inc.
for further product information see VISTAKON® Pharmaceuticals, LLC

VISTAKON®
Pharmaceuticals, LLC
7500 CENTURION PARKWAY
JACKSONVILLE, FL 32256

Direct Inquiries to:
Phone (866) 427-6815

ALAMAST®   ℞
[ă-lă-măst]
(pemirolast potassium ophthalmic solution)
0.1%

Description: ALAMAST® (pemirolast potassium ophthalmic solution) is a sterile, aqueous ophthalmic solution with a pH of approximately 8.0 containing 0.1% of the mast cell stabilizer, pemirolast potassium, for topical administration to the eyes.

Pemirolast potassium is a slightly yellow, water-soluble powder with a molecular weight of 266.3.
The chemical structure is presented below:
[See chemical structure at top of next column]
Chemical name:
9-methyl-3-(1H-tetrazol-5-yl)-4H-pyrido[1,2-α]pyrimidin-4-one potassium
Each mL contains: ACTIVE: pemirolast potassium 1 mg (0.1%); PRESERVATIVE: lauralko-

$C_{10}H_7KN_6O$

nium chloride 0.005%; INACTIVES: glycerin, dibasic sodium phosphate, monobasic sodium phosphate, phosphoric acid and/or sodium hydroxide to adjust pH, and purified water. The osmolality of ALAMAST® ophthalmic solution is approximately 240 mOsmol/kg.

Clinical Pharmacology:
Mechanism of Action: Pemirolast potassium is a mast cell stabilizer that inhibits the *in vivo* Type I immediate hypersensitivity reaction.

In vitro and *in vivo* studies have demonstrated that pemirolast potassium inhibits the antigen-induced release of inflammatory mediators (e.g., histamine, leukotriene C_4, D_4, E_4) from human mast cells.

In addition, pemirolast potassium inhibits the chemotaxis of eosinophils into ocular tissue and blocks the release of mediators from human eosinophils.

Although the precise mechanism of action is unknown, the drug has been reported to prevent calcium influx into mast cells upon antigen stimulation.

Pharmacokinetics: Topical ocular administration of one to two drops of ALAMAST® ophthalmic solution in each eye four times daily in 16 healthy volunteers for two weeks resulted in detectable concentrations in the plasma. The mean (±SE) peak plasma level of 4.7 ± 0.8 ng/mL occurred at 0.42 ± 0.05 hours and the mean $t_{1/2}$ was 4.5 ± 0.2 hours. When a single 10 mg pemirolast potassium dose was taken orally, a peak plasma concentration of 0.723 µg/mL was reached.

Following topical administration, about 10-15% of the dose was excreted unchanged in the urine.

Clinical Studies: In clinical environmental studies, ALAMAST® was significantly more effective than placebo after 28 days in preventing ocular itching associated with allergic conjunctivitis.

Indications and Usage:
ALAMAST® ophthalmic solution is indicated for the prevention of itching of the eye due to allergic conjunctivitis. Symptomatic response to therapy (decreased itching) may be evident within a few days, but frequently requires longer treatment (up to four weeks).

Contraindications:
ALAMAST® ophthalmic solution is contraindicated in patients with previously demonstrated hypersensitivity to any of the ingredients of this product.

Warnings:
For topical ophthalmic use only. Not for injection or oral use.

Precautions:
Information for patients: To prevent contaminating the dropper tip and solution, do not touch the eyelids or surrounding areas with the dropper tip. Keep the bottle tightly closed when not in use.

Patients should be advised not to wear contact lenses if their eyes are red. ALAMAST® should not be used to treat contact lens related irritation. The preservative in ALAMAST®, lauralkonium chloride, may be absorbed by soft contact lenses. Patients who wear soft contact lenses and whose eyes are not red should be instructed to wait at least ten minutes after instilling ALAMAST® before they insert their contact lenses.

Continued on next page

Alamast—Cont.

Carcinogenesis, mutagenesis, impairment of fertility: Pemirolast potassium was not mutagenic or clastogenic when tested in a series of bacterial and mammalian tests for gene mutation and chromosomal injury *in vitro* nor was it clastogenic when tested *in vivo* in rats.

Pemirolast potassium had no effect on mating and fertility in rats at oral doses up to 250 mg/kg (approximately 20,000 fold the human dose at 2 drops/eye, 40 µL/drop, QID for a 50 kg adult). A reduced fertility and pregnancy index occurred in the F_1 generation when F_0 dams were treated with 400 mg/kg pemirolast potassium during late pregnancy and lactation period (approximately 30,000 fold the human dose).

Pregnancy:
Teratogenic effects: Pregnancy Category C. Pemirolast potassium caused an increased incidence of thymic remnant in the neck, interventricular septal defect, fetuses with wavy rib, splitting of thoracic vertebral body, and reduced numbers of ossified sternebrae, sacral and caudal vertebrae, and metatarsi when rats were given oral doses ≥250 mg/kg (approximately 20,000 fold the human dose at 2 drops/eye, 40 µL/drop, QID for a 50 kg adult) during organogenesis. Increased incidence of dilation of renal pelvis/ureter in the fetuses and neonates was also noted when rats were given an oral dose of 400 mg/kg pemirolast potassium (approximately 30,000 fold the human dose). Pemirolast potassium was not teratogenic in rabbits given oral doses up to 150 mg/kg (approximately 12,000 fold the human dose) during the same time period. There are no adequate and well-controlled studies in pregnant women. Because animal reproductive studies are not always predictive of human response, ALAMAST® ophthalmic solution should be used during pregnancy only if the benefit outweighs the risk.

Non-teratogenic effects: Pemirolast potassium produced increased pre- and post-implantation losses, reduced embryo/fetal and neonatal survival, decreased neonatal body weight, and delayed neonatal development in rats receiving an oral dose at 400 mg/kg (approximately 30,000 fold the human dose). Pemirolast potassium also caused a reduction in the number of corpus lutea, the number of implantations, and number of live fetuses in the F_1 generation in rats when F_0 dams were given oral dosages ≥250 mg/kg (approximately 20,000 fold the human dose) during late gestation and the lactation period.

Nursing Mothers: Pemirolast potassium is excreted in the milk of lactating rats at concentrations higher than those in plasma. It is not known whether pemirolast potassium is excreted in human milk. Because many drugs are excreted in human milk, caution should be exercised when ALAMAST® ophthalmic solution is administered to a nursing woman.

Pediatric Use: Safety and effectiveness in pediatric patients below the age of 3 years have not been established.

Adverse Reactions:
In clinical studies lasting up to 17 weeks with ALAMAST® ophthalmic solution, headache, rhinitis, and cold/flu symptoms were reported at an incidence of 10–25%. The occurrence of these side effects was generally mild. Some of these events were similar to the underlying ocular disease being studied.

The following ocular and non-ocular adverse reactions were reported at an incidence of less than 5%:

Ocular: burning, dry eye, foreign body sensation, and ocular discomfort.

Non-Ocular: allergy, back pain, bronchitis, cough, dysmenorrhea, fever, sinusitis, and sneezing/nasal congestion.

Overdosage:
No accounts of ALAMAST® ophthalmic solution overdose were reported following topical ocular application.

Oral ingestion of the contents of a 10 mL bottle would be equivalent to 10 mg of pemirolast potassium.

Dosage and Administration:
The recommended dose is one to two drops in each affected eye four times daily.

Symptomatic response to therapy (decreased itching) may be evident within a few days, but frequently requires longer treatment (up to four weeks).

How Supplied:
ALAMAST® (pemirolast potassium ophthalmic solution) 0.1% is supplied as follows:

10 mL in a white, low density polyethylene bottle with a controlled dropper tip, and a white polyethylene screw cap.

NDC 68669-711-1010 mL fill in 11 cc container

Storage: Store at 15°–25°C (59°–77°F).

Rx only

Manufactured by:
Santen Oy, PO Box 33
FIN-33721 Tampere, Finland

Santen®

Marketed by:
VISTAKON® Pharmaceuticals, LLC
Jacksonville, FL 32256
Licensed from Mitsubishi Pharma Corporation
Tokyo, Japan
February 2005 Version
U.S. Patent No. 5,034,230
VISTAKON® Pharmaceuticals, LLC
III-03

Shown in Product Identification Guide, page 105

BETIMOL®   ℞
[bāt´-ĭ-mŏl´]
(timolol ophthalmic solution) 0.25%, 0.5%

Description: Betimol® (timolol ophthalmic solution), 0.25% and 0.5%, is a non-selective beta-adrenergic antagonist for ophthalmic use. The chemical name of the active ingredient is (S)-1-[(1, 1-dimethylethyl) amino]-3-[[4-(4-morpholinyl)-1, 2, 5-thiadiazol-3-yl]oxy]-2-propanol. Timolol hemihydrate is the levo isomer. Specific rotation is $[\alpha]^{25}_{405nm} = -16°$ (C = 10% as the hemihydrate form in 1N HCl).

The molecular formula of timolol is:

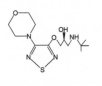

Timolol (as the hemihydrate) is a white, odorless, crystalline powder which is slightly soluble in water and freely soluble in ethanol. Timolol hemihydrate is stable at room temperature.

Betimol® is a clear, colorless, isotonic, sterile, microbiologically preserved phosphate buffered aqueous solution.

It is supplied in two dosage strengths, 0.25% and 0.5%.

Each mL of Betimol® 0.25% contains 2.56 mg of timolol hemihydrate equivalent to 2.5 mg timolol.

Each mL of Betimol® 05% contains 5.12 mg of timolol hemihydrate equivalent to 5.0 mg timolol.

Inactive ingredients: monosodium and disodium phosphate dihydrate to adjust pH (6.5 – 7.5) and water for injection, benzalkonium chloride 0.01% added as preservative.

The osmolality of Betimol® is 260 to 320 mOsmol/kg.

Clinical Pharmacology: Timolol is a non-selective beta-adrenergic antagonist.

It blocks both beta$_1$- and beta$_2$-adrenergic receptors. Timolol does not have significant intrinsic sympathomimetic activity, local anesthetic (membrane-stabilizing) or direct myocardial depressant activity.

Timolol, when applied topically in the eye, reduces normal and elevated intraocular pressure (IOP) whether or not accompanied by glaucoma. Elevated intraocular pressure is a major risk factor in the pathogenesis of glaucomatous visual field loss. The higher the level of IOP, the greater the likelihood of glaucomatous visual field loss and optic nerve damage. The predominant mechanism of ocular hypotensive action of topical beta-adrenergic blocking agents is likely due to a reduction in aqueous humor production.

In general, beta-adrenergic blocking agents reduce cardiac output both in healthy subjects and patients with heart diseases. In patients with severe impairment of myocardial function, beta-adrenergic receptor blocking agents may inhibit sympathetic stimulatory effect necessary to maintain adequate cardiac function. In the bronchi and bronchioles, beta-adrenergic receptor blockade may also increase airway resistance because of unopposed parasympathetic activity.

Pharmacokinetics
When given orally, timolol is well absorbed and undergoes considerable first pass metabolism. Timolol and its metabolites are primarily excreted in the urine. The half-life of timolol in plasma is approximately 4 hours.

Clinical Studies
In two controlled multicenter studies in the U.S., Betimol® 0.25% and 0.5% were compared with respective timolol maleate eyedrops. In these studies, the efficacy and safety profile of Betimol® was similar to that of timolol maleate.

Indications and Usage: Betimol® is indicated in the treatment of elevated intraocular pressure in patients with ocular hypertension or open-angle glaucoma.

Contraindications: Betimol® is contraindicated in patients with overt heart failure, cardiogenic shock, sinus bradycardia, second- or third-degree atrioventricular block, bronchial asthma or history of bronchial asthma, or severe chronic obstructive pulmonary disease, or hypersensitivity to any component of this product.

Warnings: As with other topically applied ophthalmic drugs, Betimol® is absorbed systemically. The same adverse reactions found with systemic administration of beta-adrenergic blocking agents may occur with topical administration. For example, severe respiratory and cardiac reactions, including death due to bronchospasm in patients with asthma, and rarely, death in association with cardiac failure have been reported following systemic or topical administration of beta-adrenergic blocking agents. Cardiac Failure: Sympathetic stimulation may be essential for support of the circulation in individuals with diminished myocardial contractility, and its inhibition by beta-adrenergic receptor blockade may precipitate more severe cardiac failure.

In patients without a history of cardiac failure, continued depression of the myocardium with beta-blocking agents over a period of time can, in some cases, lead to cardiac failure. Betimol® should be discontinued at the first sign or symptom of cardiac failure.

Obstructive Pulmonary Disease: Patients with chronic obstructive pulmonary disease (e.g. chronic bronchitis, emphysema) of mild or moderate severity, bronchospastic disease, or a history of bronchospastic disease (other than bronchial asthma or a history of bronchial asthma which are contraindications) should in general not receive beta-blocking agents.

Major Surgery: The necessity or desirability of withdrawal of beta-adrenergic blocking agents prior to a major surgery is controversial. Beta-adrenergic receptor blockade impairs the ability of the heart to respond to beta-adrenergically mediated reflex stimuli. This may augment the risk of general anesthesia in surgical procedures. Some patients receiving beta-adrenergic receptor blocking agents have been subject to protracted severe hypotension during anesthesia. Difficulty in restarting and maintaining the heartbeat has also been reported. For these reasons, in patients undergoing elective surgery, gradual withdrawal of beta-adrenergic receptor blocking agents is recommended. If necessary during surgery, the effects of beta-adrenergic blocking agents may be reversed by sufficient doses of beta-adrenergic agonists.

Diabetes Mellitus: Beta-adrenergic blocking agents should be administered with caution in patients subject to spontaneous hypoglycemia or to diabetic patients (especially those with labile diabetes) who are receiving insulin or oral hypoglycemic agents. Beta-adrenergic receptor blocking agents may mask the signs and symptoms of acute hypoglycemia.

Thyrotoxicosis: Beta-adrenergic blocking agents may mask certain clinical signs (e.g. tachycardia) of hyperthyroidism. Patients suspected of developing thyrotoxicosis should be managed carefully to avoid abrupt withdrawal of beta-adrenergic blocking agents which might precipitate a thyroid storm.

Precautions:
General
Because of the potential effects of beta-adrenergic blocking agents relative to blood pressure and pulse, these agents should be used with caution in patients with cerebrovascular insufficiency. If signs or symptoms suggesting reduced cerebral blood flow develop following initiation of therapy with Betimol®, alternative therapy should be considered.

There have been reports of bacterial keratitis associated with the use of multiple dose containers of topical ophthalmic products. These containers had been inadvertently contaminated by patients who, in most cases, had a concurrent corneal disease or a disruption of the ocular epithelial suface. (See PRECAUTIONS, Information for Patients.)

Muscle Weakness: Beta-adrenergic blockade has been reported to potentiate muscle weakness consistent with certain myasthenic symptoms (e.g. diplopia, ptosis, and generalized weakness). Beta-adrenergic blocking agents have been reported rarely to increase muscle weakness in some patients with myasthenia gravis or myasthenic symptoms.

In angle-closure glaucoma, the goal of the treatment is to reopen the angle. This requires constricting the pupil. Betimol® has no effect on the pupil. Therefore, if timolol is used in angle-closure glaucoma, it should always be combined with a miotic and not used alone.

Anaphylaxis: While taking beta-blockers, patients with a history of atopy or a history of severe anaphylactic reactions to a variety of allergens may be more reactive to repeated accidental, diagnostic, or therapeutic challenge with such allergens. Such patients may be unresponsive to the usual doses of epinephrine used to treat anaphylactic reactions.

The preservative benzalkonium chloride may be absorbed by soft contact lenses. Patients who wear soft contact lenses should wait 5 minutes after instilling Betimol® before they insert their lenses.

Information for Patients
Patients should be instructed to avoid allowing the tip of the dispensing container to contact the eye or surrounding structures.

Patients should also be instructed that ocular solutions can become contaminated by common bacteria known to cause ocular infections. Serious damage to the eye and subsequent loss of vision may result from using contaminated solutions. (See PRECAUTIONS, General.)

Patients requiring concomitant topical ophthalmic medications should be instructed to administer these at least 5 minutes apart.

Patients with bronchial asthma, a history of bronchial asthma, severe chronic obstructive pulmonary disease, sinus bradycardia, second- or third-degree atrioventricular block, or cardiac failure should be advised not to take this product (See CONTRAINDICATIONS.)

Drug Interactions
Beta-adrenergic blocking agents: Patients who are receiving a beta-adrenergic blocking agent orally and Betimol® should be observed for a potential additive effect either on the intraocular pressure or on the known systemic effects of beta-blockade.

Patients should not usually receive two topical ophthalmic beta-adrenergic blocking agents concurrently.

Catecholamine-depleting drugs: Close observation of the patient is recommended when a beta-blocker is administered to patients receiving catecholamine-depleting drugs such as reserpine, because of possible additive effects and the production of hypotension and/or marked bradycardia, which may produce vertigo, syncope, or postural hypotension.

Calcium antagonists: Caution should be used in the co-administration of beta-adrenergic blocking agents and oral or intravenous calcium antagonists, because of possible atrioventricular conduction disturbances, left ventricular failure, and hypotension. In patients with impaired cardiac function, co-administration should be avoided.

Digitalis and calcium antagonists: The concomitant use of beta-adrenergic blocking agents with digitalis and calcium antagonists may have additive effects in prolonging atrioventricular conduction time.

Injectable Epinephrine: (See PRECAUTIONS, General, Anaphylaxis.)

Carcinogenesis, Mutagenesis, Impairment of Fertility
Carcinogenicity of timolol (as the maleate) has been studied in mice and rats. In a two-year study orally administrated timolol maleate (300mg/kg/day) (approximately 42,000 times the systemic exposure following the maximum recommended human ophthalmic dose) in male rats caused a significant increase in the incidence of adrenal pheochromocytomas; the lower doses, 25 mg or 100 mg/kg daily did not cause any changes.

In a life span study in mice the overall incidence of neoplasms was significantly increased in female mice at 500 mg/kg/day (approximately 71,000 times the systemic exposure following the maximum recommended human ophthalmic dose). Furthermore, significant increases were observed in the incidences of benign and malignant pulmonary tumors, benign uterine polyps, as well as mammary adenocarcinomas. These changes were not seen at the daily dose level of 5 or 50 mg/kg (approximately 700 or 7,000, respectively, times the systemic exposure following the maximum recommended human ophthalmic dose). For comparison, the maximum recommended human oral dose of timolol maleate is 1 mg/kg/day.

Mutagenic potential of timolol was evaluated in vivo in the micronucleus test and cytogenetic assay and in vitro in the neoplastic cell transformation assay and Ames test, In the bacterial mutagenicity test (Ames test) high concentrations of timolol maleate (5000 and 10,000 g/ plate) statistically significantly increased the number of revertants in *Salmonella typhimurium* TA100, but not in the other three strains tested. However, no consistent dose-response was observed nor did the number of revertants reach the double of the control value, which is regarded as one of the criteria for a positive result in the Ames test. *In vivo* genotoxicity tests (the mouse micronucleus test and cytogenetic assay) and *in vitro* the neoplastic cell transformation assay were negative up to dose levels of 800 mg/kg and 100 g/mL, respectively.

No adverse effects on male and female fertility were reported in rats at timolol oral doses of up to 150 mg/kg/day (21,000 times the systemic exposure following the maximum recommended human ophthalmic dose).

Pregnancy Teratogenic effects:
Category C: Teratogenicity of timolol (as the maleate) after oral administration was studied in mice and rabbits. No fetal malformations were reported in mice or rabbits at a daily oral dose of 50 mg/kg (7,000 times the systemic exposure following the maximum recommended human ophthalmic dose). Although delayed fetal ossification was observed at this dose in rats, there were no adverse effects on postnatal development of offspring. Doses of 1000 mg/kg/ day (142,000 times the systemic exposure following the maximum recommended human ophthalmic dose) were maternotoxic in mice and resulted in an increased number of fetal resorptions. Increased fetal resorptions were also seen in rabbits at doses of 14,000 times the systemic exposure following the maximum recommended human ophthalmic dose in this case without apparent maternotoxicity.

There are no adequate and well-controlled studies in pregnant women. Betimol® should be used during pregnancy only it the potential benefit justifies the potential risk to the fetus.

Nursing mothers:
Because of the potential for serious adverse reactions in nursing infants from timolol, a decision should be made whether to discontinue nursing or to discontinue the drug, taking into account the importance of the drug to the mother.

Pediatric use:
Safety and efficacy in pediatric patients have not been established.

Adverse Reactions:
The most frequently reported ocular event in clinical trials was burning/stinging on instillation and was comparable between Betimol® and timolol maleate (approximately one in eight patients).

The following adverse events were associated with use of Betimol® in frequencies of more than 5% in two controlled, double-masked clinical studies in which 184 patients received 0.25% or 0.5% Betimol®:

OCULAR:
Dry eyes, itching, foreign body sensation, discomfort in the eye, eyelid erythema, conjunctival injection, and headache.

BODY AS A WHOLE:
Headache.

The following side effects were reported in frequencies of 1 to 5%:

OCULAR:
Eye pain, epiphora, photophobia, blurred or abnormal vision, corneal fluorescein staining, keratitis, blepharitis and cataract.

BODY AS A WHOLE:
Allergic reaction, asthenia, common cold and pain in extremities.

CARDIOVASCULAR:
Hypertension.

DIGESTIVE:
Nausea.

METABOLIC/NUTRITIONAL:
Peripheral edema.

Continued on next page

Betimol—Cont.

NERVOUS SYSTEM/PSYCHIATRY:
Dizziness and dry mouth.
RESPIRATORY:
Respiratory infection and sinusitis.
In addition, the following adverse reactions have been reported with ophthalmic use of beta blockers:
OCULAR:
Conjunctivitis, blepharoptosis, decreased corneal sensitivity, visual disturbances including refractive changes, diplopia and retinal vascular disorder.
BODY AS A WHOLE:
Chest pain.
CARDIOVASCULAR:
Arrhythmia, palpitation, bradycardia, hypotension, syncope, heart block, cerebral vascular accident, cerebral ischemia, cardiac failure and cardiac arrest.
DIGESTIVE:
Diarrhea.
ENDOCRINE:
Masked symptoms of hypoglycemia in insulin dependent diabetics (See WARNINGS).
NERVOUS SYSTEM/PSYCHIATRY:
Depression, impotence, increase in signs and symptoms of myasthenia gravis and paresthesia.
RESPIRATORY:
Dyspnea, bronchospasm, respiratory failure and nasal congestion.
SKIN:
Alopecia, hypersensitivity including localized and generalized rash, urticaria.
Overdosage: No information is available on overdosage with Betimol®. Symptoms that might be expected with an overdose of a beta-adrenergic receptor blocking agent are bronchospasm, hypotension, bradycardia, and acute cardiac failure.
Dosage and Administration: Betimol® Ophthalmic Solution is available in concentrations of 0.25 and 0.5 percent. The usual starting dose is one drop of 0.25 percent Betimol® in the affected eye(s) twice a day. If the clinical response is not adequate, the dosage may be changed to one drop of 0.5 percent solution in the affected eye(s) twice a day.
If the intraocular pressure is maintained at satisfactory levels, the dosage schedule may be changed to one drop once a day in the affected eye(s). Because of diurnal variations in intraocular pressure, satisfactory response to the once-a-day dose is best determined by measuring the intraocular pressure at different times during the day.
Since in some patients the pressure-lowering response to Betimol® may require a few weeks to stabilize, evaluation should include a determination of intraocular pressure after approximately 4 weeks of treatment with Betimol®.
Dosages above one drop of 0.5 percent Betimol® twice a day generally have not been shown to produce further reduction in intraocular pressure, If the patient's intraocular pressure is still not at a satisfactory level on this regimen, concomitant therapy with pilocarpine and other miotics, and/or epinephrine, and/or systemically administered carbonic anhydrase inhibitors, such as acetazolamide can be instituted.
How Supplied: Betimol® (timolol ophthalmic solution) is a clear, colorless solution.
Betimol® 0.25% is supplied in a white, opaque, plastic, ophthalmic dispenser bottle with a controlled drop tip as follows:
NDC 68669-522-05 5.0mL fill in 5 cc container
NDC 68669-522-1010mL fill in 11 cc container
NDC 68669-522-1515mL fill in 15 cc container
Betimol® 0.5% is supplied in a white, opaque, plastic, ophthalmic dispenser bottle with a controlled drop tip as follows:
NDC 68669-525-055.0mL fill in 5 cc container

NDC 68669-525-1010mL fill in 11 cc container
NDC 68669-525-1515mL fill in 15 cc container
Rx Only
STORAGE
Store between 15-30°C (59-86°F). Do not freeze. Protect from light.
MARKETED BY:
VISTAKON® Pharmaceuticals, LLC
Jacksonville, FL 32256 USA
MANUFACTURED BY:
Santen Oy, P.O. Box 33
FIN-33721 Tampere, Finland
Santen®
VISTAKON® Pharmaceuticals, LLC
Shown in Product Identification Guide, page 105

QUIXIN®

℞

[*quik-sin*]
(levofloxacin ophthalmic solution) 0.5%

Description: QUIXIN® (levofloxacin ophthalmic solution) 0.5% is a sterile topical ophthalmic solution. Levofloxacin is a fluoroquinolone antibacterial active against a broad spectrum of Gram-positive and Gram-negative ocular pathogens. Levofloxacin is the pure (-)-(S)-enantiomer of the racemic drug substance, ofloxacin. It is more soluble in water at neutral pH than ofloxacin.

Structural formula

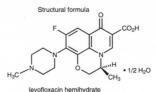

levofloxacin hemihydrate

$C_{18}H_{20}FN_3O_4 \cdot 1/2 H_2O$ Mol Wt 370.38

[See chemical structure at top of next column]
Chemical Name: (-)-(S)-9-fluoro-2, 3-dihydro-3-methyl-10-(4-methyl-1-piperazinyl)-7-oxo-7H-pyrido [1, 2, 3-*de*]-1, 4 benzoxazine-6-carboxylic acid hemihydrate.
Levofloxacin (hemihydrate) is a yellowish-white crystalline powder.
Each mL of QUIXIN® contains 5.12 mg of levofloxacin hemihydrate equivalent to 5 mg levofloxacin.
Contains:
Active: Levofloxacin 0.5% (5 mg/mL); **Preservative:** benzalkonium chloride 0.005%; **Inactives:** sodium chloride and water. May also contain hydrochloric acid and/or sodium hydroxide to adjust pH.
QUIXIN® solution is isotonic and formulated at pH 6.5 with an osmolality of approximately 300 mOsm/kg. Levofloxacin is a fluorinated 4-quinolone containing a six-member (pyridobenzoxazine) ring from positions 1 to 8 of the basic ring structure.
Clinical Pharmacology:
Pharmacokinetics:
Levofloxacin concentration in plasma was measured in 15 healthy adult volunteers at various time points during a 15-day course of treatment with QUIXIN® solution. The mean levofloxacin concentration in plasma 1 hour postdose, ranged from 0.86 ng/mL on Day 1 to 2.05 ng/mL on Day 15. The highest maximum mean levofloxacin concentration of 2.25 ng/mL was measured on Day 4 following 2 days of dosing every 2 hours for a total of 8 doses per day. Maximum mean levofloxacin concentrations increased from 0.94 ng/mL on Day 1 to 2.15 ng/mL on Day 15, which is more than 1,000 times lower than those reported after standard oral doses of levofloxacin.
Levofloxacin concentration in tears was measured in 30 healthy adult volunteers at various time points following instillation of a single drop of QUIXIN® solution. Mean levofloxacin

concentrations in tears ranged from 34.9 to 221.1 µg/mL during the 60-minute period following the single dose. The mean tear concentrations measured 4 and 6 hours postdose were 17.0 and 6.6 µg/mL. The clinical significance of these concentrations is unknown.
Microbiology:
Levofloxacin is the *L*-isomer of the racemate, ofloxacin, a quinolone antimicrobial agent. The antibacterial activity of ofloxacin resides primarily in the *L*-isomer. The mechanism of action of levofloxacin and other fluoroquinolone antimicrobials involves the inhibition of bacterial topoisomerase IV and DNA gyrase (both of which are type II topoisomerases), enzymes required for DNA replication, transcription, repair, and recombination.
Levofloxacin has *in vitro* activity against a wide range of Gram-negative and Gram-positive microorganisms and is often bactericidal at concentrations equal to or slightly greater than inhibitory concentrations.
Fluoroquinolones, including levofloxacin, differ in chemical structure and mode of action from β-lactam antibiotics and aminoglycosides, and therefore may be active against bacteria resistant to β-lactam antibiotics and aminoglycosides. Additionally, β-lactam antibiotics and aminoglycosides may be active against bacteria resistant to levofloxacin.
Resistance to levofloxacin due to spontaneous mutation *in vitro* is a rare occurrence (range: 10^{-9} to 10^{-10}).
Levofloxacin has been shown to be active against most strains of the following microorganisms, both *in vitro* and in clinical infections as described in the INDICATIONS AND USAGE section:
AEROBIC GRAM-POSITIVE MICROORGANISMS
Corynebacterium species*
Staphylococcus aureus
Staphylococcus epidermidis
Streptococcus pneumoniae
Streptococcus (Groups C/F)
Streptococcus (Group G)
Viridans group streptococci
AEROBIC GRAM-NEGATIVE MICROORGANISMS
*Acinetobacter lwoffii**
Haemophilus influenzae
*Serratia marcescens**

---

*Efficacy for this organism was studied in fewer than 10 infections.
The following *in vitro* data are also available, but their clinical significance in ophthalmic infections is unknown. The safety and effectiveness of levofloxacin in treating ophthalmological infections due to these microorganisms have not been established in adequate and well-controlled trials.
These organisms are considered susceptible when evaluated using systemic breakpoints. However, a correlation between the *in vitro* systemic breakpoint and ophthalmological efficacy has not been established. The list of organisms is provided as guidance only in assessing the potential treatment of conjunctival infections. Levofloxacin exhibits *in vitro* minimal inhibitory concentrations (MICs) of 2 µg/mL or less (systemic susceptible breakpoint) against most (≥90%) strains of the following ocular pathogens.
AEROBIC GRAM-POSITIVE MICROORGANISMS
Enterococcus faecalis
Staphylococcus saprophyticus
Streptococcus agalactiae
Streptococcus pyogenes
AEROBIC GRAM-NEGATIVE MICROORGANISMS
Acinetobacter anitratus
Acinetobacter baumannii
Citrobacter diversus
Citrobacter freundii
Enterobacter aerogenes
Enterobacter agglomerans

Enterobacter cloacae
Escherichia coli
Haemophilus parainfluenzae
Klebsiella oxytoca
Klebsiella pneumoniae
Legionella pneumophila
Moraxella catarrhalis
Morganella morganii
Neisseria gonorrhoeae
Proteus mirabilis
Proteus vulgaris
Providencia rettgeri
Providencia stuartii
Pseudomonas aeruginosa
Pseudomonas fluorescens

Clinical Studies: In randomized, double-masked, multicenter controlled clinical trials where patients were dosed for 5 days, QUIXIN® demonstrated clinical cures in 79% of patients treated for bacterial conjunctivitis on the final study visit day (day 6-10). Microbial outcomes for the same clinical trials demonstrated an eradication rate for presumed pathogens of 90%.

Indications and Usage: QUIXIN® solution is indicated for the treatment of bacterial conjunctivitis caused by susceptible strains of the following organisms:

AEROBIC GRAM-POSITIVE MICROORGANISMS

*Corynebacterium species**
Staphylococcus aureus
Staphylococcus epidermidis
Streptococcus pneumoniae
Streptococcus (Groups C/F)
Streptococcus (Group G)
Viridans group streptococci

AEROBIC GRAM-NEGATIVE MICROORGANISMS

*Acinetobacter Iwoffii**
Haemophilus influenzae
*Serratia marcescens**

---

*Efficacy for this organism was studied in fewer than 10 infections.

Contraindications: QUIXIN® solution is contraindicated in patients with a history of hypersensitivity to levofloxacin, to other quinolones, or to any of the components in this medication.

Warnings: NOT FOR INJECTION.

QUIXIN® solution should not be injected subconjunctivally, nor should it be introduced directly into the anterior chamber of the eye.

In patients receiving systemic quinolones, serious and occasionally fatal hypersensitivity (anaphylactic) reactions have been reported, some following the first dose. Some reactions were accompanied by cardiovascular collapse, loss of consciousness, angioedema (including laryngeal, pharyngeal or facial edema), airway obstruction, dyspnea, urticaria, and itching. If an allergic reaction to levofloxacin occurs, discontinue the drug. Serious acute hypersensitivity reactions may require immediate emergency treatment. Oxygen and airway management should be administered as clinically indicated.

Precautions:
General:
As with other anti-infectives, prolonged use may result in overgrowth of non-susceptible organisms, including fungi. If superinfection occurs, discontinue use and institute alternative therapy. Whenever clinical judgment dictates, the patient should be examined with the aid of magnification, such as slit-lamp biomicroscopy, and, where appropriate, fluorescein staining.

Patients should be advised not to wear contact lenses if they have signs and symptoms of bacterial conjunctivitis.

Information for Patients:
Avoid contaminating the applicator tip with material from the eye, fingers or other source. Systemic quinolones have been associated with hypersensitivity reactions, even following a single dose. Discontinue use immediately and contact your physician at the first sign of a rash or allergic reaction.

Drug Interactions:
Specific drug interaction studies have not been conducted with QUIXIN®. However, the systemic administration of some quinolones has been shown to elevate plasma concentrations of theophylline, interfere with the metabolism of caffeine, and enhance the effects of the oral anticoagulant warfarin and its derivatives, and has been associated with transient elevations in serum creatinine in patients receiving systemic cyclosporine concomitantly.

Carcinogenesis, Mutagenesis, Impairment of Fertility:
In a long term carcinogenicity study in rats, levofloxacin exhibited no carcinogenic or tumorigenic potential following daily dietary administration for 2 years; the highest dose (100 mg/kg/day) was 875 times the highest recommended human ophthalmic dose.

Levofloxacin was not mutagenic in the following assays: Ames bacterial mutation assay (*S. typhimurium* and *E. coli*), CHO/HGPRT forward mutation assay, mouse micronucleus test, mouse dominant lethal test, rat unscheduled DNA synthesis assay, and the *in vivo* mouse sister chromatid exchange assay. It was positive in the *in vitro* chromosomal aberration (CHL cell line) and *in vitro* sister chromatid exchange (CHL/IU cell line) assays.

Levofloxacin caused no impairment of fertility or reproduction in rats at oral doses as high as 360 mg/kg/day, corresponding to 3,150 times the highest recommended human ophthalmic dose.

Pregnancy: Teratogenic Effects. Pregnancy Category C:
Levofloxacin at oral doses of 810 mg/kg/day in rats, which corresponds to approximately 7,000 times the highest recommended human ophthalmic dose, caused decreased fetal body weight and increased fetal mortality.

No teratogenic effect was observed when rabbits were dosed orally as high as 50 mg/kg/day, which corresponds to approximately 400 times the highest recommended maximum human ophthalmic dose, or when dosed intravenously as high as 25 mg/kg/day, corresponding to approximately 200 times the highest recommended human ophthalmic dose.

There are, however, no adequate and well-controlled studies in pregnant women. Levofloxacin should be used during pregnancy only if the potential benefit justifies the potential risk to the fetus.

Nursing Mothers:
Levofloxacin has not been measured in human milk. Based upon data from ofloxacin, it can be presumed that levofloxacin is excreted in human milk. Caution should be exercised when QUIXIN® is administered to a nursing mother.

Pediatric Use:
Safety and effectiveness in infants below the age of one year have not been established. Oral administration of quinolones has been shown to cause arthropathy in immature animals. There is no evidence that the ophthalmic administration of levofloxacin has any effect on weight bearing joints.

Geriatric Use:
No overall differences in safety or effectiveness have been observed between elderly and other adult patients.

Adverse Reactions: The most frequently reported adverse events in the overall study population were transient decreased vision, fever, foreign body sensation, headache, transient ocular burning, ocular pain or discomfort, pharyngitis and photophobia. These events occurred in approximately 1-3% of patients. Other reported reactions occurring in less than 1% of patients included allergic reactions, lid edema, ocular dryness, and ocular itching.

Dosage and Administration:
Days 1 and 2:
Instill one to two drops in the affected eye(s) every 2 hours while awake, up to 8 times per day.

Days 3 through 7:
Instill one to two drops in the affected eye(s) every 4 hours while awake, up to 4 times per day.

How Supplied: QUIXIN® (levofloxacin ophthalmic solution) 0.5% is supplied in a white, low density polyethylene bottle with a controlled dropper tip and a tan, high density polyethylene cap in the following size:
5 mL fill in 5 cc container - NDC 68669-135-05

Storage:
Store at 15° – 25°C (59° – 77°F).
Rx Only.

Manufactured by:
Santen Oy, P.O. Box 33, FIN-33721 Tampere, Finland
Licensed from:
Daiichi Pharmaceutical Co., Ltd., Tokyo, Japan
U.S. PAT. NO. 5,053,407

Marketed by:
VISTAKON® Pharmaceuticals, LLC
Jacksonville, FL 32256 USA
VISTAKON® Pharmaceuticals, LLC
March 2004 Version
Shown in Product Identification Guide, page 105

POISON CONTROL CENTERS

The American Association of Poison Control Centers (AAPCC) uses a single, nationwide emergency number to automatically link callers with their regional poison center. This toll-free number, **800-222-1222**, also works for **teletype lines (TTY)** for the hearing-impaired and **telecommunication devices (TTD)** for individuals who are deaf. However, a few local poison centers and the ASPCA/Animal Poison Control Center are not part of this nationwide system and continue to use separate numbers.

Most of the centers listed below are certified by the AAPCC. **Certified centers are marked by an asterisk after the name**. Each has to meet certain criteria.

It must, for example, serve a large geographic area; it must be open 24 hours a day and provide direct-dial or toll-free access; it must be supervised by a medical director; and it must have registered pharmacists or nurses available to answer questions from the public.

Within each state, centers are listed alphabetically by city. Some state poison centers also list their original emergency numbers (including TTY/TDD) that only work within that state. For these listings, callers may use either the state number or the nationwide 800 number.

ALABAMA

BIRMINGHAM

Regional Poison Control Center, The Children's Hospital of Alabama (*)

1600 7th Ave. South
Birmingham, AL 35233-1711
Business: 205-939-9201
Emergency: 800-222-1222
www.chsys.org

TUSCALOOSA

Alabama Poison Center (*)

2503 Phoenix Dr.
Tuscaloosa, AL 35405
Business: 205-345-0600
Emergency: 800-222-1222
          800-462-0800
          (AL)
www.alapoisoncenter.org

ALASKA

JUNEAU

Alaska Poison Control System

Section of Community Health and EMS
410 Willoughby Ave., Room 103
Box 110616
Juneau, AK 99811-0616
Business: 907-465-3027
Emergency: 800-222-1222
www.chems.alaska.gov

(PORTLAND, OR)

Oregon Poison Center (*) Oregon Health Sciences University

3181 SW Sam Jackson
Park Rd. CB550
Portland, OR 97239
Business: 503-494-8311
Emergency: 800-222-1222
www.oregonpoison.com

ARIZONA

PHOENIX

Banner Poison Control Center (*) Banner Good Samaritan Medical Center

901 E. Willetta St.
Room 2701
Phoenix, AZ 85006
Business: 602-495-4884
Emergency: 800-222-1222
www.bannerpoisoncontrol.com

TUCSON

Arizona Poison and Drug Information Center (*) Arizona Health Sciences Center

1501 N. Campbell Ave.
Room 1156
Tucson, AZ 85724
Business: 520-626-7899
Emergency: 800-222-1222

ARKANSAS

LITTLE ROCK

Arkansas Poison and Drug Information Center College of Pharmacy - UAMS

4301 West Markham St.
Mail Slot 522-2
Little Rock, AR 72205-7122
Business: 501-686-5540
Emergency: 800-222-1222
          800-376-4766
          (AR)
TDD/TTY: 800-641-3805

ASPCA/ANIMAL POISON CONTROL CENTER

1717 South Philo Rd.
Suite 36
Urbana, IL 61802
Business: 217-337-5030
Emergency: 888-426-4435
          800-548-2423
www.napcc.aspca.org

CALIFORNIA

FRESNO/MADERA

California Poison Control System-Fresno/Madera Div.(*) Children's Hospital of Central California

9300 Valley Children's Place
MB 15
Madera, CA 93638-8762
Business: 559-622-2300
Emergency: 800-222-1222
          800-876-4766
          (CA)
TDD/TTY: 800-972-3323
www.calpoison.org

SACRAMENTO

California Poison Control System-Sacramento Div.(*) UC Davis Medical Center

Room HSF 1024
2315 Stockton Blvd.
Sacramento, CA 95817
Business: 916-227-1400
Emergency: 800-222-1222
          800-876-4766
          (CA)
TDD/TTY: 800-972-3323
www.calpoison.org

SAN DIEGO

California Poison Control System-San Diego Div. (*) UC San Diego Medical Center

200 West Arbor Dr.
San Diego, CA 92103-8925
Business: 858-715-6300
Emergency: 800-222-1222
          800-876-4766
          (CA)
TDD/TTY: 800-972-3323
www.calpoison.org

SAN FRANCISCO

California Poison Control System-San Francisco Div.(*) San Francisco General Hospital University of California San Francisco

Box 1369
San Francisco, CA 94143-1369
Business: 415-502-6000
Emergency: 800-222-1222
          800-876-4766
          (CA)
TDD/TTY: 800-972-3323
www.calpoison.org

COLORADO

DENVER

Rocky Mountain Poison and Drug Center (*)

777 Bannock St.
Mail Code 0180
Denver CO 80204-4507
Business: 303-739-1100
Emergency: 800-222-1222
TDD/TTY: 303-739-1127
          (CO)
www.RMPDC.org

CONNECTICUT

FARMINGTON

**Connecticut Regional Poison Control Center (*)
University of Connecticut Health Center**

263 Farmington Ave.
Farmington, CT 06030-5365
Business: 860-679-4540
Emergency: 800-222-1222
TDD/TTY: 866-218-5372
http://poisoncontrol.uchc.edu

DELAWARE

(PHILADELPHIA, PA)

**The Poison Control Center (*)
Children's Hospital of Philadelphia**

34th St. & Civic Center Blvd.
Philadelphia, PA 19104-4303
Business: 215-590-2003
Emergency: 800-222-1222
                800-722-7112
                (DE)
TDD/TTY: 215-590-8789
www.poisoncontrol.chop.edu

DISTRICT OF COLUMBIA

WASHINGTON, DC

National Capital Poison Center (*)

3201 New Mexico Ave., NW
Suite 310
Washington, DC 20016
Business: 202-362-3867
Emergency: 800-222-1222
www.poison.org

FLORIDA

JACKSONVILLE

**Florida Poison Information Center-Jacksonville (*)
SHANDS Hospital**

655 West 8th St.
Jacksonville, FL 32209
Business: 904-244-4465
Emergency: 800-222-1222
http://fpicjax.org

MIAMI

**Florida Poison Information Center-Miami (*)
University of Miami–Department of Pediatrics**

P.O. Box 016960 (R-131)
Miami, FL 33101
Business: 305-585-5250
Emergency: 800-222-1222
www.miami.edu/poison-center

TAMPA

**Florida Poison Information Center-Tampa (*)
Tampa General Hospital**

P.O. Box 1289
Tampa, FL 33601-1289
Business: 813-844-7044
Emergency: 800-222-1222
www.poisoncentertampa.org

GEORGIA

ATLANTA

**Georgia Poison Center (*)
Hughes Spalding Children's Hospital, Grady Health System**

80 Jesse Hill Jr. Dr., SE
P.O. Box 26066
Atlanta, GA 30303-3050
Business: 404-616-9237
Emergency: 800-222-1222
                404-616-9000
                (Atlanta)
TDD: 404-616-9287
www.georgiapoisoncenter.org

HAWAII

(DENVER, CO)

Rocky Mountain Poison and Drug Center (*)

777 Bannock St.
Mail Code 0180
Denver CO 80204-4507
Business: 303-739-1100
Emergency: 800-222-1222
www.RMPDC.org

IDAHO

(DENVER, CO)

Rocky Mountain Poison and Drug Center (*)

777 Bannock St.
Mail Code 0180
Denver CO 80204-4507
Business: 303-739-1100
Emergency: 800-222-1222
www.RMPDC.org

ILLINOIS

CHICAGO

Illinois Poison Center (*)

222 South Riverside Plaza
Suite 1900
Chicago, IL 60606
Business: 312-906-6136
Emergency: 800-222-1222
TDD/TTY: 312-906-6185
www.illinoispoisoncenter.org

INDIANA

INDIANAPOLIS

**Indiana Poison Control Center (*)
Clarian Health Partners Methodist Hospital**

I-65 at 21st St.
Indianapolis, IN 46206-1367
Business: 317-962-2335
Emergency: 800-222-1222
                800-382-9097
                317-962-2323
                (Indianapolis)
TTY: 317-962-2336
www.clarian.org/poisoncontrol

IOWA

SIOUX CITY

**Iowa Statewide Poison Control Center
Iowa Health System and the University of Iowa Hospitals and Clinics**

401 Douglas St., Suite 402
Sioux City, IA 51101
Business: 712-279-3710
Emergency: 800-222-1222
                712-277-2222
                (IA)
www.iowapoison.org

KANSAS

KANSAS CITY

**Mid-America Poison Control Center
University of Kansas Medical Center**

3901 Rainbow Blvd.
Room B-400
Kansas City, KS 66160-7231
Business   913-588-6638
Emergency: 800-222-1222
                800-332-6633
                (KS)
TDD: 913-588-6639
www.kumc.edu/poison

KENTUCKY

LOUISVILLE

Kentucky Regional Poison Center (*)

PO Box 35070
Louisville, KY 40232-5070
Business: 502-629-7264
Emergency: 800-222-1222
                502-589-8222
                (Louisville)
www.krpc.com

LOUISIANA

MONROE

**Louisiana Drug and Poison Information Center (*)
University of Louisiana at Monroe**

700 University Ave.
Monroe, LA 71209-6430
Business: 318-342-3648
Emergency: 800-222-1222
www.lapcc.org

MAINE

PORTLAND

Northern New England Poison Center

Maine Medical Center
22 Bramhall St.
Portland, ME 04102
Business: 207-662-7220
Emergency: 800-222-1222
                207-871-2879
                (ME)
TDD/TTY: 877-299-4447
                (ME)
                207-871-2879
                (ME)
www.nnepc.org

MARYLAND

BALTIMORE

**Maryland Poison Center (*)
University of Maryland at Baltimore
School of Pharmacy**

20 North Pine St., PH 772
Baltimore, MD 21201
Business: 410-706-7604
Emergency: 800-222-1222
TDD: 410-706-1858
www.mdpoison.com

(WASHINGTON, DC)

National Capital Poison Center (*)

3201 New Mexico Ave., NW
Suite 310
Washington DC 20016
Business: 202-362-3867
Emergency: 800-222-1222
TDD/TTY: 202-362-8563
                (MD)
www.poison.org

MASSACHUSETTS

BOSTON

Regional Center for Poison Control and Prevention (*)
(Serving Massachusetts and Rhode Island)

300 Longwood Ave.
Boston, MA 02115
Business: 617-355-6609
Emergency: 800-222-1222
TDD/TTY: 888-244-5313
www.maripoisoncenter.com

MICHIGAN

DETROIT

Regional Poison Control Center (*) Children's Hospital of Michigan

4160 John R. Harper
Professional Office Bldg.
Suite 616
Detroit, MI 48201
Business: 313-745-5335
Emergency: 800-222-1222
TDD/TTY: 800-356-3232
www.mitoxic.org/pcc

GRAND RAPIDS

DeVos Children's Hospital Regional Poison Center (*)

100 Michigan St., NE
Grand Rapids, MI 49503
Business: 616-391-3690
Emergency: 800-222-1222
http://poisoncenter.
     devoschildrens.org

MINNESOTA

MINNEAPOLIS

Minnesota Poison Control System (*) Hennepin County Medical Center

701 Park Ave.
Mail Code RL
Minneapolis, MN 55415
Business: 612-873-3144
Emergency: 800-222-1222
www.mnpoison.org

MISSISSIPPI

JACKSON

Mississippi Regional Poison Control Center, University of Mississippi Medical Center

2500 North State St.
Jackson, MS 39216
Business: 601-984-1680
Emergency: 800-222-1222

MISSOURI

ST. LOUIS

Missouri Regional Poison Center (*) Cardinal Glennon Children's Hospital

7980 Clayton Rd.
Suite 200
St. Louis, MO 63117
Business: 314-772-5200
Emergency: 800-222-1222
TDD/TTY: 314-612-5705
www.cardinalglennon.com

MONTANA

(DENVER, CO)

Rocky Mountain Poison and Drug Center (*)

777 Bannock St.
Mail Code 0180
Denver CO 80204-4507
Business: 303-739-1100
Emergency: 800-222-1222
TDD/TTY: 303-739-1127
www.RMPDC.org

NEBRASKA

OMAHA

The Poison Center (*) Children's Hospital

8401 W. Dodge St., Suite 115
Omaha, NE 68114
Business: 402-955-5555
Emergency: 800-222-1222
www.nebraskapoison.com

NEVADA

(DENVER, CO)

Rocky Mountain Poison and Drug Center (*)

777 Bannock St.
Mail Code 0180
Denver CO 80204-4507
Business: 303-739-1100
Emergency: 800-222-1222
www.RMPDC.org

(PORTLAND, OR)

Oregon Poison Center (*) Oregon Health Sciences University

3181 SW Sam Jackson
Park Rd.
Portland, OR 97201
Business: 503-494-8600
Emergency: 800-222-1222
www.oregonpoison.com

NEW HAMPSHIRE

(PORTLAND, ME)

Northern New England Poison Center

Maine Medical Center
22 Bramhall St.
Portland, ME 04102
Business: 207-662-7220
Emergency: 800-222-1222
www.nnepc.org

NEW JERSEY

NEWARK

New Jersey Poison Information and Education System (*) UMDNJ

65 Bergen St.
Newark, NJ 07101
Business: 973-972-9280
Emergency: 800-222-1222
TDD/TTY: 973-926-8008
www.njpies.org

NEW MEXICO

ALBUQUERQUE

New Mexico Poison and Drug Information Center (*)

MSC09-5080
1 University of New Mexico
Albuquerque, NM 87131-0001
Business: 505-272-4261
Emergency: 800-222-1222
http://HSC.UNM.edu/pharmacy/
     poison

NEW YORK

BUFFALO

Western New York Regional Poison Control Center (*) Children's Hospital of Buffalo

219 Bryant St.
Buffalo, NY 14222
Business: 716-878-7654
Emergency: 800-222-1222
www.fingerlakespoison.org

MINEOLA

Long Island Regional Poison and Drug Information Center (*) Winthrop University Hospital

259 First St.
Mineola, NY 11501
Business: 516-663-2650
Emergency: 800-222-1222
TDD: 516-747-3323
     (Nassau)
     516-924-8811
     (Suffolk)

www.lirpdic.org

NEW YORK CITY

New York City Poison Control Center (*) NYC Dept. of Health

455 First Ave., Room 123
New York, NY 10016
Business: 212-447-8152
Emergency: 800-222-1222
(English) 212-340-4494
     212-POISONS
     (212-764-7667)

Emergency: 212-VENENOS
(Spanish) (212-836-3667)
TDD: 212-689-9014

ROCHESTER

Finger Lakes Regional Poison and Drug Information Center (*) University of Rochester Medical Center

601 Elmwood Ave.
Box 321
Rochester, NY 14642
Business: 585-273-4155
Emergency: 800-222-1222
TTY: 585-273-3854

SYRACUSE

Central New York Poison Center (*) SUNY Upstate Medical University

750 East Adams St.
Syracuse, NY 13210
Business: 315-464-7078
Emergency: 800-222-1222
www.cnypoison.org

NORTH CAROLINA

CHARLOTTE

Carolinas Poison Center (*) Carolinas Medical Center

PO Box 32861
Charlotte, NC 28232
Business: 704-512-3795
Emergency: 800-222-1222
TDD: 800-735-8262
TTY: 800-735-2962
www.ncpoisoncenter.org

NORTH DAKOTA

(MINNEAPOLIS, MN)

Minnesota Poison Control System (*) Hennepin County Medical Center

701 Park Ave.
Mail Code 820
Minneapolis, MN 55415
Business: 612-873-3144
Emergency: 800-222-1222
www.ndpoison.org

OHIO

CINCINNATI

Cincinnati Drug and Poison Information Center (*) Regional Poison Control System

3333 Burnet Ave.
Vernon Place, 3rd Floor
Cincinnati, OH 45229
Business: 513-636-5111
Emergency: 800-222-1222
TDD/TTY: 800-253-7955
www.cincinnatichildrens.org/dpic

CLEVELAND

Greater Cleveland Poison Control Center

11100 Euclid Ave.
MP 6007
Cleveland, OH 44106-6007
Business: 216-844-1573
Emergency: 800-222-1222
216-231-4455
(OH)

COLUMBUS

Central Ohio Poison Center (*)

700 Children's Dr.
Room L032
Columbus, OH 43205-2696
Business: 614-722-2635
Emergency: 800-222-1222
TTY: 614-228-2272
www.bepoisonsmart.com

OKLAHOMA

OKLAHOMA CITY

Oklahoma Poison Control Center (*) Children's Hospital at OU Medical Center

940 Northeast 13th St.
Room 3510
Oklahoma City, OK 73104
Business: 405-271-5062
Emergency: 800-222-1222
www.oklahomapoison.org

OREGON

PORTLAND

Oregon Poison Center (*) Oregon Health Sciences University

3181 S.W. Sam Jackson
Park Rd., CB550
Portland, OR 97239
Business: 503-494-8968
Emergency: 800-222-1222
www.oregonpoison.com

PENNSYLVANIA

PHILADELPHIA

The Poison Control Center (*) Children's Hospital of Philadelphia

34th Street & Civic Center Blvd.
Philadelphia, PA 19104-4399
Business: 215-590-2003
Emergency: 800-222-1222
215-386-2100
(PA)
TDD/TTY: 215-590-8789
www.poisoncontrol.chop.edu

PITTSBURGH

Pittsburgh Poison Center (*) Children's Hospital of Pittsburgh

3705 Fifth Ave.
Pittsburgh, PA 15213
Business: 412-390-3300
Emergency: 800-222-1222
412-681-6669
www.chp.edu/clinical/03a_
poison.php

PUERTO RICO

SANTURCE

San Jorge Children's Hospital Poison Center

268 San Jorge St.
Santurce, PR 00912
Business: 787-726-5660
Emergency: 800-222-1222
TTY: 787-641-1934
www.poisoncenter.net

RHODE ISLAND

(BOSTON, MA)

Regional Center for Poison Control and Prevention (*)
(Serving Massachusetts and Rhode Island)

300 Longwood Ave.
Boston, MA 02115
Business: 617-355-6609
Emergency: 800-222-1222
TDD/TTY: 888-244-5313
www.maripoisoncenter.com

SOUTH CAROLINA

COLUMBIA

Palmetto Poison Center (*) College of Pharmacy University of South Carolina

Columbia, SC 29208
Business: 803-777-7909
Drug Info: 800-777-7805
Emergency: 800-222-1222
803-922-1117
(SC)
www.pharm.sc.edu/PPS/pps.htm

SOUTH DAKOTA

(MINNEAPOLIS, MN)

Hennepin Regional Poison Center (*) Hennepin County Medical Center

701 Park Ave.
Minneapolis, MN 55415
Business: 612-873-3144
Emergency: 800-222-1222
www.mnpoison.org

SIOUX FALLS

Provides education only— Does not manage exposure cases.

Sioux Valley Poison Control Center (*)

1305 W. 18th St.
Box 5039
Sioux Falls, SD 57117-5039
Business: 605-328-6670
www.sdpoison.org

TENNESSEE

NASHVILLE

Tennessee Poison Center (*)

1161 21st Ave. South
501 Oxford House
Nashville, TN 37232-4632
Business: 615-936-0760
Emergency: 800-222-1222
www.poisonlifeline.org

TEXAS

AMARILLO

Texas Panhandle Poison Center (*) Northwest Texas Hospital

1501 S. Coulter Dr.
Amarillo, TX 79106
Business: 806-354-1630
Emergency: 800-222-1222
www.poisoncontrol.org

DALLAS

North Texas Poison Center (*) Texas Poison Center Network Parkland Health and Hospital System

5201 Harry Hines Blvd.
Dallas, TX 75235
Business: 214-589-0911
Emergency: 800-222-1222
www.poisoncontrol.org

EL PASO

West Texas Regional Poison Center (*) Thomason Hospital

4815 Alameda Ave.
El Paso, TX 79905
Business 915-534-3800
Emergency: 800-222-1222
www.poisoncontrol.org

GALVESTON

Southeast Texas Poison Center (*) The University of Texas Medical Branch

3.112 Trauma Bldg.
301 University Ave.
Galveston, TX 77555-1175
Business: 409-766-4403
Emergency: 800-222-1222
www.poisoncontrol.org

SAN ANTONIO

South Texas Poison Center (*) The University of Texas Health Science Center–San Antonio

7703 Floyd Curl Dr., MC 7849
San Antonio, TX 78229-3900
Business: 210-567-5762
Emergency: 800-222-1222
www.poisoncontrol.org

TEMPLE

Central Texas Poison Center (*) Scott & White Memorial Hospital

2401 South 31st St.
Temple, TX 76508
Business: 254-724-7401
Emergency: 800-222-1222
www.poisoncontrol.org

UTAH

SALT LAKE CITY

Utah Poison Control Center (*)

585 Komas Dr.
Suite 200
Salt Lake City, UT 84108
Business: 801-587-0600
Emergency: 800-222-1222
                 801-587-0600
                 (UT)
http://uuhsc.utah.edu/poison

VERMONT

(PORTLAND, ME)

**Northern New England
Poison Center**

Maine Medical Center
22 Bramhall St.
Portland, ME 04102
Business: 207-662-7220
Emergency: 800-222-1222
www.nnepc.org

VIRGINIA

CHARLOTTESVILLE

**Blue Ridge Poison Center (*)
University of Virginia Health
System**

PO Box 800774
Charlottesville, VA 22908-0774
Business: 434-924-0347
Emergency: 800-222-1222
www.healthsystem.virginia.edu.
  brpc

RICHMOND

**Virginia Poison Center (*)
Virginia Commonwealth
University**

P.O. Box 980522
Richmond, VA 23298-0522
Business: 804-828-4780
Emergency: 800-222-1222
                 804-828-9123
www.vcu.edu/mcved/vpc

WASHINGTON

SEATTLE

**Washington Poison
Center (*)**

155 NE 100th St.
Suite 400
Seattle, WA 98125-8011
Business: 206-517-2350
Emergency: 800-222-1222
                 206-526-2121
                 (WA)
TDD: 800-572-0638
                 (WA)
www.wapc.org

WEST VIRGINIA

CHARLESTON

**West Virginia
Poison Center (*)**

3110 MacCorkle Ave. SE
Charleston, WV 25304
Business: 304-347-1212
Emergency: 800-222-1222
www.wvpoisoncenter.org

WISCONSIN

MILWAUKEE

**Children's Hospital
of Wisconsin Statewide
Poison Center**

9000 W. Wisconsin Ave.
P.O. Box 1997, Mail Station
677A
Milwaukee, WI 53226
Business: 414-266-2952
Emergency: 800-222-1222
TDD/TTY: 414-266-2542
www.chw.org

WYOMING

(OMAHA, NE)

**The Poison Center (*)
Children's Hospital**

8401 W. Dodge St., Suite 115
Omaha, NE 68114
Business: 402-955-5555
Emergency: 800-222-1222
www.nebraskapoison.com

DRUG INFORMATION CENTERS

ALABAMA

BIRMINGHAM

Drug Information Service
University of Alabama
UAB Hospital Pharmacy
Drug Information-JT1720
619 S. 19th St.
Birmingham, AL 35249-6860
Mon.-Fri. 8 AM-5 PM
205-934-2162
www.health.uab.edu/pharmacy

Global Drug
Information Service
Samford University
McWhorter School
of Pharmacy
800 Lakeshore Dr.
Birmingham, AL 35229-7027
Mon.-Wed. 8 AM-9 PM
Thurs.-Fri. 8 AM-4:30 PM
205-726-2519 or 2891
www.samford.edu/schools/
pharmacy/dic/index.html

HUNTSVILLE

Huntsville Hospital Drug
Information Center
101 Sivley Rd.
Huntsville, AL 35801
Mon.-Fri. 7 AM-3:30 PM
256-265-8284

ARIZONA

TUCSON

Arizona Poison and Drug
Information Center
Arizona Health
Sciences Center
University Medical Center
1501 N. Campbell Ave.
Room 1156
Tucson, AZ 85724
7 days/week, 24 hours
520-626-6016
800-222-1222
(Emergency)
www.pharmacy.arizona.edu

ARKANSAS

LITTLE ROCK

Arkansas Drug Information
Center
4301 W. Markham St.
Slot 522-2
Little Rock, AR 72205
Mon.-Fri. 8:30 AM-5 PM
501-686-5072
(Little Rock area only -
for healthcare
professionals only)
800-228-1233
(AR only - **for healthcare**
professionals only)

CALIFORNIA

LOS ANGELES

Los Angeles Regional
Drug Information Center
LAC & USC Medical Center
1200 N. State St.
Trailer 25
Los Angeles, CA 90033
Mon.-Fri. 8 AM-4 PM
Closed 12 PM to 1 PM
323-226-7741

SAN DIEGO

Drug Information Service
University of California
San Diego Medical Center
200 West Arbor Dr.
MC 8925
San Diego, CA 92103-8925
Mon.-Fri. 9 AM-5 PM
619-543-6971
(for healthcare
professionals only)

SAN FRANCISCO

Drug Information Analysis
Service
University of California,
San Francisco
533 Parnassus Ave.
Room U12
San Francisco, CA 94143-0622
Mon.-Fri. 8:30 AM-4:30 PM
415-502-9540
(for healthcare
professionals only)

STANFORD

Drug Information Center
University of California
Stanford Hospital and Clinics
300 Pasteur Dr.
Room H-0301
Stanford, CA 94305
Mon.-Fri. 8 AM-4 PM
650-723-6422

COLORADO

DENVER

Rocky Mountain Poison
and Drug Center
990 Bannock St.
(Physical address)
777 Bannock St.
(Mailing address)
Denver, CO 80264
303-739-1123
800-222-1222
(Emergency)
www.rmpdc.org

CONNECTICUT

FARMINGTON

Drug Information Service
University of Connecticut
Health Center
263 Farmington Ave.
Farmington, CT 06030
Mon.-Fri. 7:30 AM-4 PM
860-679-2783

HARTFORD

Drug Information Center
Hartford Hospital
P.O. Box 5037
80 Seymour St.
Hartford, CT 06102
Mon.-Fri. 8:30 AM-5 PM
860-545-2221
860-545-2961 (After 5 PM)
www.hartfordhospital.org

NEW HAVEN

Drug Information Center
Yale-New Haven Hospital
20 York St.
New Haven, CT 06540-3202
Mon.-Fri. 8:30 AM-5 PM
203-688-2248
www.ynhh.org

DISTRICT OF COLUMBIA

Drug Information Service
Howard University Hospital
Room BB06
2041 Georgia Ave. NW
Washington, DC 20060
Mon.-Fri. 8:30 AM-4 PM
202-865-1325
800-222-1222
(Emergency)
www.huhosp.org/patientpublic/
pharmacy.htm

FLORIDA

FT. LAUDERDALE

Nova Southeastern University
College of Pharmacy
Drug Information Center
3200 S. University Dr.
Ft. Lauderdale, FL 33328
Mon.-Fri. 9 AM-5 PM
954-262-3103
http://pharmacy.nova.edu

GAINESVILLE

Drug Information &
Pharmacy Resource Center
Shands Hospital at
University of Florida
P.O. Box 100316
Gainesville, FL 32610-0316
Mon.-Fri. 9 AM-5 PM
352-265-0408
(for healthcare
professionals only)
http://shands.org/professional/
drugs

JACKSONVILLE

Drug Information Service
Shands Jacksonville
655 W. 8th St.
Jacksonville, FL 32209
Mon.-Fri. 8:30 AM-5 PM
904-244-4185
(for healthcare
professionals only)
904-244-4700
(for consumers,
Mon.-Fri. 9:30 AM-4 PM)

ORLANDO

Orlando Regional Drug Information Service
Orlando Regional Healthcare System
1414 Kuhl Ave., MP 192
Orlando, FL 32806
Mon.-Fri. 8 AM-4 PM
  321-841-8717

TALLAHASSEE

Drug Information Education Center
Florida Agricultural and Mechanical University College of Pharmacy and Pharmaceutical Sciences
Tallahassee, FL 32307
Mon.-Fri. 9 AM-5 PM
  850-488-5239

WEST PALM BEACH

Drug Information Center
Nova Southeastern University, West Palm Beach
3970 RCA Blvd., Suite 7006A
Palm Beach Gardens, FL 33410
Mon.-Fri. 9 AM-5 PM
  561-622-0658
  (for healthcare professionals only)

GEORGIA

ATLANTA

Emory University Hospital
Dept. of Pharmaceutical Services-Drug Information
1364 Clifton Rd. NE
Atlanta, GA 30322
Mon.-Fri. 8 AM-1 PM
  404-712-4644
  (for healthcare professionals only)

Drug Information Service
Northside Hospital
1000 Johnson Ferry Rd. NE
Atlanta, GA 30342
Mon.-Fri. 9 AM-5 PM
  404-851-8676 (GA only)

AUGUSTA

Drug Information Center
Medical College of Georgia Hospital and Clinic
BI2101
1120 15th St.
Augusta, GA 30912
Mon.-Fri. 8:30 AM-5 PM
  706-721-2887

COLUMBUS

Columbus Regional Drug Information Center
710 Center St.
Columbus, GA 31902
Mon.-Fri. 8 AM-5 PM
  706-571-1934
  (for healthcare professionals only)

IDAHO

POCATELLO

Drug Information Center
Idaho State University School of Pharmacy
970 S. 5th St.
Campus Box 8092
Pocatello, ID 83209
Mon.-Thur. 8:30 AM-5 PM
Fri. 8:30 AM-3 PM
  208-282-4689
  800-334-7139 (ID only)
http://pharmacy.isu.edu

ILLINOIS

CHICAGO

Drug Information Center
Northwestern Memorial Hospital
Feinberg Pavilion, LC 700
251 E. Huron St.
Chicago, IL 60611
Mon.-Fri. 8:30 AM-5 PM
  312-926-7573

Drug Information Services
University of Chicago Hospitals
5841 S. Maryland Ave.
MC 0010
Chicago, IL 60637-1470
Mon.-Fri. 9 AM-5 PM
  773-702-1388

Drug Information Center
University of Illinois at Chicago
833 S. Wood St.
MC 886
Chicago, IL 60612-7231
Mon.-Fri. 8 AM-4 PM
  312-996-5332
  (for healthcare professionals only)
  312-996-3682
  (for consumers, Mon.-Fri. 9 AM-12 PM)
www.uic.edu/pharmacy/services/di/index.html

HARVEY

Drug Information Center
Ingalls Memorial Hospital
1 Ingalls Dr.
Harvey, IL 60426
Mon.-Fri. 8 AM-4:30 PM
  708-333-2300

HINES

Drug Information Service
Hines Veterans Administration Hospital
2100 S. 5th Ave.
Pharmacy Services
MC119
P.O. Box 5000
Hines, IL 60141-5000
Mon.-Fri. 8 AM-4:30 PM
  708-202-8387,
    ext. 23780

PARK RIDGE

Drug Information Center
Advocate Lutheran General Hospital
1775 Dempster St.
Park Ridge, IL 60068
Mon.-Fri. 7:30 AM-4 PM
  847-723-8128
  (for healthcare professionals only)

INDIANA

INDIANAPOLIS

Drug Information Center
St. Vincent Hospital and Health Services
2001 W. 86th St.
Indianapolis, IN 46260
Mon.-Fri. 8 AM-4 PM
  317-338-3200
  (for healthcare professionals only)
Drug Information Service
Clarian Health Partners

Pharmacy Department I-65
at 21st St.
Room CG04
Indianapolis, IN 46202
Mon.-Fri. 8 AM-4:30 PM
  317-962-1750

MUNCIE

Drug Information Center
Ball Memorial Hospital
2401 University Ave.
Muncie, IN 47303
Mon.-Fri. 8 AM-4:30 PM
  765-747-3035

IOWA

DES MOINES

Regional Drug Information Center
Mercy Medical Center-Des Moines
1111 Sixth Ave.
Des Moines, IA 50314
Mon.-Fri. 8 AM-4:30 PM
  (regional service; in-house service answered 7 days/ week, 24 hours)
  515-247-3286

IOWA CITY

Drug Information Center
University of Iowa Hospitals and Clinics
200 Hawkins Dr.
Iowa City, IA 52242
Mon.-Fri. 8 AM-4:30 PM
  319-356-2600

KANSAS

KANSAS CITY

Drug Information Center
University of Kansas Medical Center
3901 Rainbow Blvd.
Kansas City, KS 66160
Mon.-Fri. 8:30 AM-4:30 PM
  913-588-2328
  (for healthcare professionals only)

KENTUCKY

LEXINGTON

University of Kentucky Central Pharmacy
Chandler Medical Center
800 Rose St., C-114
Lexington, KY 40536-0293
7 days/week, 24 hours
  859-323-5642

LOUISIANA

MONROE

Louisiana Drug and Poison Information Center
University of Louisiana at Monroe College of Pharmacy
Sugar Hall
Monroe, LA 71209-6430
Mon.-Fri. 8 AM-4:30 PM
  318-342-1710

NEW ORLEANS

Xavier University Drug Information Center
Tulane University Hospital and Clinic
1440 Canal St.
Suite 808
New Orleans, LA 70112
Mon.-Fri. 9 AM-5 PM
504-588-5670

MARYLAND

ANDREWS AFB

Drug Information Services
79 MDSS/SGQP
1050 W. Perimeter Rd.
Suite D1-119
Andrews AFB, MD 20762-6660
Mon.-Fri. 7:30 AM-5 PM
240-857-4565

BALTIMORE

Drug Information Service
Johns Hopkins Hospital
600 N. Wolfe St.
Carnegie 180
Baltimore, MD 21287-6180
Mon.-Fri. 8:30 AM-5 PM
410-955-6348

Drug Information Service
University of Maryland
School of Pharmacy
Pharmacy Hall Room 760
20 North Pine St.
Baltimore, MD 21201
Mon.-Fri. 8:30 AM-5 PM
410-706-7568
(consumers only)
410-706-0898
**(for healthcare
professionals only)**
www.pharmacy.umaryland.
edu/umdi

EASTON

**Drug Information
Pharmacy Dept.
Memorial Hospital**
219 S. Washington St.
Easton, MD 21601
7 days/week, 7 AM-5:30 PM
410-822-1000, ext. 5645

MASSACHUSETTS

BOSTON

Drug Information Services
**Brigham and Women's
Hospital**
75 Francis St.
Boston, MA 02115
Mon.-Fri. 7 AM-3 PM
617-732-7166

WORCESTER

Drug Information Pharmacy
**UMass Memorial
Medical Center
Healthcare Hospital**
55 Lake Ave. North
Worcester, MA 01655
Mon.-Fri. 8:30 AM-5 PM
508-856-3456
508-856-2775 (24-hour)

MICHIGAN

ANN ARBOR

Drug Information Service
Dept. of Pharmacy Services
**University of Michigan
Health System**
1500 East Medical
Center Dr.
UH B2D301
Box 0008
Ann Arbor, MI 48109-0008
Mon.-Fri. 8 AM-5 PM
734-936-8200

DETROIT

Drug Information Center
**Department of Pharmacy
Services**
**Detroit Receiving Hospital
and University Health Center**
4201 St. Antoine Blvd.
Detroit, MI 48201
Mon.-Fri. 9 AM-5 PM
313-745-4556
www.dmcpharmacy.org

LANSING

Drug Information Services
Sparrow Hospital
1215 East Michigan Ave.
Lansing, MI 48912
7 days/week, 24 hours
517-364-2444

PONTIAC

Drug Information Center
St. Joseph Mercy Oakland
44405 Woodward Ave.
Pontiac, MI 48341
Mon.-Fri. 8 AM-4:30 PM
248-858-3055

ROYAL OAK

Drug Information Services
William Beaumont Hospital
3601 West 13 Mile Rd.
Royal Oak, MI 48073-6769
Mon.-Fri. 8 AM-4:30 PM
248-898-4077

SOUTHFIELD

Drug Information Service
Providence Hospital
16001 West 9 Mile Rd.
Southfield, MI 48075
Mon.-Fri. 8 AM-4 PM
248-849-3125

MISSISSIPPI

JACKSON

Drug Information Center
**University of Mississippi
Medical Center**
2500 N. State St.
Jackson, MS 39216
Mon.-Fri. 8 AM-4:30 PM
601-984-2060

MISSOURI

KANSAS CITY

**University of
Missouri-Kansas City
Drug Information Center**
2411 Holmes St., MG-200
Kansas City, MO 64108
Mon.-Fri. 9 AM-4 PM
816-235-5490
http://druginfo.umkc.edu/

SPRINGFIELD

Drug Information Center
St. John's Hospital
1235 E. Cherokee St.
Springfield, MO 65804
Mon.-Fri. 8 AM-4:30 PM
417-820-3488

ST. JOSEPH

**Regional Medical Center
Pharmacy**
5325 Faraon St.
St. Joseph, MO 64506
7 days/week, 24 hours
816-271-6141

MONTANA

MISSOULA

Drug Information Service
**University of Montana School
of Pharmacy and Allied Health
Sciences**
32 Campus Dr.
1522 Skaggs Bldg.
Missoula, MT 59812-1522
Mon.-Fri. 8 AM-5 PM
406-243-5254
800-501-5491
www.umt.edu/druginfo

NEBRASKA

OMAHA

Drug Informatics Service
School of Pharmacy
Creighton University
2500 California Plaza
Health Science Library
Room 204
Omaha, NE 68178
Mon.-Fri. 8:30 AM-4:30 PM
402-280-5101
http://druginfo.creighton.edu

NEW JERSEY

NEWARK

**New Jersey Poison
Information and Education
System**
65 Bergen St.
Newark, NJ 07107
Mon.-Fri. 8 AM- 5 PM
973-972-9280
800-222-1222
(Emergency)
www.njpies.org

NEW BRUNSWICK

Drug Information Service
**Robert Wood Johnson
University Hospital**
Pharmacy Department
1 Robert Wood Johnson Pl.
New Brunswick, NJ 08901
Mon.-Fri. 8:30 AM-4:30 PM
732-937-8842

NEW MEXICO

ALBUQUERQUE

New Mexico Poison Center
**University of New Mexico
Health Sciences Center**
MSC09 5080
1 University of New Mexico
Albuquerque, NM 87131
7 days/week, 24 hours
505-272-4261
800-222-1222
(Emergency)
http://hsc.unm.edu/pharmacy/
poison

NEW YORK

BROOKLYN

International Drug Information Center
Long Island University
Arnold & Marie Schwartz
College of Pharmacy &
Health Sciences
75 DeKalb Ave.
RM-HS509
Brooklyn, NY 11201
Mon.-Fri. 9 AM-5 PM
      718-488-1064
www.liu.edu

NEW HYDE PARK

Drug Information Center
St. John's University at Long
Island Jewish Medical Center
270-05 76th Ave.
New Hyde Park, NY 11040
Mon.-Fri. 8 AM-3 PM
      718-470-DRUG (3784)

NEW YORK CITY

Drug Information Center
Memorial Sloan-Kettering
Cancer Center
1275 York Ave.
RM S-702
New York, NY 10021
Mon.-Fri. 9 AM-5 PM
      212-639-7552

Drug Information Center
Mount Sinai Medical Center
1 Gustave Levy Pl.
New York, NY 10029
Mon.-Fri. 9 AM-5 PM
      212-241-6619
      (for in-house healthcare
      professionals only)

Drug Information Service
New York Presbyterian
Hospital
Room K04
525 E. 68th St.
New York, NY 10021
Mon.-Fri. 9 AM-5 PM
      212-746-0741

ROCHESTER

Finger Lakes
Poison and Drug
Information Center
University of Rochester
601 Elmwood Ave.
Rochester, NY 14642
Mon.-Fri. 8 AM-5 PM
      585-275-3718

ROCKVILLE CENTER

Drug Information Center
Mercy Medical Center
1000 North Village Ave.
Rockville Center, NY
11571-9024
Mon.-Fri. 8 AM-4 PM
      516-705-1053

NORTH CAROLINA

BUIES CREEK

Drug Information Center
School of Pharmacy
Campbell University
P.O. Box 1090
Buies Creek, NC 27506
Mon.-Fri. 8:30 AM-4:30 PM
      910-893-1200
      x2701
      800-760-9697 (Toll free)
      x2701
      800-327-5467 (NC only)

CHAPEL HILL

University of North
Carolina Hospitals
Drug Information Center
Dept. of Pharmacy
101 Manning Dr.
Chapel Hill, NC 27514
Mon.-Fri. 8 AM-4:30 PM
      919-966-2373

DURHAM

Drug Information Center
Duke University Health
Systems
DUMC Box 3089
Durham, NC 27710
Mon.-Fri. 8 AM-5 PM
      919-684-5125

GREENVILLE

Eastern Carolina Drug
Information Center
Pitt County
Memorial Hospital
Dept. of Pharmacy Service
P.O. Box 6028
2100 Stantonsburg Rd.
Greenville, NC 27835
Mon.-Fri. 8 AM-5 PM
      252-847-4257

WINSTON-SALEM

Drug Information
Service Center
Wake-Forest University
Baptist Medical Center
Medical Center Blvd.
Winston-Salem, NC 27157
Mon.-Fri. 8 AM-5 PM
      336-716-2037
      (for healthcare
      professionals only)

OHIO

ADA

Drug Information Center
Raabe College of Pharmacy
Ohio Northern University
Ada, OH 45810
Mon.-Thurs. 8:30 AM-5 PM,
      7-10 PM
Fri. 8:30 AM- 4 PM;
Sun. 2 PM-10 PM
      419-772-2307
www.onu.edu/pharmacy/
druginfo

CINCINNATI

Drug and Poison
Information Center
Children's Hospital
Medical Center
3333 Burnet Ave. VP-3
Cincinnati, OH 45229
Mon.-Fri. 9 AM-5 PM
      513-636-5054
      (Administration)
      513-636-5111
      (7 days/week, 24 hours)

CLEVELAND

Drug Information Service
Cleveland Clinic Foundation
9500 Euclid Ave.
Cleveland, OH 44195
Mon.-Fri. 8:30 AM-4:30 PM
      216-444-6456
      (for healthcare
      professionals only)

COLUMBUS

Drug Information Center
Ohio State University Hospital
Dept. of Pharmacy
Doan Hall 368
410 W. 10th Ave.
Columbus, OH 43210-1228
7 days/week, 24 hours
      614-293-8679
      (for in-house healthcare
      professionals only)

Drug Information Center
Riverside Methodist Hospital
3535 Olentangy River Road
Columbus, OH 43214
7 days/week, 24 hours
      614-566-5425

TOLEDO

Drug Information Services
St. Vincent Mercy Medical
Center
2213 Cherry St.
Toledo, Ohio 43608-2691
Mon.-Fri. 7 AM-5 PM
      419-251-4227
www.rx.medctr.ohio-state.edu

OKLAHOMA

OKLAHOMA CITY

Drug Information Service
Integris Health
3300 Northwest Expressway
Oklahoma City, OK 73112
Mon.-Fri. 8 AM-4:30 PM
      405-949-3660

Drug Information Center
OU Medical Center
Presbyterian Tower
700 NE 13th St.
Oklahoma City, OK 73104
Mon.-Fri. 8 AM-4:30 PM
      405-271-6226
Fax: 405-271-6281

TULSA

Drug Information Center
Saint Francis Hospital
6161 S. Yale Ave.
Tulsa, OK 74136
Mon.-Fri. 8 AM-4:30 PM
      918-494-6339
      (for healthcare
      professionals only)

PENNSYLVANIA

PHILADELPHIA

Drug Information Center
Temple University Hospital
Dept. of Pharmacy
3401 N. Broad St.
Philadelphia, PA 19140
Mon.-Fri. 8 AM-4:30 PM
      215-707-4644

Drug Information Service
Tenet Health System
Hahnemann University
Hospital
Department of Pharmacy
MS 451
Broad and Vine Streets
Philadelphia, PA 19102
Mon.-Fri. 8 AM-4 PM
      215-762-DRUG (3784)
      (for healthcare
      professionals only)

Drug Information Service
Dept. of Pharmacy
Thomas Jefferson
University Hospital
111 S. 11th St.
Philadelphia, PA 19107-5089
Mon.-Fri. 8 AM-5 PM
      215-955-8877

University of Pennsylvania
Health System Drug
Information Service
Hospital of the University of
Pennsylvania
Department of Pharmacy
3400 Spruce St.
Philadelphia, PA 19104
Mon.-Fri. 8:30 AM-4 PM
215-662-2903

PITTSBURGH

Pharmaceutical
Information Center
Mylan School of Pharmacy
Duquesne University
431 Mellon Hall
Pittsburgh, PA 15282
Mon.-Fri. 8 AM-4 PM
412-396-4600

Drug Information Center
University of Pittsburgh
302 Scaife Hall
200 Lothrop St.
Pittsburgh, PA 15213
Mon.-Fri. 8:30 AM-4:30 PM
412-647-3784
**(for healthcare
professionals only)**

UPLAND

Drug Information Center
Crozer-Chester Medical
Center
Dept. of Pharmacy
1 Medical Center Blvd.
Upland, PA 19013
Mon.-Fri. 8 AM-4:30 PM
610-447-2851
**(for in-house healthcare
professionals only)**

PUERTO RICO

PONCE

Centro Informacion
Medicamentos
Escuela de Medicina de
Ponce
P.O. Box 7004
Ponce, PR 00732-7004
Mon.-Fri. 8 AM-4:30 PM
787-840-2575

SAN JUAN

Centro de Informacion de
Medicamentos-CIM
Escuela de Farmacia-RCM
P.O. Box 365067
San Juan, PR 00936-5067
Mon.-Fri. 8 AM-5:30 PM
787-758-2525, ext. 1516

SOUTH CAROLINA

CHARLESTON

Drug Information Service
Medical University of
South Carolina
150 Ashley Ave.
Rutledge Tower Annex
Room 604
P.O. Box 250584
Charleston, SC 29425-0810
Mon.-Fri. 9 AM-5:30 PM
843-792-3896
800-922-5250

COLUMBIA

Drug Information Service
University of South Carolina
College of Pharmacy
Columbia, SC 29208
Mon.-Fri. 8 AM-5 PM
803-777-7804
www.pharm.sc.edu

SPARTANBURG

Drug Information Center
Spartanburg Regional
Healthcare System
101 E. Wood St.
Spartanburg, SC 29303
Mon.-Fri. 8 AM-4:30 PM
864-560-6910

TENNESSEE

KNOXVILLE

Drug Information Center
University of Tennessee
Medical Center at Knoxville
1924 Alcoa Highway
Knoxville, TN 37920-6999
Mon.-Fri. 8 AM-4:30 PM
865-544-9124

MEMPHIS

South East Regional Drug
Information Center
VA Medical Center
1030 Jefferson Ave.
Memphis, TN 38104
Mon.-Fri. 6:30 AM-4 PM
901-523-8990, ext. 6720

Drug Information Center
University of Tennessee
875 Monroe Ave.
Suite 116
Memphis, TN 38163
Mon.-Fri. 8 AM-5 PM
901-448-5556

TEXAS

AMARILLO

Drug Information Center
Texas Tech Health
Sciences Center
School of Pharmacy
1300 Coulter Rd.
Amarillo, TX 79106
Mon.-Fri. 8 AM-5 PM
806-356-4008

GALVESTON

Drug Information Center
University of Texas
Medical Branch
301 University Blvd.
Galveston, TX 77555-0701
Mon.-Fri. 8 AM-5 PM
409-772-2734

HOUSTON

Drug Information Center
Ben Taub General Hospital
Texas Southern
University/HCHD
1504 Taub Loop
Houston, TX 77030
Mon.-Fri. 8:30 AM-5 PM
713-873-3710

LACKLAND A.F.B.

Drug Information Center
Dept. of Pharmacy
Wilford Hall Medical Center
2200 Bergquist Dr.
Suite 1
Lackland A.F.B., TX 78236
7 days/week, 24 hours
210-292-5414

LUBBOCK

Drug Information and
Consultation Service
Covenant Medical Center
3615 19th St.
Lubbock, TX 79410
Mon.-Fri. 8 AM-5 PM
806-725-0408

SAN ANTONIO

Drug Information Service
University of Texas
Health Science Center
at San Antonio
Department of Pharmacology
7703 Floyd Curl Drive
San Antonio, TX 78229-3900
Mon.-Fri. 8 AM-4 PM
210-567-4280

TEMPLE

Drug Information Center
Scott and White
Memorial Hospital
2401 S. 31st St.
Temple, TX 76508
Mon.-Fri. 8 AM-5 PM
254-724-4636

UTAH

SALT LAKE CITY

Drug Information Service
University of Utah Hospital
421 Wakara Way
Suite 204
Salt Lake City, UT 84108
Mon.-Fri. 7 AM-5 PM
801-581-2073

VIRGINIA

HAMPTON

Drug Information Center
Hampton University School
of Pharmacy
Hampton Harbors Annex
Hampton, VA 23668
Mon.-Fri. 9 AM-4 PM
757-728-6693

WEST VIRGINIA

MORGANTOWN

West Virginia Center for
Drug and Health Information
West Virginia University
Robert C. Byrd
Health Sciences Center
1124 HSN, P.O. Box 9520
Morgantown, WV 26506
Mon.-Fri. 8:30 AM-5 PM
304-293-6640
800-352-2501 (WV)
www.hsc.wvu.edu/SOP

WYOMING

LARAMIE

Drug Information Center
University of Wyoming
P.O. Box 3375
Laramie, WY 82071
Mon.-Fri. 8:30 AM-4:30 PM
307-766-6988

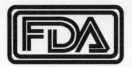

U.S. FOOD AND DRUG ADMINISTRATION

Medical Product Reporting Programs

MedWatch (24-hour service) **800-332-1088**
*Reporting of problems with drugs, devices, biologics (except vaccines), medical foods,
and dietary supplements.*

Vaccine Adverse Event Reporting System (24-hour service) **800-822-7967**
Reporting of vaccine-related problems.

Mandatory Medical Device Reporting **240-276-3000**
*Reporting required from user facilities regarding device-related deaths
and serious injuries.*

Veterinary Adverse Drug Reaction Program **888-332-8387**
Reporting of adverse drug events in animals.

Division of Drug Marketing, Advertising, and Communication (DDMAC) **301-796-1200**
Inquiries from health professionals regarding product promotion.

USP Medication Errors **800-233-7767**
*Reporting of medication errors or near-errors to help avoid future problems
through improvement in product names and packaging.*

Information for Health Professionals

Center for Drug Evaluation and Research Drug Information Hotline **301-827-4573**
Information on human drugs including hormones.

Center for Biologics Office of Communications **301-827-2000**
Information on biological products including vaccines and blood.

Center for Devices and Radiological Health **800-638-2041**
Automated request for information on medical devices and radiation-emitting products.

Emergency Operations **301-443-1240**
*Emergencies involving FDA-regulated products, tampering reports,
and emergency Investigational New Drug requests.*

Office of Orphan Products Development **301-827-3666**
Information on products for rare diseases.

General Information

General Consumer Inquiries **888-463-6332**
Consumer information on regulated products/issues.

Freedom of Information **301-827-6500**
Requests for publicly available FDA documents.

Office of Public Affairs **301-827-6250**
Interviews/press inquiries on FDA activities.

Center for Food Safety and Applied Nutrition **888-723-3366**
*Information on food safety, seafood, dietary supplements, women's nutrition,
and cosmetics.*

Consumer Information Service, Center for Devices and Radiological Health **800-638-2041**
*Information on medical devices, mammography facilities, and
radiation-emitting products.*

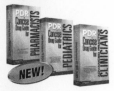